Muscle Aging, Inclusion-Body Myositis and Myopathies

Muscle Aging, Inclusion-Body Myositis and Myopathies

EDITED BY

Valerie Askanas, MD, PhD

Departments of Neurology and Pathology, University of Southern California Neuromuscular Center, University of Southern California Keck School of Medicine, Good Samaritan Hospital, Los Angeles, CA, USA

and

W. King Engel, MD

Departments of Neurology and Pathology, University of Southern California Neuromuscular Center, University of Southern California Keck School of Medicine, Good Samaritan Hospital, Los Angeles, CA, USA

WILEY-BLACKWELL

A John Wiley & Sons, Ltd., Publication

This edition first published 2012 © 2012 by Blackwell Publishing Ltd

Blackwell Publishing was acquired by John Wiley & Sons in February 2007. Blackwell's publishing program has been merged with Wiley's global Scientific, Technical and Medical business to form Wiley-Blackwell.

Registered office: John Wiley & Sons, Ltd, The Atrium, Southern Gate, Chichester, West Sussex, PO19 8SQ, UK

Editorial offices: 9600 Garsington Road, Oxford, OX4 2DQ, UK
The Atrium, Southern Gate, Chichester, West Sussex, PO19 8SQ, UK
111 River Street, Hoboken, NJ 07030-5774, USA

For details of our global editorial offices, for customer services and for information about how to apply for permission to reuse the copyright material in this book please see our website at www.wiley.com/wiley-blackwell

The right of the author to be identified as the author of this work has been asserted in accordance with the UK Copyright, Designs and Patents Act 1988.

Library of Congress Cataloging-in-Publication Data

Muscle aging : inclusion-body myositis and myopathies / edited by Valerie Askanas and King Engel.
  p. ; cm.
 Includes bibliographical references and index.
 ISBN-13: 978-1-4051-9646-8 (hardcover : alk. paper)
 ISBN-10: 1-4051-9646-7
 I. Askanas, Valerie. II. Engel, King.
 [DNLM: 1. Myositis, Inclusion Body–physiopathology. 2. Aging. WE 544]
 LC classification not assigned
 612.3–dc23
                                                                                      2011029718

A catalogue record for this book is available from the British Library.

Wiley also publishes its books in a variety of electronic formats. Some content that appears in print may not be available in electronic books.

Set in 9/12pt Meridien by Thomson Digital, Noida, India
Printed and bound in Singapore by Markono Print Media Pte Ltd

1   2012

Contents

List of contributors

Zohar Argov, MD
Department of Neurology
Hadassah Hebrew University Medical Center
Ein Kerem
Jerusalem, Israel

Valerie Askanas, MD, PhD
Departments of Neurology and Pathology
University of Southern California Neuromuscular Center
University of Southern California Keck School of Medicine
Good Samaritan Hospital
Los Angeles, CA, USA

Mallikarjun Badadani
Division of Genetics and Metabolism
Department of Pediatrics and Center for Molecular and
Mitochondrial Medicine and Genetics
University of California
Irvine, CA, USA

Nisha M. Badders
Department of Developmental Neurobiology
St. Jude Children's Research Hospital
Memphis, TN, USA

Aldobrando Broccolini, MD
Department of Neuroscience
Catholic University School of Medicine
Rome, Italy

Vincent Caiozzo
Department of Orthopedic Surgery
University of California
Irvine, CA, USA

Marinos C. Dalakas, MD
Neuroimmunology Unit
Department of Pathophysiology
National University of Athens Medical School
Athens, Greece

Kelvin J. A. Davies, PhD, DSc
James E. Birren Chair of Gerontology
Professor of Molecular Biology and Computational Biology
Andrus Gerontology Center
The University of Southern California
Los Angeles, CA, USA

Eric Dec
Division of Genetics and Metabolism
Department of Pediatrics and Center for Molecular
and Mitochondrial Medicine and Genetics
University of California
Irvine, CA, USA

Salvatore DiMauro, MD
Department of Neurology
Columbia University Medical Center
New York, NY, USA

Micah J. Drummond, PhD
Department of Physical Therapy
University of Utah
Salt Lake City, UT, USA

W. King Engel, MD
Departments of Neurology and Pathology
University of Southern California Neuromuscular Center
University of Southern California Keck School of Medicine
Good Samaritan Hospital
Los Angeles, CA, USA

Michio Hirano, MD
Department of Neurology
Columbia University Medical Center
New York, NY, USA

Virginia E. Kimonis, MD, MRCP
Department of Pediatrics
University of California Irvine School of Medicine
Orange, CA, USA

Shalini Mahajan, MD
Good Samaritan Hospital
Los Angeles, CA, USA

May Christine V. Malicdan, MD
Department of Neuromuscular Research
National Institute of Neuroscience
National Center of Neurology and Psychiatry
Tokyo, Japan

Barbara Martin
Department of Neurology
University of Kentucky Medical School
Lexington, KY, USA

Frank L. Mastaglia, MD
Centre for Neuromuscular and
Neurological Disorders
University of Western Australia
Queen Elizabeth II Medical Centre
Perth, WA, Australia

Massimiliano Mirabella, MD
Department of Neuroscience
Catholic University School of Medicine
Rome, Italy

Angele Nalbandian
Division of Genetics and Metabolism
Department of Pediatrics and Center for Molecular
and Mitochondrial Medicine and Genetics
University of California
Irvine, CA, USA

Jenny K. Ngo, PhD
Davis School of Gerontology, Ethel Percy Andrus
Gerontology Center
University of Southern California
Los Angeles, CA, USA

Ichizo Nishino, MD, PhD
Department of Neuromuscular Research
National Institute of Neuroscience
National Center of Neurology and Psychiatry
Tokyo, Japan

Anna Nogalska, PhD
Department of Neurology
University of Southern California Neuromuscular Center
University of Southern California Keck School of Medicine
Good Samaritan Hospital
Los Angeles, CA, USA

Satoru Noguchi, PhD
Department of Neuromuscular Research
National Institute of Neuroscience
National Center of Neurology and Psychiatry
Tokyo, Japan

Ikuya Nonaka, MD
Department of Neuromuscular Research
National Institute of Neuroscience
National Center of Neurology and Psychiatry
Tokyo, Japan

Blake B. Rasmussen, PhD
Department of Nutrition & Metabolism
Division of Rehabilitation Sciences
Sealy Center on Aging
University of Texas Medical Branch
Galveston, TX, USA

Eric Schon, PhD
Departments of Neurology, and
Genetics and Development
Columbia University Medical Center
New York, NY, USA

Charles Smith
Department of Neurology
University of Kentucky Medical School
Lexington, KY, USA

J. Paul Taylor
Department of Developmental Neurobiology
St. Jude Children's Research Hospital
Memphis, TN, USA

Jouni Vesa
Division of Genetics and Metabolism
Department of Pediatrics and Center for Molecular
and Mitochondrial Medicine and Genetics
University of California
Irvine, CA, USA

Douglas Wallace
Division of Genetics and Metabolism
Department of Pediatrics and Center for Molecular
and Mitochondrial Medicine and Genetics;
Department of Biological Chemistry,
Departments of Ecology and
Evolutionary Biology
University of California
Irvine, CA, USA

Giles D. Watts
School of Medicine, Cell Biology and Biochemistry
Health Policy and Practice
University of East Anglia
Norwich, Norfolk, UK

Cezary Wójcik, MD, PhD, DSc
Department of Anatomy and Cell Biology
Indiana University School of Medicine
Evansville Center for Medical Education
Evansville, IN, USA

Preface

This book contains chapters by internationally recognized experts and covers two currently very important topics: muscle aging, and sporadic inclusion-body myositis, the most common aging-associated muscle disease. Also described are hereditary inclusion-body myopathies, which are genetically determined disorders pathologically rather similar to sporadic inclusion-body myositis but which become clinically manifest in early, or sometimes later, adulthood.

Human muscle aging causes a gradual enfeeblement of older persons, and is progressively evident from about age 40 onwards. It causes muscle weakness and frailty of the elderly, resulting in falling and ensuing complications. The cost of caring for weakening older persons in the USA and around the world is escalating. There is a striking paucity of information related to human muscle aging.

This book is focused on various aging-associated neuromuscular disorders at the cellular and clinical levels. These are exemplified by the characteristic histochemical abnormalities seen in older patients' muscle biopsies, and in a number of clinical vignettes of representative aging patients.

Emphasis is given to various treatable, and not-yet-treatable, human conditions associated with aging. We stress that the phrase "you are just getting old" is not an acceptable medical diagnosis, and that aging is not a satisfactory explanation for the cause of neuromuscular symptoms. Nevertheless, *aging certainly is a risk factor* for a number of disorders. A full *neuromuscular evaluation* is needed to properly analyze and diagnose a neuromuscular problem in an aging patient, as the basis for providing the *best possible treatment*. Herein we describe some examples of successful treatments, but much more remains to be done to help aging neuromuscular

patients. Presented are the current knowledge of these aspects and new concepts intended to help development of innovative treatments. For the not-yet-treatable neuromuscular disorders associated with aging, the goal should be to not only stop their relentless progressive weakness, but to *provide enduring improvement*.

Sporadic inclusion-body myositis is the most common progressive muscle disease of older persons, age 50 and above. As the world population ages, sporadic inclusion-body myositis is becoming more prevalent and a significant health hazard. It causes *increasingly severe muscle weakness*, leading relentlessly to pronounced disability, including frequent falls and resultant injuries, inability to arise from a chair or toilet, or to grip a fork, spoon, or drinking glass. Swallowing difficulties and choking can occur. Sporadic inclusion-body myositis is generally underdiagnosed, and it is often misdiagnosed.

In this book are presented numerous details of the newest molecular mechanisms involved in the pathogenesis of sporadic inclusion-body myositis. These remarkable discoveries have not yet led to enduring treatment, but they are providing important leads toward that goal. Of urgent importance, therefore, is further clarification of the molecular pathogenesis of this disease, including learning the *ultimate upstream cause*, as well as details of the downstream *muscle-destroying cellular molecular mechanisms*.

Also of special interest – to general neurologists, neuroscientists, and gerontologists, as well as to internists and general physicians, nurses, and physical therapists, and to especially-curious patients, caregivers, and members of the general public – are the very intriguing, remarkable *similarities* between the special pathologic features of *muscle fibers in sporadic inclusion-body myositis* and pathologic features of *brains of patients with Alzheimer disease and Parkinson disease*. The similarities between sporadic inclusion-body myositis and those two most common neurodegenerative diseases of older persons suggest that aspects of the molecular pathogenic mechanisms may be extremely similar, or even in some aspects the same.

Specifically, the similarities of sporadic inclusion-body myositis with the Alzheimer brain include accumulations of amyloid-β, phosphorylated tau and numerous other "Alzheimer disease-characteristic" proteins. The similarities of inclusion-body myositis with Parkinson disease include accumulations of α-synuclein, parkin, DJ-1, and other abnormalities. These similarities suggest that (a)   the aging-associated degenerative-muscle and degenerative-brain diseases may share certain pathogenic steps and (b)   knowledge of one disease might help elucidate the cause and treatment of the others. And, despite the remarkable molecular sim-ilarities in those very different tissues, muscles and brain (the movers and the thinker), the separate muscle and brain diseases appear to never cross into the territory of the other. *What protects the sporadic inclusion-body myositis patient's brain from succumbing to the same degeneration as in his muscle fibers, and what protects Alzheimer and Parkinson patients from having the same abnormalities in their muscles as in their brain?* These are dramatic, very intriguing phenomena, understanding of which might very well contribute to finding cures.

The Editors are pleased to acknowledge their gratitude to various collaborators, including many clinical and research fellows, whose dedication and hard work greatly contributed to the results described in this book.

Valerie Askanas, MD, PhD
W. King Engel, MD

PART 1
Muscle Aging

CHAPTER 1

Aging of the human neuromuscular system: pathological aspects

W. King Engel and Valerie Askanas

Departments of Neurology and Pathology, University of Southern California Neuromuscular Center,
University of Southern California Keck School of Medicine, Good Samaritan Hospital, Los Angeles, CA, USA

Introduction

This chapter discusses both our original findings and concepts, as well as some data of others from the literature. It is not able to cover all aspects of this broad topic. Selected references are presented to stimulate further exploration of the various points discussed.

Succinct introduction to the biology of the neuromuscular system, for clinicians

Aging persons often have progressive *fatigability*, *weakness*, *slowness*, and *general frailty*, accompanied by visible atrophy of limb muscles. The weakness frequently is a cause of *falling*, which can result in serious injury, and sometimes death. *Healthy muscle* is maintained by: (a) its own salutary trophic metabolic processes; (b) multifactorial trophic influences dispensed from its innervating lower motor neuron (LMN) that are received at each muscle fiber's single neuromuscular junction; and (c) circulating trophic influences. The LMN itself is interdependent both (a) on normal trophic factors from the numerous myelin-containing Schwann cells surrounding its long axonal process like oblong beads on a string, and (b) on retrograde trophic influences acquired from its numerous muscle fibers at the neuromuscular junctions. Each LMN in the

human biceps is responsible for activating about 200 muscle fibers and for the continuing trophic nurturing of good health of those muscle fibers. A *motor unit* refers to one LMN, its Schwann cells, and the muscle fibers it innervates. A *neuromuscular disorder*, or disease, is one arising from abnormality of any part of the motor unit.

The LMNs and lower sensory neurons have a vital interdependence with the Schwann cells that coat and nurture their axonal extensions: the neurons cannot survive without the Schwann cells, and vice versa. Just as trophic factors "emitting" from LMNs induce and control the special *type-1* versus *type-2* characteristics of the muscle fibers they innervate, the LMNs probably also induce and maintain hypothetically different sets of "type-1" and "type-2" Schwann cells, respectively, on themselves. And, probably the Schwann cells on sensory neurons are different from ones on motor neurons, because clinically there can be anti-Schwann-cell dysimmune diseases that rather preferentially affect either motor or sensory neurons, and even preferentially involve selectively large-diameter sensory nerve fibers (faster-conducting, conveying position, vibration, and touch sensations) or small-diameter sensory nerve fibers (slower-conducting, conveying pain signals).

A *motor unit*, with its arborizations, has been likened to a *tree*, the leaves being compared to the muscle fibers (I think that I shall always see, a motor unit as a tree; with apologies to Joyce Kilmer).

Muscle Aging, Inclusion-Body Myositis and Myopathies, First Edition. Edited by Valerie Askanas and W. King Engel.
© 2012 Blackwell Publishing Ltd. Published 2012 by Blackwell Publishing Ltd.

In regard to its loss of "leaves," a tree in autumn, or a waning motor unit, can be affected *in toto* or *in portio* [1, 2]. *In toto* reflects all of the leaves becoming "malnurtured" at about the same time, and *in portio* is manifested as leaves on the more distal twigs being affected first, showing the first autumnal color changes (as is characteristic of maple trees).

The clinically evident muscle atrophy of elderly persons, which we call *atrophy of aging muscle (AAM)* (an intentionally general descriptive term), is often assumed to be strictly *myogenous* (defined as meaning a process involving only muscle, but not LMNs or their peripherally extending axons). However, based on our evidence, it is likely that *in a number of circumstances AAM is ultimately neurogenic*, i.e. caused by malfunction of the LMNs, or antecedently by impaired trophic influence of the Schwann cells on their LMNs. Because of its clinical, social, and economic importance, AAM will be discussed in regard to some facets of the known and putative malfunctions of the motor unit components, their causes, and their possible treatments.

Note that we use AAM instead of the term sarcopenia. "Sarcopenia" sounds like a definitive diagnosis but *it is not*. It is often erroneously interpreted as designating a singular pathogenesis. Sarcopenia simply refers, imprecisely, to muscle atrophy in aged animals; it does not indicate or imply any pathogenic mechanism, of which there are a number of possibilities. *AAM is usually manifest as type-2 fiber atrophy.* A further critique of "sarcopenia" is presented below.

AAM *is not a definitive clinical diagnosis*, no more than is anemia, or jaundice, or stroke; it is a reason to look carefully, *in each individual patient*, for a cause, and especially for a *treatable cause*. Several known causes are described below and in Chapters 2 and 3 in this volume. Whether there is also an as-yet-unidentified general pervasive cause (or causes) that eventually harms the muscles of every aging person is not known. Biochemical studies seeking a general, nearly universal cause typically do not intensively seek, in individual patients and in experimental animals, the possible presence of an identifiable and potentially treatable primary cause (such as peripheral neuropathy, nerve-root radicu-lopathy, malnutrition, hyperparathyroidism, or a myovascular component).

Aging is a risk factor for AAM, but it is *not an ultimate cause*. "You're just getting old" is not a cause of AAM, and clinically it certainly should not be used as a dismissive diagnosis of an older patient.

Cellular aging, in general

Despite a vast literature on cellular aging, the causes and mechanisms are still poorly understood, and treatment non-existent. Mature, post-mitotic muscle fibers, similarly to post-mitotic neurons, seem to be more susceptible to a *chronic cellular aging* than are dividing cells. Cellular aging involves abnormalities of various subcellular aspects, such as nuclei, mitochondria, endoplasmic reticulum, Golgi, and structural and aqueous components. Proteasome and lysosome degradations are especially important. Oxidative stress and endoplasmic reticulum stress are also proposed to play important roles. The *"proteome"* designates the large and varied family of proteins of a cell, the profile of which is cell-type-specific.

One can wonder whether the general aging changes of cells are due to effects of a still-obscure omnipotent *"master vitalostat,"* such as a *"master gene"* acting like a rheostat that gradually turns down the vitality of the cell. If there is a master vitalostat. What initiates the turning-down, what are the key steps by which it executes that turn-down, and how can it be controlled? What are the underlying *genetic* factors, and/or important *epigenetic* mechanisms? (Philosophically, why are all living creatures programmed from "conception" to die?) In the atrophy process, there might be multiple stages and pathways participating, some of which, if identifiable, could become amenable to not-yet-developed treatments. Hypothetically, for skeletal muscle there might be at least two so-called master genes, *Fiber2atrophin* and *Fiber1atrophin*, that are normally inhibited, but when activated by an atrophy-promoting factor they instigate cascades of other genetic activations and inhibitions, resulting in preferential atrophy of type-2 or type-1 muscle fibers respectively. Preferential type-2 fiber atrophies are discussed below. (Preferential atrophy of type-1 fibers is seen in myotonic dystrophy type-1, a disease caused by expansion of CTG trinucleotide repeats of the gene *DMPK*; and in preferential "congenital type-1 fiber hypotrophy with central nuclei" [3], which in some patients is attributable to a genetic mutation of *myotubularin*, *myogenic-factor-6*, or *dynamin-1*.)

Some unanswered questions

Is the muscle frailty associated with AAM universally inevitable, like the aging-related, more-visible frailty and atrophy of skin, like the failure of estrogen in menopausal women and the gradual petering-out of testosterone in aging men, like scalp follicles disappearing or producing only non-pigmented hairs, like vascular sclerosis, like accumulation of "wear-and-tear" lipofuscin pigment within lower-motor neurons, other neurons, and muscle fibers? What is the most essential mechanism that starts and perpetuates AAM? Is it something we all ingest, or do not ingest; is it the cumulative solar or cosmic irradiation, or Mother Earth's constant radon emission; or perhaps there is something else to which we all are exposed? Is there a gradual cellular accumulation of something cumulatively more toxic than the accumulating lipofuscin – such as oxidatively damaged or otherwise-toxified misfolded proteins – that gradually "rusts" beneficent cellular functions and activates "atrophy processes"? Why can't any of the pathogenic mechanisms putatively contributing to AAM be prevented or treated *now*? Much work needs to be done before we can prescribe an elixir to make the elderly intellectually brilliant and vigorous.

Indefinable are the terms "normal aged person" or "normal-control aged person." In muscle biopsies of aging persons we nearly always have observed different combinations and various degrees of denervation atrophy and/or type-2 fiber atrophy (see below).

Neuromuscular histology

Normal skeletal muscle is the most abundant of human tissues. It is composed of muscle fibers that are very long cylinders. Their length is about 1000 times their typical diameter of about 45–65 µm (in the biceps). Transverse histochemical sections of muscle biopsies are diagnostically more informative than longitudinal ones. The universally used stain for general evaluation of muscle-biopsy histochemistry is the Engel trichrome [4, 5]. (It stains myofibrils green and their Z-disks red; mitochondria, t-tubules, longitudinal endoplasmic reticulum, and plasmalemma red; and DNA and RNA dark blue. It also stains the protein component of Schwann cell myelin red and neuronal axons green.) The histochemical types of human muscle fibers are most distinctively delineated by two myofibrillar ATPase reactions: (a) the regular ATPase (reg-ATPase) incubated at pH 9.4 [6], and (b) the acid-preincubated reverse-ATPase (rev-ATPase) [7]. (Some myopathologists also use antibodies against different types of myosin for fiber-type definition.) In normal adult human and mammalian animal muscle, fibers lightly stained with reg-ATPase and reciprocally dark with rev-ATPase are arbitrarily designated *type-1 fibers* [4, 7–10], while the fibers oppositely stained are *type-2 fibers*. The type-1 fibers are high in most of the mitochondrial oxidative-enzyme activities (e.g. cytochrome oxidase (COX), succinate dehydrogenase (SDH), and hydroxybuty-rate dehydrogenase), as well as myoglobin and triglyceride droplets; and they are low in the anerobic glycolysis enzymes myophosphorylase and UDPG-glycogen transferase, in glycogen, and in the aqueous sarcoplasmic enzyme lactate dehydrogenase. The type-2 fibers are oppositely stained with those reactions. (Interestingly, the very useful mitochondrial oxidative enzyme menadione-mediated α-glycerophosphate dehydrogenase (men-αGPDH) is stronger in type-2 fibers.) Type-1 fibers have more capillaries adjacent to them and are better equipped for oxidative metabolism, and clinically are utilized for prolonged muscle activity. The type-2 fibers are better equipped for anaerobic glycolysis, and clinically are utilized for short bursts of more intense activity. In some neuromuscular disorders there is a rather selective involvement of one fiber type, and in other disorders the involvement is nonselective [11]. (A muscle biopsy, done as an outpatient procedure with local, not general anesthesia, must be from a muscle *not recently needled* for electromyography, therapeutic injection, or "acupuncture therapy": these can produce confounding focal myopathy [12].)

During normal development, *each LMN* induces and trophically maintains the distinctiveness and uniformity of histochemical and functional fiber type and subtype of its approximately 200 muscle fibers controlled by it as members of its motor unit. We have therefore hypothesized that there are, respectively, type-1 and type-2 LMNs, and A and B subtypes of each. (In the cat anterior horns, we were not able to histochemically distinguish the different types of LMNs from each other [13–15] but we could demonstrate that the large α-motor neurons are rich in phosphorylase and glycogen and poor in mitochondrial SDH, while the small neurons, namely the gamma efferents, renshaw neurons and interneurons have the opposite histochemical profile.) Muscle fibers denervated from any cause gradually atrophy. If only some fibers in a muscle are denervated, they become *small angular fibers* when viewed in transverse sections (Figure 1.1a–e), progressing to become *pyknotic nuclear clumps* (Figure 1.2a). At some indefinable point, the atrophying fibers become incapable of attracting and/or accepting reinnervating nerve sprouts, but before that point of no return, they can be rescued by reinnervation. Muscle fibers can "switch" their histochemical type when denervated and then reinnervated by the type of LMN opposite to their original type of innervating LMN (i.e., *foreign reinnervation*) [16]. Denervated muscle fibers apparently can promiscuously accept comforting reinnervation from any type or subtype of LMN, a phenomenon commonly occurring in chronic neurogenic diseases that we have demonstrated experimentally in nerve-crush + reinnervation experiments [16–20]. In human muscle, This seemingly random foreign reinnervation results in *type-grouping* (Figure 1.3), which is evident as smaller or larger groups of the same histochemical fiber type replacing the normal, rather even inter-mixture of type-2 and type-1 fibers. When seen in a patient's diagnostic muscle biopsy, type-grouping is considered a manifestation of "established reinnervation" (Figure 1.3), namely previously denervated orphaned muscle fibers having been successfully reinnervated by

neurite sprouts from nearby relatively healthy LMN axons of the opposite (foreign) type.

In abnormal human muscle, two situations produce muscle fibers of intermediate degree of staining with both ATPases: (a) partially converted fibers that are in the process of being "switched" due to foreign reinnervation, which is typically a neuropathic phenomenon (although in a myopathy there can sometimes be "myogenous de-innervation" due to muscle-fiber abnormality at or near the neuromuscular junction with survival of the more distal portion of the fiber thereby cut off from the innervation influence and thus able to accept foreign reinnervation); and (b) regenerating/degenerating ("regen-degen") muscle fibers (RNA-positive, often alkaline-phosphatase-positive, and sometimes slightly acid-phosphatase-positive), which are usually evident in the setting of a myopathy, although a few of them can occur in the setting of prominent denervation (Engel, unpublished results) and in infantile spinal muscular atrophy [21].

Physiologically, *type-1 fibers* are considered to be *slow-twitch* and rather fatigue-resistant, while the *type-2 fibers* are *fast-twitch* and fast-fatiguing, as found in normal mammalian muscle [22, 23] and corroborated in human muscle [24, 25]. The designations slow-twitch and fast-twitch were introduced [4, 8, 9, 26] to distinguish the twitch properties of mammalian twitch-muscle fibers from amphibian non-twitch, extremely slow tonic fibers of the thigh adductor clasp muscles.

Relative paucity of one type of muscle fiber in a patient's biopsy can be caused, hypothetically, by (a) *preferential impairment* of the corresponding type of LMNs or Schwann cells; (b) if both LMN types are equally abnormal, *preferentially more successful sprouting* and reinnervation ability of the opposite type of LMNs; (c) if there are large groups of both types of muscle fibers in a chronic reinnervation situation, *biopsy sampling* could produce a non-representative impression of paucity; or (d) preferential myopathic loss of that type of muscle fiber. (We use the term fiber-type paucity and not fiber-type predominance because it is more likely that the muscle fibers that are *too few* reflect the abnormal status.)

In our muscle biopsies of elderly patients, we have observed that type-1 fiber paucity (Figure 1.3d) is

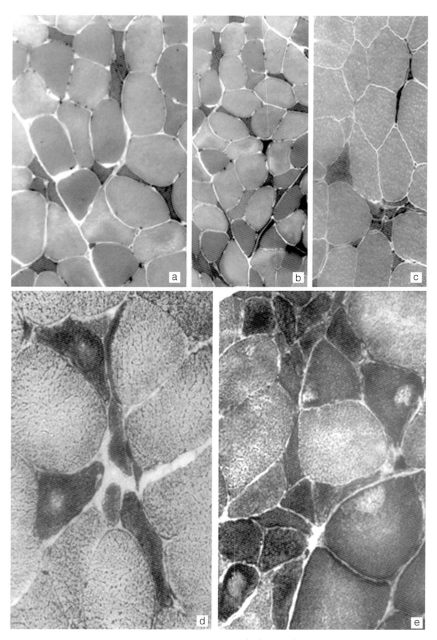

Figure 1.1 (a–e) Recent denervation without innervation, evidenced by small dark angular muscle fibers; (a,b) amyotrophic lateral sclerosis; (c–e) dysimmune peripheral neuropathy. Also, moderately atrophic muscle target fibers each with a pale small central regions and often having three concentric zones of staining; (d,e) one large two-zoned muscle targetoid-core fiber (possibly a pre-target fiber); Dark dots within some normal fibers in (a) indicate esterase-positive lipofuscin collections. (a–c) Pan-esterase staining; (d,e) NADH-tetrazolium reductase staining. Magnification: (a) ×2000; (b) ×1330; (c) ×1830; (d) ×4330; (e) ×4170. Note that Figures 1.1–1.4, except Figure 1.2b, are transverse sections of fresh-frozen human biopsies. Muscle fibers are stained with various histochemical reactions.

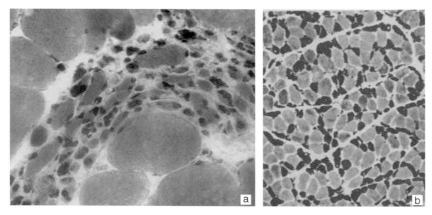

Figure 1.2 (a) End stage of "recent" denervation, evidenced by very atrophic muscle fibers with their clumps of pyknotic nuclei (with the NADH-TR stain such end-stage atrophic fibers typically would show high activity), peripheral neuropathy, Engel trichrome stain. (b) Greater atrophy of the dark type-2 fibers 27 weeks following experimental denervation, guinea pig [22], regular ATPase. Magnification: (a) ×3330; (b) ×500.

evident more often than type-2 fiber paucity. In aging humans it is uncertain whether there is a gradual loss of spinal cord LMNs. If there is, possibly the type-1 fiber paucity could be due to an aging-associated gradual loss preferentially of type-1 LMNs.

More structurally labile are the type-2 muscle fibers, and especially the type-2B fibers. In human skeletal muscle: (a) they are more prone to selectively atrophy, which occurs in various conditions such as experimental pan-denervation [19, 20] (Figure 1.2b), glucocorticoid toxicity, disuse, cachexia, remote-effect of a neoplasm, and male castration; and (b) they are more prone to hypertrophy with work, especially in men. In normal young adult men the diameter of type-2 fibers is larger than of type-1 fibers, but in normal young adult women type-2 fibers are smaller (the gender difference has been attributed to more testosterone in men). There are two subtypes of normal type-2 fibers, 2A and 2B [27]. The 2B fibers are the more labile regarding atrophy and hypertrophy. At a less acidic acid-pre-incubation for rev-ATPase staining, the 2B fibers have properties intermediate between the 2A fibers and the type-1 fibers. In some type-2-fiber atrophies the subtype-2B fibers are the more prone to atrophy. There are also two subtypes of type-1 fibers, 1A and 1B [28].

Atrophy in aging human muscle: description and new concepts

The topic of *type-2 fiber atrophy* is large, multifaceted, and complex, and the subject of numerous experimental animal studies (selected references are given). Some of our personal concepts and general principles will be discussed here, but this is not a complete review of all possibly pertinent studies. The causes of type-2 atrophy are multiple, and even in an individual patient the cause can be multifactorial.

In contrast to a large body of literature regarding muscle aging in animals, there is a paucity of information regarding human muscle aging. The clinical and experimental muscle atrophies associated with cachexia, hyponutrition (starvation), remote (para-neoplastic) neoplasm, experimental (and probably human) total denervation without successful reinnervation (Figure 1.2b), glucocorticoid "myotoxicity", and disuse all involve *preferential type-2 fiber atrophy,* and they have a number of their molecular degradative steps in common [29–37].

General questions include: what makes the type-2 fibers relatively susceptible to these atrophogenic processes? And what relatively protects type-1 fibers from them? Another question is why do muscle fibers (cells) have such an *elaborate protein-catabolizing*

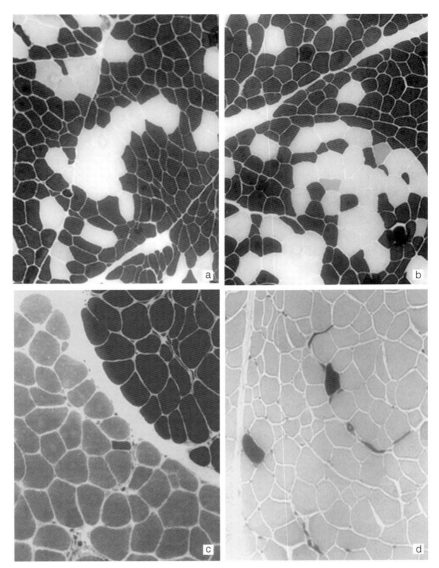

Figure 1.3 (a–c) Established reinnervation, indicated by muscle fiber type-grouping, in three adult males with chronic dysimmune peripheral neuropathy. Darkly-stained type-2 fibers and lightly-stained type-1 fibers are type-grouped, in contrast to what normally would be a rather even intermixture of fiber types (not illustrated). The successfully "foreign reinnervated" fibers among the type-grouped type-1 fibers have retained, or re-achieved, their normal diameter. In (a,b) there is also rather diffuse type-2 fiber atrophy of moderate degree, because in these adult males the dark type-2 fibers normally would have been of somewhat larger diameter than the light type-1 fibers. (c) Very large type-groupings, and also a very few tiny atrophic muscle fibers. (d) Prominent paucity of type-1 fibers (dark), possibly caused by a sampling phenomenon of a very large type-grouping (or, hypothetically, by a selective loss of type-1 lower motor neurons or type-1 Schwann cells). (a–c) Regular ATPase, incubated at pH 9.4 [4–6]; (d) acid-preincubated at pH 4.35 and then the ATPase staining at pH 9.4 [7]. Magnification: (a,b) ×830; (c) ×1500; (d) ×1330.

complex, namely to unleash "atrogenes" controlling *self-destructing molecular systems*? Is it to provide rapid-response hypertrophy, or atrophy martyring? Most important medically, can we prevent or treat the crippling atrophy in aging persons?

There are two major categories of muscle-fiber atrophy: (a) ordinary denervation atrophy (Figures 1.1–1.3) and (b) type-2 muscle fiber atrophy (Figure 1.4), and other less frequently seen atrophies, including vacuolar atrophies. Conceptu-

ally, type-2 fiber atrophy can be either *neurogenous* or *myogenous*, or both. Determining which applies to each specific patient is essential to establishing patient-specific treatments. We propose that the putatively neurogenous type is much more common (see below).

Mechanisms of muscle-fiber atrophy involve:
• Greater catabolism than synthesis of muscle-fiber proteins, especially catabolism of myofibrillar proteins, which occurs mainly through two subsystems:

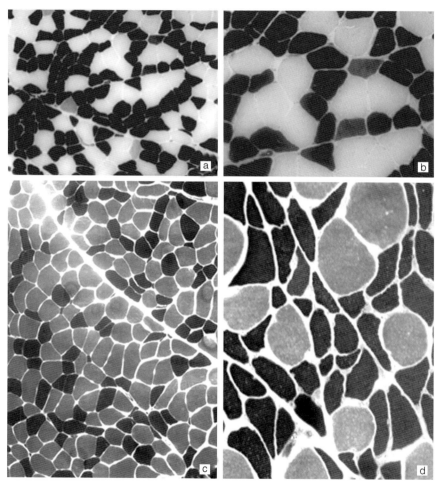

Figure 1.4 Type-2 fiber atrophy in four males. Many of the darker-stained type-2 fibers are of smaller diameter than the lighter-stained type-1 fibers, whereas in normal men the type-2 fibers should have a larger diameter than the type-1 fibers There is also a concurrent slight type-grouping in (a) and slight paucity of type-1 fibers in (d). The patients in (a–c) have a chronic dysimmune peripheral neuropathy, and in (d) a chronic glucocorticoid toxicity. Regular myofibrillar ATPase, pH 9.4. Magnification: (a) ×830; (b) ×2000; (c) ×830; (d) ×2500.

proteasomes involving ubiquitinated proteins and autophagy/lysosomes (see Chapter 7 for details).

• Less certain is the possibility that there might also be decreased synthesis of muscle protein in the atrophy of aging, as occurs in some forms of "cellular senescence."

Neurogenic atrophy

Neurogenic changes include denervation, "dysinnervation," and reinnervation. While these are not restricted to older persons, they are the most common pathologic changes found in the atrophying muscle of aging persons.

Denervation

This is a *complete loss* of LMN influences on its muscle fibers, and that produces weakness.

Dysinnervation

This is our hypothetical concept of only partially impaired, incomplete loss of neural influence, especially of molecular neurotrophic factors, some of which are still able to be produced from crippled but alive motor neurons. Our putative "dysinnervation" phenomenon can be conceptualized as having some aspects similar to a persistence of the early stages of ordinary "recent denervation," to which it appears histochemically similar.

Pan-denervations and pan-dysinnervations in regard to type-2 fiber atrophy

These are postulated as adversely influencing mainly the type-2 fibers (or sub-preferentially the type-2B fibers). Hypothetically, "pan-denervations" are due to (a) abnormality of *both* type-2 and type-1 LMNs or of their intimately related, respectively type-2 and type-1 Schwann cells (which are nurturing the LMNs and being nurtured by them). This results in lack of trophic influence on "all" the muscle fibers, either: (i) fully (in pan-denervations) or (ii) partially deficient – quantitatively or qualitatively – (in pan-dysinnervations), to which the type-2 muscle fibers (or sub-preferentially type-2B fibers) are more susceptible; or (b) hypothetically, relatively selective abnormality at the level of the presumed type-2 LMNs, or of their closely associated Schwann cells that we designate as "type-2 (or type-2B) Schwann cells." Whereas in *denervation* diseases the loss of each individual LMN's trophic influence on its muscle fibers is, by this definition, total. In dysinnervations there can be a hypothetical *quantitative partial loss* impairing *all* of the LMN's trophic influences to some degree or *qualitative loss* affecting only a fraction of the presumably several "trophic factors" originating from the affected LMNs. Denervation always produces weakness, the degree being related to the number of muscle fibers denervated.

The dysinnervations can occur in disorders of the following.

• LMNs, at the level of the soma, axon, root, proximal axon or distal axonal twigs. One putative example is "axonal" *hyperactivity*, which produces fasciculations, macrocramps, and multi-microcramps [38]. The discomforting and disabling multi-microcramps are presumably due to lability and persistent aberrant firings of distal axonal twigs – each twig innervating a few abnormally contracting/microcramping muscle fibers – caused by molecular abnormality essentially at (a) the axons themselves, or (b) at their enveloping Schwann cells. Dysinnervations can produce fatigue and weakness in relation to the quantity and quality of the neural impairment.

• Schwann cells: Schwann cell trophism to LMNs is vital for the normal function and survival of those LMNs. *Dysschwannian peripheral neuropathies* are the result of abnormal Schwann cells causing a secondary involvement of the proximal or distal portions of their encompassed axons, retrograde of the neuronal somas. Examples of dysschwannian neuropathies include: (a) diabetes-2 (type-2 diabetes) dysimmune neuropathies, (2) genetico-diabetoid-2 dysimmune neuropathies, (3) other dysimmune dysschwannian neuropathies, and (4) various non-dysimmune neuropathies (such as genetic and toxic ones). The first three are types of chronic immune dysschwannian polyneuropathy (CIDP).

Recent denervation without reinnervation compared to type-2 fiber atrophy

When slightly to moderately evolved, *recent denervation without reinnervation* (Figure 1.1a–e) is manifest (in transversely cut muscle fibers) as small angular-contoured ("angular") fibers, which are often, but not always, excessively dark with the NADH-TR and/or pan-esterase and/or the men-αGPDH reaction; sometimes those fibers are low in myophosphorylase and/or COX reactivity (Askanas and Engel, unpublished results) [4]. (The denervated type-1 fibers are more likely to be excessively dark with the NADH-TR, SDH, and pan-esterase reactions and the denervated type-2 fibers more likely excessively dark with the men-αGPDH reaction.) Slightly or moderately small "roungulated" (shape between rounded and angulated) (Figure 1.4a–c), often "pre-angular," muscle fibers can indicate either early recent denervation or type-2 fiber atrophy, the latter evidenced in its early and mid stages as more roungulated than angular atrophy. Three-zone "target fibers" (Figure 1.1d,e) in muscle are another sign of impaired innervation [4, 39], and they are often associated with an improvable dysschwannian neuropathy (Engel, unpublished results). Two-zone "targetoid fibers" (Figure 1.1e) are probably of the same neurogenic pathogenesis as target fibers but, because they are, individually, often histochemically indistinguishable from central-core disease fibers, they are called "targetoid-core fibers."

In early and mid stages of recent denervation, e.g. from amyotrophic lateral sclerosis (ALS) or peripheral neuropathy, on transverse sections typically there are scattered (not grouped) small, angular-contoured fibers, whose angularity seems to be due to their being slightly indented by the adjacent normal fibers, which apparently have greater internal hydrostatic turgidity pressure than the denervated fibers. By contrast, in early and mid stages of type-2 fiber atrophy, many of the type-2 fibers (or the 2B subset of fibers) are in about the same stage atrophy, and they are more likely to be roungulated. In nearly total recent denervation (pan-denervation), e.g. in the acute neuropathy of Guillian–Barré disease, the denervated fibers are roungulated, probably because there are no normally turgid muscle fibers to compress them. The ultrastructure of type-2 fiber atrophy resembles that of denervation atrophy [40].

(Regarding type-2 fiber atrophy, in what seem to be an advanced stage of atrophy, some fibers have become very small, dark and angular. Arbitrarily, in a setting of type-2 fiber atrophy we consider those small angular fibers and pyknotic nuclear clumps as evidence of a denervation aspect. In the advanced stage of type-2 fiber atrophy associated with small dark angular muscle fibers, the situation in that biopsy sample can be proposed to reflect (a) that all those atrophic type-2 fibers are the result of a dysinnervation process, which we favour or (b) it is "strictly a myogenous" process (if such actually exists) eventuating into atrophic fibers with denervation-like properties.) Seemingly relevant is that Goldberg et al. has reported that in rodents biochemical changes are similar between denervation atrophy and atrophy caused by cancer cachexia, starvation, disuse, and corticosteroid atrophy [29–37]. It should also be emphasized that experimental surgical pan-denervation of a muscle, plus preventing reinnervation, produces type-2 fiber atrophy, as we have shown [19, 20] (see below).

Accordingly, the neurogenic kind of type-2 fiber atrophy is proposed to be a *dysinnervation evolving into denervation*.

Pan-denervation or pan-dysinnervation hypothetically can be manifest as type-2 fiber atrophy

This can be without or with manifestation of associated ordinary recent denervation and/or established reinnervation. When there is coexisting type-2 fiber atrophy and atrophic small dark angular fibers like those of recent denervation, it can be difficult to decide whether the interpretation is: (a) two separate processes consisting of type-2 fiber atrophy plus recent denervation, or (b) the small angular fibers represent the advanced state of the type-2 fiber atrophy. The latter interpretation would be especially likely if that patient's type-2 fiber atrophy is considered to be the result of a neurogenic pan-denervation or pan-dysinnervation process. In the early and mid stages of type-2 fiber atrophy the atrophying type-2 fibers retain their normal, relative lighter-staining with NADH-TR vis-à-vis the darker type-1 fibers, for example in glucocorticoid-induced atrophy of humans, and they retain their distinctive reg-ATPase and rev-ATPase appearances throughout the type-2 atrophy [4, 9, 41–43].

Both type-2 fiber atrophy and recent denervation

Both type-2 fiber atrophy (which often seems to be due to dysinnervation) and recent denervation (with or without established reinnervation) exist *concurrently* in muscle biopsies of many aging patients (see details above and below).

Established reinnervation following previous denervation

This is manifest by muscle fiber type-grouping (detailed above) [4, 9, 16–18, 42, 43].

End-stage non-reinnervation following previous denervation

This is evident as "pyknotic nuclear clumps" (Figure 1.2a) of extremely atrophic muscle fibers. With the NADH-TR stain such "end-stage" atrophic fibers typically show high activity, indicating that they are still alive. These end-stage, apparently alive atrophic fibers can have long-persisting pyknotic nuclei, some of which can show certain features of apoptosis, such as DNA fragmentation by Tunel staining [44]. Because this atrophying process is extremely slow compared to the rapid cellular deterioration of ordinary apoptosis, we have called it "apoptosis lente."

Hypoactivity ("disuse atrophy") is manifest as type-2 fiber atrophy

This atrophy can be attributed to net reduction of overall neural activation, which triggers catabolic processes within the muscle fibers. Causes include: supra-segmental central nervous system disorders, experimental de-afferentation of LMNs, general illnesses, cast on a limb, arthritic joint pains, and psychosocial factors, such as depression or interminable television.

General neuropathic mechanisms that could cause type-2 fiber atrophy

Because the neuromuscular system is complex, there are several hypothetical neuropathic mechanisms:

1 *unlimited* pan-neuropathic: disorders (including supra-segmental disorders) affecting *all* type-2 LMNs plus all type-1 LMNs, but a disorder to which the type-2 fibers are more susceptible;

2 *unlimited* dysschwannian pan-neurogenic: LMN malfunction secondary to disorders affecting *all* type-2 plus type-1 Schwann-cells, but disorders to which the type-2 muscle fibers are more susceptible (Figure 1.2b) [19, 20];

3 *limited* type-2 neurogenic: disorders affecting *only* type-2 LMNs;

4 *limited* dysschwannian neurogenic: secondary to disorders affecting *only* type-2 Schwann-cells.

In each of these four situations, the disorder of each individual cell involved (LMN or Schwann cell) can be *complete* (resulting in denervation) or *partial* (resulting in dysinnervation).

Type-2 fiber atrophy is, after ordinary denervation and reinnervation, the second most common pathology we find in muscle atrophy of the aging. Different human conditions are associated with type-2 fiber atrophy, implying various possible pathogenic mechanisms. In the individual patient, determining which cause of the type-2 atrophy is most influential might lead to an appropriate treatment.

In the various conditions, is there a "final common path" to the type-2 fiber atrophy? This is not certain, but several of the conditions associated with type-2 fiber atrophy have the same major players, such as: ubiquitin ligases and the ubiquitin-proteasome proteolytic system; the autophagy proteolytic system; the FoxO3 system that coordinates the two proteolytic systems [32, 34, 35, 45]; JunB [29]; and myostatin (see below). Even if there is a final common pathogenic path, finding a final common elixir must be a long and winding road.

Experimentally, certain maneuvers have been reported to allegedly prevent or retard, or even reverse, type-2 fiber-associated atrophy, such as: peroxisome proliferator-activated receptor (PPAR) co-activator 1α or 1β overexpression [32]; probably increasing puromycin-sensitive aminopeptidase [30]; decreasing insulin-like growth factor 1 (IGF-1)-phosphinositide 3-kinase (PI3K)-Akt signaling and its activation of mammalian target of rapamycin (mTOR) and FoxO3 pathways [33]; increasing peroxisome proliferator-activated receptor γ coactivator 1α (PGC-1α; by suppressing FoxO3 action and atrophy-specific gene transcriptions [34]); enhancing JunB transcription factor [29]; and antagonizing ActRIIB [31]. If confirmed, these might provide clinical therapeutic leads.

Type-2 fiber atrophy: further comments

In an individual patient the cause of type-2 fiber atrophy can be multifactorial. For example, possibilities are: (a) in arthritic muscle atrophy, in which the commonly associated muscle-fiber atrophy is typically type-2 fiber atrophy [46], but whether the mechanism(s) is, speculatively, related to hypofunction/disuse, or a putative pain reflex decreasing LMN function, and/or, in rheumatoid arthritis, a concomitant dysimmune mechanism; (b) in HIV the atrophy could be dysschwannian dysimmune neuropathic, dysneuronal neuropathotoxic, cachectic, or possibly viral-myotoxic, or a combination of these.

Neuropathic mechanisms causing type-2 fiber atrophy are discussed above.

"Myopathic" mechanisms causing type-2 fiber atrophy

General comments

"Atrogenes" are a common set of genes whose expression is coordinately induced or suppressed in muscle during generalized wasting states (such as fasting, cancer cachexia, renal failure, and diabetes) [36, 45]. These can be activated by intrinsic or extrinsic muscle-fiber abnormalities.

Atrophy: "Protectosome" Versus Atrogenes
Hypothetically, aging changes might be considered a "wearing out" or a "weariness" of the cellular protective mechanisms. The normal muscle fiber, like all cells, has what we are calling a *protectosome*, i.e. a group of factors that normally inhibit expression of atrophy-producing "atrogenes;" thereby the protectosome is holding in abeyance the *atrophogenic mechanisms* with which the muscle fibers of all of us are normally equipped. However, those atrophogenic factors are constantly ready to be unleashed to produce self-erosion, self-catabolization, a sort of self-cannibalization; this putatively occurs when a

beneficent protective system falters in an aging cellular environment, or other circumstances that cause type-2 fiber atrophy. The myofiber's internal protective systems include control of endogenous free radicals and of misfolded proteins.

Myostatin
Myostatin is a negative regulator of muscle mass in normal development, and it is an important factor limiting the size of mature muscle fibers [47–53]. A normal level of myostatin is sufficient to inhibit myofibrillar synthesis rate and phosphorylation of S6K and rpS6 [54]. In normal human muscle, it is not known which fiber type expresses more myostatin, because with the antibodies used no immunoreactive myostatin was detectable in normal fibers of either type. In human type-2 muscle fiber atrophy associated with aging, myostatin protein/precursor–protein (Mstn/MstnPP), but not the mRNA, was quantitatively increased, and it was immunohistochemically increased preferentially in the atrophying type-2 muscle fibers [55]. It was also increased quantitatively in the weakening muscle of sporadic inclusion-body myositis (s-IBM), which is an aging-associated myopathy (see [55]). We propose that increased myostatin is an important pathogenic component of the type-2 fiber atrophy associated with "aging," but of yet-undetermined mechanism. Mstn/MstnPP might play an adverse role in the pathogenic cascade of type-2 muscle fiber atrophy in various situations. Quantitative increase of myostatin and its mRNA has been reported by others in human atrophic muscle associated with arthritis, with HIV, and with glucocorticoid myotoxic type-2 fiber atrophy (see [55]). Elevated serum myostatin levels occur in end-stage liver diseases, in which patients have profound muscle wasting [56]. In normal animal muscle there seems to be a pool of extracellular pro-myostatin [57]. In animal models of chronic heart failure, skeletal muscle myostatin is increased, and treadmill exercise can mitigate that myosin protein expression [58]. The actual mechanisms by which myostatin protein is pathologically increased could be a therapeutic target. IGF-1 inhibits the effects of myostatin and tends to preserve skeletal muscle in mouse models of cachexia. Administration of

ACVR2B-Fc inhibited myostatin and muscle wasting in two models of cancer cachexia, without affecting tumor growth [59]. Three days of lower-limb suspension in humans causes the unloaded ("disused") muscles to increase myostatin mRNA and protein [60], and acute antibody-directed myostatin inhibition atenuated similar disuse muscle atrophy and weakness in mice [61].

In aneurally cultured muscle fibers, tumor necrosis factor alpha (TNFα)-induced expression of myostatin through a p38 mitogen-activated protein kinase (MAPK)-dependent pathway [58]. In rats, fenfibrate, a PPARα agonist, reportedly decreased atrogenes and myostatin expression, and improved adjuvant-arthritis-induced muscle atrophy: not discussed was the hypothetical possibility that the adjuvant, collaterally, also has an unrecognized myotoxic effect [62]. That adjuvant-arthritis-associated muscle atrophy could also be attenuated by systemically administrated IGF-1, which also decreased atrogin-1 and insulin-like growth factor-binding protein 3 (IGFBP3) [63].

Clinical arthritis is associated with muscle atrophy, which may be multifactorial, involving disuse and perhaps myotoxic cytokines [46]. Terracciano et al. [46] found type-2 fiber atrophy in patients with osteoporosis or osteoarthritis (more prominent in the former), that was associated with increased circulating "inflammatory mediators," namely interleukin-6, C-reactive protein, and TNFα.

Ubiquitin-proteasome System
This is considered a major site of protein catabolism in muscle-fiber atrophies, and the activity is upregulated by ubiquitin ligases: muscle RING-finger 1 (MuRF1) and MAFbx (atrogen-1). They target particular protein substrates for degradation via the ubiquitin-proteasome pathway. The growth factor IGF-1 can block that upregulation. MuRF substrates include components of the muscle sarcomeric thick filaments, especially the myosin heavy chain. In denervation or fasting muscle atrophy, there is loss of: myosin-binding protein c and myosin light chains 1 and 2 from the myofibrils before any measurable decrease of myosin heavy chain. This selective loss requires MuRF1. Myosin heavy chain (MyHC) in myofibrils is relatively protected from

ubiquitination by its associated proteins. Because the targeted proteins stabilize the myosin-containing thick filaments, their selective ubiquitination may facilitate thick filament disassembly (the filament components are decreased by a mechanism not requiring MuRF) [37]. Others agree that during muscle atrophy, thick (myosin), but not thin (act), filaments are degraded by MuRF1-dependent ubiquitination.

FoxO3 Signaling
This coordinates activation of both autophagy/lysosomal and the proteasome catabolic pathways by FoxO3, a transcription factor that produces rapid loss of muscle mass with disuse, and systemically with fasting, cancer, and other disorders due to its causing overall accelerated breakdown of muscle proteins [33, 64–69]. Activation of the transcription factor FoxO3 is essential for muscle atrophy, via transcription of a set of atrophy-related genes (*atrogenes*) including critical ubiquitin ligases, as well as autophagy-related genes. FoxO3 coordinately activates both proteolytic systems, but especially *autophagy/lysosomal proteolysis*. FoxO3 is necessary and sufficient for the induction of autophagy in skeletal muscle, and FoxO3 is said to control the transcription of autophagy-related genes *Bnip3* and *LC3*. Activated FoxO3 stimulates autophagy through, transcription-dependent mechanisms, increasing transcription of many autophagy-related genes, which are also induced in mouse muscle atrophying due to denervation or fasting. In atrophying muscle, decreased IGF-1-PI3K-Akt signaling stimulates autophagy not only through TOR, but also more slowly by FoxO3-dependent transcription, thereby coordinating regulation of proteasome and lysosome systems. Elevated PGC-1α or PGC-1β [34, 70, 71] was reportedly "therapeutic," as manifested in several ways. It prevented the accelerated proteolysis induced by starvation or by FoxO3 transcription factors. In mouse muscle, it inhibited denervation atrophy by preventing FoxO's induction of autophagy and atrophy-specific ubiquitin ligases, and it decreased inhibition of ubiquitin ligase's induction of transcription by nuclear factor κB (NFκB). In myotubes, it caused increased protein content

and decreased overall protein degradation without altering protein synthesis.

Altruistic martyring

The type-2 fibers, and especially the 2B fibers, more readily atrophy in a number of different clinical situations, but the reasons are not known. In general, atrophying type-2 fibers are undergoing self-cannibalization and can be considered either *victims* or *martyrs*.

Martyring type-2 fibers can be thought of as, survivalistically, selflessly giving up their protein, especially their myofibrillar protein, to be broken down into its component amino acids, which then are utilized by other cells that are more essential for survival of the patient or animal, such as brain, liver, kidney, and blood cells. The muscle amino acids are used (a) via the alanine shunt, for synthesis by the liver into glucose that is circulated for wider utilization, or (b) for building cellular peptides and proteins. This martyring occurs in states of hyponutrition and cachexia, which are often induced by a chronic illness such as cancer or renal, pulmonary, cardiac or infectious disease. Autophagy, through bulk degradation of muscle-fiber protein and organelles by lysosomal enzymes and proteasomal proteolysis, helps other cells and the animal to survive during starvation.

Cancer cachexia (cachexia being the loss of lean body mass) impairs the patient's quality of life and response to antineoplastic therapies, and reportedly accounts for a least 20% of the deaths in cancer patients. Cachectic atrophy is, controversally, defined by some as muscle wasting that cannot be reversed nutritionally, while others, and ourselves, consider malnutrition muscle atrophy also as cachexia. One analytical difficulty clinically is that many cachectic patients are undernourished due to decreased food intake, which they often deny. Provoked by a cancer or other chronic disease, toxic cytokines can be released into the circulation and then probably can: (a) have a direct toxic/cachectic effect on muscle fibers; (b) acting via intermediate cells, including LMNs, have an indirect myoatrophying effect; and (c) suppress the appetite. Cachectogenic toxic cytokines include TNFα and interleukins 1β, 6, 8, 12, and 23, and these can be released by neoplastic cells, macrophages, and adipocytes. Released by adipocytes, leptin is appetite-suppressing and adiponectin is appetite-stimulating. Some of these factors in some test systems can be blocked by the following: an NFκB inhibitor SN50; anti-TNFα drugs etanercept, infliximab, and adalimumab; an anticytokine effect of thalidomide; and anti-IL12 and anti-IL23 drug ustekinumab (independently of a TNFα effect).

Treatment of cancer cachexia experimentally is to attack: the mediators, including cytokines and tumor-derived factors including TNFα and their *receptors*; androgen receptor inhibitors; proteolytic pathways (ubiquitin-proteasome and autophagy paths), intracellular signaling pathways NFκB, AP1, FoxO, and PKP, and the negative modulators of muscle growth/hypertrophy (myostatin, glycogen synthase kinase 3β (GSK3-β)) [72]. In tumor-bearing mice, there is marked muscle wasting and weight loss, associated with increased phospho-extracellular-signal-regulated kinase (pERK) and decreased myosin heavy chain: this is prevented by ERK inhibition and return of atrogin-1 expression to normal [73]. But despite "benefits" to some experimental animals, there is no good treatment for cachectic muscle atrophy in patients (see IGF-1, below).

Is there a hypothetical *cachexia lente* in many aging persons, due to a variable, additive multifactorial combination of low-grade systemic illness, hyponutrition, hypoactivity, and, possibly low-grade ischemia from anywhere in the vascular tree, including the capillaries?

Myotoxic phenomena: glucocorticoid atrophy

Muscle biopsies of glucocorticoid (corticosteroid)-treated patients having muscle weakness show what we first identified as preferential atrophy of type-2 fibers (the glycolytic, fast-twitch fibers) [4, 8, 10, 41]. In animal experiments, glucocorticoid is considered to act directly on muscle fibers to cause the now well-known type-2 fiber atrophy. (Hypothetically, perhaps with glucocorticoid toxicity there could also be a concurrent toxic neuropathic mechanism contributing directly to the atrophy, including the possibility of neuropathically susceptibilizing the muscle fiber to the glucocorticoid toxicity.)

Glucocorticoid treatment can cause insulin resistence of muscle fibers, and often aggravates diabetes-2 or makes manifest type-2 diabetes in genetically predisposed and/or obese patients.

In glucocorticoid atrophy, muscle proteolysis is especially through the ubiquitin-proteasome system, which is considered to have the major role in that catabolism. It is mediated through increased expression of several atrogenes, genes involved in muscle atrophy (such as *atrogen1* and *MuRF1*, which are two ubiquitin ligases involved in targeting proteins to be degraded by the proteasome machinery). Glucocorticoids are, according to some investigators, also anti-anabolic, blunting muscle protein synthesis. Some aspects of the glucocorticoid atrophy may result from a demonstrated decreased production of IGF-1 and increased myostatin. IGF-1, by inhibition through the PI3K-Akt pathway, antagonizes the catabolic action of glucocorticoid. The activity of the transcription factor FoxO is a major activation switch for the stimulation of several atrogenes [74]. Glucocorticoid increases myostatin expression, and in mice myostatin gene deletion prevents glucocorticoid-induced muscle atrophy. Glucocorticoid increases mRNA of enzymes involved in proteolytic pathways (atrogen1, MuRF1, and cathepsin-L), and it increases chymotrypsin-like proteasomal activity [48, 52, 75]. Glucocorticoid- and sepsis-induced muscle wasting are associated with down-regulating the expression of the nuclear cofactor PGC-1β in skeletal muscle, suggesting that this contributes to the muscle wasting [71]. In glucocorticoid-linked muscle atrophy, the myosin heavy chain is preferentially lost.

Other extrinsic triggering mechanisms or associations of muscle atrophy in aging persons

- Hormonal abnormalities: high glucocorticoid; low androgen; high parathyroid hormone; low growth hormone; insulin resistance (e.g. from high glucocorticoid); high thyroid hormone; diabetes-2 dysimmune and genetico-diabetoid-2 dysimmune neuropathic mechanisms; possibly high parathyroid-related-protein (sometimes released from tumor cells).
- Abnormal immune complexes and/or toxic antibodies, as follows.

1 In dermatomyositis we have described deposition of toxic immune complexes in small blood vessels of muscle, which is typically associated with perifascicular atrophy (meaning the atrophic muscle fibers, which are often vacuolated, tend to be located at the periphery of fascicles of muscle fibers), and location of that atrophy is probably due to ischemia, caused by those vascular deposits.
2 In myasthenia gravis, which is caused by toxic antibodies against the nicotinic receptor at the post-synaptic (muscle side) part of the neuromuscular junction, we have found muscle-biopsy features of recent denervation and/or type-2 fiber atrophy in every myasthenia gravis patient [76]. This mechanism of atrophy is literally a *myopathic dysreception* and might be multifactorial, resulting from both hypoactivity and possibly impaired concurrent dysreception of trophic-factors from the LMN. Additionally, there is probably some binding of toxic antibody to the nicotinic receptors located at the pre-synaptic neural tips of the LMNs, evident by α-bungarotoxin binding [77], thereby causing an additional true neuropathic component. (Those pre-synaptic acetylcholine receptors are probably the mediators of pyridostigmine-provoked fasciculations in myasthenics and normals; Engel, unpublished results.) (Two other possibly pathogenically relevant phenomena are α-bungarotoxin-delineated: (a) neo-appearance of nicotinic receptors on denervated human muscle fibers [78], and (b) presence of nicotinic receptors on human thymic epithelial cells [79].)
3 Circulating toxic auto-antibodies can result in type-2 fiber atrophy in dysimmune neuropathies: these are dysschwannian more often than dysneuronal type (see above).
- Putative prion, or "prionoid", and other misfolded, "sticky" abnormal proteins, originating intracellularly or extracellularly, could be capable of disrupting normal cellular function.
- Neurogenic "susceptibilization:" in individual persons with "*elder-atrophy*," it is unknown whether or not hypothetical denervation or dysinnervation is occurring and susceptibilizing the muscle fibers to undergo atrophy from a concurrent myopathic mechanism.
- Other external hypothetical susceptibilization mechanisms for muscle atrophy. These could

include impaired supply of blood, oxygen, glucose, or other vital factors.

The speculative likelihood of type-2 fiber atrophy "altruism" being important in different conditions

Likely
Hyponutrition/starvation: the mechanism, in principle, could be increased catabolism affecting: (a) an aspect that is more active in type-2 fibers, or decrease of a normal mechanism that is more important in type-2 fibers (such as anerobic glycolysis or mitochondrial α-glycerolphosphate dehydrogenase); or (b) an aspect having a narrower margin of error in type-2 fibers, meaning being closer to being insufficient (for example, mitochondrial oxidative metabolism, such as affecting COX or SDH).

Uncertain
In HIV there is often a complex pathogenesis of the muscle atrophy, which histochemically is type-2 fiber atrophy with or without denervation atrophy. It can have five components: (a) neuropathic, *viz.* dysimmune dysschwannian denervation neuropathy early in the course of the disease, and virogenic toxicity causing dysneuronal neuropathy later; (b) often cachexia; (c) hypomotility/disuse; (d) possible nerve toxicity of anti-HIV drugs; (e) infrequently, myotoxicity from viral products. With HIV, type-2 fiber atrophy in response to a hyponutritional/cachectic aspect would be altruistic, but when in response to the other causes it would not be.

Probably not likely
 (a) Hypoactivity from lassitude, or immobilization in a cast or brace; (b) atrogenic toxins attributed to a remote neoplasm (unless it is acting via hyponutrition); (c) glucocorticoid toxicity (possibly by causing insulin resistance, more so in type 2-fibers); (d) HIV viral toxicity.

Not likely
 (a) Myotoxins; (b) denervation/dysinnervation diseases (e.g., ALS, peripheral neuropathy, root/nerve mechanical pressure), although they secondarily cause dysphagia and hyponutrition; (c) myasthenia gravis (before hyponutrition), possibly involving both hypoactivity and insufficient neurotrophic factors; (d) pain, local or regional (arthritis, osteo- and rheumatoid, causing hypoactivity and/or a putative "*dolorogenic atrophy*"); (e) surgical or pharmacological castration of normal males; and (f) the "feminosity" aspect of normal women having type-2 fibers smaller than type-1 fibers. (We do not know the gender-specific diameters of muscle fibers in species of spiders in which the female is much larger and typically eats the male right after copulation.)

Other changes in aging muscle

Mitochondrial abnormalities: histochemical aspects

Diminished COX staining
Specifically this is the absence, or prominent decrease, of COX staining at a given transverse level of a muscle fiber and often segmentally distributed as multifocal absences along the long individual muscle fibers (Figure 1.5b) (see [80]). These foci are often increased in aging human muscle, without an identified mitochondria-related mitochondrial DNA (mtDNA) or nuclear DNA defect (Engel, unpublished results) [80]. They indicate mitochondrial abnormality, and we suggest that they might be only the tip of the iceberg, evoking the possibility of an accompanying, histochemically inapparent crippling reduction or absence of COX in a portion of the muscle fiber's multitudinous mitochondria. Because type-2 fibers normally have considerably less COX activity (and perhaps less "COX reserve"), hypothetically they might be more likely to atrophy from a partial impairment of COX activity. The specific pathogenesis of *multifocal COX deficiency* and other mitochondrial abnormalities in aging muscle fibers is unknown, and treatment not established.

Specific or not-yet-specific mitochondrial myopathies
Primary defects of mtDNA, or nuclear DNA, affecting muscle mitochondria (with or without other cells),

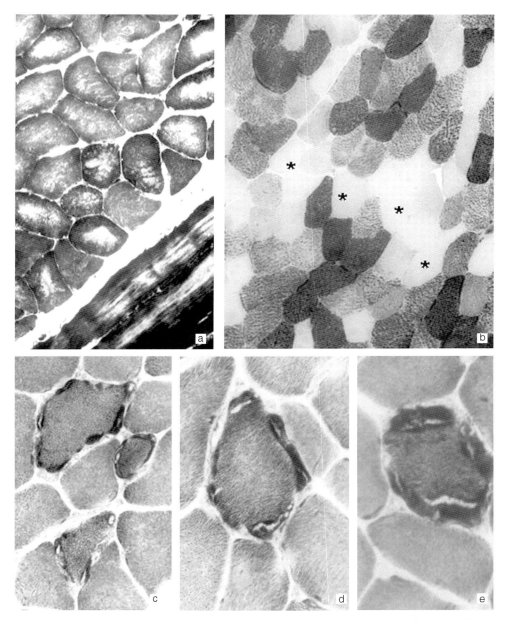

Figure 1.5 Disturbed mitochondrial activity in patients over age 70. (a) "Moth-eaten" and "large central pallor" patterns in various muscle fibers stained for cytochrome-oxidase activity. At the lower right are two longitudinally cut muscle fibers showing a very elongated distribution of central pallor within those fibers; these are an occasional finding in a chronic peripheral neuropathy patient. (b,c) Many normal-diameter muscle fibers (some indicated by asterisks) have complete absence of cytochrome oxidase staining (white fibers in this photograph), intermingled with normal type-1 (very dark) and type-2 (slightly dark) fibers. (c–e) Several "ragged-red" type of muscle fibers, actually "ragged-blue" fibers in these succinate dehydrogenase stainings of mitochondria. They are excessively stained in comparison to the other surrounding normally stained fibers. Magnification: (a) ×2000; (b) ×1670; (c) ×3000; (d) ×3670; (e) ×3670.

associated with characteristic clinical syndromes, can be highlighted by muscle biopsy histochemistry, but identifying the specific defect requires special biochemical techniques (see Chapter 4 in this volume). Not-yet-specific defects presumably underlie the more commonly seen muscle fibers having either absent, diminished or, infrequently, excessive, staining with COX or SDH, and they are more abundant in aging human muscle (Figures 1.5a and Figure 1.6a–c). When unassociated with a specific clinical syndrome, aging human muscle can have increasingly abnormal mitochondrial biochemical functions, to various degrees [81, 82]. Some mitochondrially focused investigators have deemed the general aging of muscle a "mitochondrial myopathy" (see Chapter 4) [83]. Like aging humans, "otherwise normal" aging animals have more fatigable muscle associated with mitochondrial biochemical abnormalities [84]. Mitochondrial abnormalities of aging humans are not yet treatable.

Ragged-red fibers and rugged-red fibers

In both of these, the accumulations of abnormal mitochondria are bright red with the Engel trichrome stain [4, 5, 85–87], and their mitochondriality can be demonstrated histochemically by abnormally dark (Figure 1.5c–e), or sometimes concurrently absent, staining with one of these: SDH, COX, β-hydroxybutyrate dehydrogenase, or men-αGPDH: they are sometimes deficient in one mitochondrial enzyme accompanied by an increased amount of others. The overall cytoarchitecture of the *ragged-red fibers* (which we first described [88]) appears abnormally loose, while the *rugged-red fibers* have a firm, fully-packed appearance. Molecular genetic analyses in special laboratories can sometimes identify the exact mtDNA or nuclear DNA defect crippling the mitochondria (see Chapter 4). These mitochondrial accumulations are often, but not always, more evident in type-1 fibers (which normally have more mitochondria). Ragged-red fibers are more frequent in aging human muscle, and especially in s-IBM (an aging-associated muscle disease) (see Chapter 7 in this volume).

A normal variation can be the *rugged-red* appearance of a bright red rim of packed mitochondria in many of the type-1 fibers, especially in some persons

doing very vigorous prolonged endurance exercising such as frequent long-distance cycling. In normal human muscle, histochemistry demonstrates that the mitochondria are *qualitatively different* between type-1 and type-2 muscle fibers: mitochondria in type-1 fibers have stronger SDH and weaker men-αGPDH activities, and type-2 fibers show the converse [4, 8–10].

"One-way streaks" and "increase-decrease fibers"

These "mitochondrial pattern abnormalities" (Figure 1.6) are based on rearrangements of the normal orderly array of mitochondria in a delicate pattern amongst the myofibrils. These pattern abnormalities probably reflect myofibrillar abnormality and/or mitochondrial abnormality.

Secondary mitochondriopathy

This hypothetical pathogenesis might occur in an unrecognized "noxious neighborhood," *viz.* an abnormal milieu within muscle fibers that affects mitochondrial function; for example, one involving a glycolytic enzyme, or another nonmitochondrial defect.

In *adult-onset muscle phosphorylase deficiency* there are prominent histochemically-evident mitochondrial disturbances. An example was our patient (the first identified) who had clinical onset of fatigue and weakness at age 48. Her muscle biopsy showed prominent patchy absence of mitochondrial oxidative enzyme activity histochemically (Figure 1.6d) [89]. We now hypothesize that the mitochondria were secondarily impaired due to intracellular lack of ATP consequent to defective anaerobic glycolysis caused by the myophosphorylase deficiency. By analogy, possibly other, or even many, mitochondrial abnormalities might be due to damage inflicted by a glycolytic or other nonmitochondrial biochemical abnormality (things one sees are not always what at first they seem to be). For example, possibly the patchy mitochondrial activity loss in other aging patients (Figures 1.5a,b and Figure 1.6a–c) could have an underlying aspect of insufficient glycolysis-generated ATP. Therapeutically speculating, patients like ours with late-onset myophosphorylase deficiency, and perhaps ones

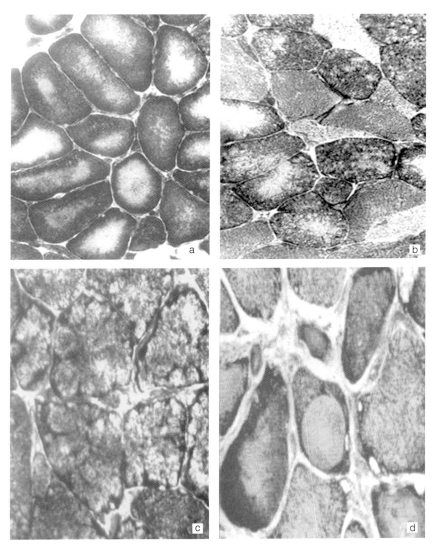

Figure 1.6 Loss of mitochondrial cytochrome oxidase activity in various patterns of distribution, in patients over age 70. (a) Regions of "large central pallor" (which are much larger than the pale regions of targetoid-core fibers); this is an occasional finding, as in this chronic peripheral neuropathy patient. (Apparently-identical changes were evident in muscle 14 days following suprasegmental cordotomy [21].) (b,c) "Decrease-increase" pattern in type-1 fibers: this is a disturbed arrangement of mitochondrial staining, due probably to abnormality of both mitochondria and myofibrils, and possibly also of stabilizing desmin filaments. This looks like a "myopathic" phenomenon, but it can be accompanying recent denervation, or type-2 fiber atrophy (evidenced by the small angular lightly stained fibers in panel b). (d) Muscle fibers showing regions of complete or moth-eaten absence of mitochondrial staining, in a patient with *adult-onset myophosphorylase activity* deficiency (completely absent myophosphorylase was proved histochemically and biochemically). This suggests that the manifested mitochondrial abnormality may be secondary to the glycolytic defect. Magnification: (a) ×2170; (b) ×2000; (c) ×4000; (d) ×3170.

with another glycolytic defect, might benefit from a putative "mitochondrial therapy," such as L-carnitine or CoQ10, or another that in the future will be found more beneficial.

In most cases of type-2 fiber atrophy we have observed histochemically that the atrophic type-2 fibers seem to have somewhat reduced oxidative enzyme activity, while maintaining the usual abundant myophosphorylase activity typical of type-2 fibers. Possible caveat: there could be impairment of an unstudied glycolytic or other non-mitochondrial enzyme involved in ATP production (or other important mitochondrial-supporting function).

Intracellular amyloid-β oligomers in s-IBM: in s-IBM, ragged-red fibers are somewhat more abundant than in similarly aged non-IBM patients, and mitochondrial functional defects occur (see Chapters 7 and 10). From Askanas' studies, the earliest identifiable pathogenic step in s-IBM is intracellular increase of amyloid-β oligomers, which are considered to be *mitotoxic* because their over-expression within cultured human muscle fibers produces mitochondrial abnormalities (see Chapters 7 and 10).

Uncontrolled free radicals can also damage mitochondria.

Other histochemical changes in aging muscle fibers

Increased acid phosphatase staining, a marker of lysosomal activity

Histochemically, the major amount of enzymatically active acid phosphatase is associated with accumulations of lipofuscin granules, typically located beneath the plasmalemma at the periphery of muscle fibers, and especially adjacent to nuclei (Figure 1.7b,c) (including being adjacent to any internal nuclei). There is also a delicate multipunctate distribution of acid phosphatase (without histochemically discernable lipofuscin granules) throughout the muscle-fiber cytoplasm. Acid phosphatase *at both of these sites increases with aging* in everyone, but the amount in aging muscle varies quantitatively from person to person (Engel, unpublished results). It is not established whether the gradual increase of the lysosomal acid phosphatase is

beneficial, neutral, or detrimental. It could be a signal that various invisible, possibly toxic, misfolded and indigestible molecules are gradually accumulating in the aging muscle fiber. The lipofuscin itself is thought to be *indigestible cellular detritus.*

Triglyceride lipid droplets are sometimes increased in muscle fibers

These droplets (Figure 1.7a), which do not seem to be aging-related, can result from excessive circulating triglycerides, or from impairment of their catabolism within the muscle fibers, including the mitochondrial phase of their utilization for ATP/energy fuel. They also seem to be more numerous in obese persons (Engel and Askanas, unpublished results).

Vacuolar myopathies of adult onset

These include the following: (a) s-IBM is a vacuolar myopathy with protein aggregates (inclusions), which include aggregates containing amyloid-β, phosphorylated-tau, α-synuclein, parkin, and many other Alzheimer- and Parkinson-type proteins in those accumulations (see Chapters 7 and 10). s-IBM still lacks a definitive treatment (see Chapter 7). (b) Hereditary inclusion-body myopathy is due to mutation of the *GNE* or *VCP* gene (see Chapters 12 and 15). (c) Adult-onset acid-maltase deficiency. (d) Dermatomyositis often well-treatable (see above and Chapter 3).

Amyloid

Abnormal aggregations of misfolded protein molecules stainable with the fluorescence Congo red method of Askanas [90], or more simply but less inclusively with crystal violet, are called "amyloid." The amyloid in skeletal muscle tissue can be: (a) *extracellular,* usually in muscle connective tissue regions or in blood-vessel walls. including blood vessels of peripheral nerves; or (b) *intracellular* (within muscle fibers) of s-IBM (see Chapters 7 and 10). Muscle extracellular amyloid is often composed of the variable portion of an immunoglobulin light chain, or mutant transthyretin, but sometimes other proteins are involved primarily or secondarily. (Extracellular amyloid can be clinically identified, noninvasively, by Mibi radioisotope scanning [91]). We have previously postulated that *cyto-disturbance*

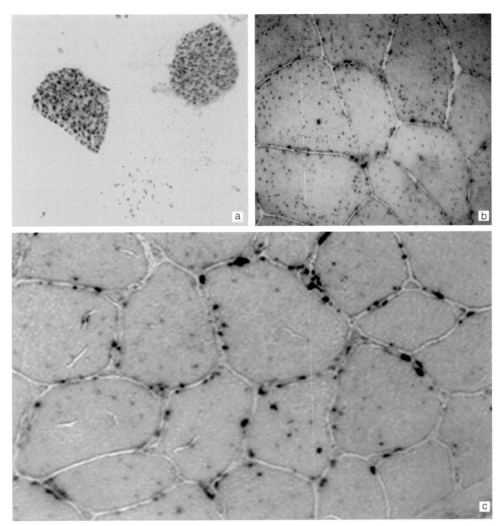

Figure 1.7 (a) Excessive triglyceride droplets in two normal-size muscle fibers. With this photographic exposure, the staining of normal fibers is only faintly evident in the lower part of the figure. Oil red O stain. (b,c) Excessive staining of acid phosphatase activity in the form of multiple tiny dots. The larger clumps of staining, usually peripherally located, are closely associated with lipofuscin granules. Although the acid-phosphatase staining in everyone gradually increases with aging, this amount of staining is excessive for this man's age of 45 (it is more like that of someone age 85). Magnification: (a) ×3330; (b) ×4500; (c) ×5830.

from extracellular amyloid [92] and from intracellular amyloid (see Chapters 7 and 10) is not due to space-occupying mechanical pressure of the visible deposits, but rather a molecular *cytotoxic affinity* of the misfolded amyloid precursor molecules existing as toxic oligomers and monomers.

Rods

In adult-onset rod myopathy, which we now designate as "*adult-onset rod myopathy syndrome*" because of its association with a monoclonal gammopathy [93–95], with or without dysschwannian, probably dysimmune, neuropathy [96]. Recently, we have successfully treated a patient with intravenous im-munoglobulin (IVIG) [94], and even more effectively when rituximab was added [96]. Interestingly, rods in animal muscle fibers can be produced by tenot-omy [97]. Perhaps in the patients the autoimmune attack is on the tendons.

Vascular aspects of aging muscle

These are discussed in Chapter 2 of this volume.

Putative animal "models" of human "AAM": biochemical studies

Such studies are numerous. They will not be re-viewed in detail, partly because it is not certain which are directly relevant to the complex human problem. Because therapy for patients is the ultimate goal, biochemical studies of aging human muscle would be relevant to understanding the pathogen-esis of aging atrophy if, in the patients studied, the disorder is actually primary within their muscle fibers. But if the problem is caused by a dysinnerva-tion or denervation phenomenon, the essential trouble needing repair is located elsewhere, farther upstream in the motor unit.

"Sarcopenia": critique of the term, concept, and "diagnosis"

"Sarcopenia" simply refers to muscle atrophy in aged animals, and it is often considered to be manifest typically as type-2 fiber atrophy. However, sarcopenia is a term we never use because it is imprecise: it is not a definite pathogenic diagnosis. It is often erroneously interpreted as designating a singular pathogenesis, but it still is enigmatic. The designation "sarcopenia" is commonly employed in experimental work, in which it is sometimes used, pseudoprecisely, for the broad topic of muscle atrophy in aged animals, a phenomenon for which we prefer to use the more direct, non-specific designation AAM. For an aging patient complaining of muscle weakness and atrophy, stating a diagnosis of sarcopenia is meaningless: it adds nothing beyond the patient's chief complaint.

So-called "sarcopenia" seems more neuropathic than purely myopathic

If, as we postulate, there is a significant neuropathic component in "sarcopenia," analyses of homoge-nized muscle are actually *looking only at the train wreck but not seeking the upstream cause of the derailment.* If a denervation/dysinnervation component is indeed present, that would require moving the focus of pathogenic interest and analysis upstream to the LMNs, their Schwann cells, and possibly to their pre-synaptic afferent neurons.

Because muscle of "sarcopenic" animals report-edly shows, typically, type-2 fiber atrophy, the fol-lowing comments are relevant.

• "Dysinnervation" is our concept of partially im-paired neurotrophic influence from crippled but still-alive motor neurons. In human type-2 fiber atrophies, including those of aged persons, histo-chemically we often (a) identify a subtle partial- or pan-denervation or (b) suspect a dysinnervation, neither being primarily myogenous. In this respect, we have strikingly demonstrated type-2 atrophy in experimental animals by acute pan-denervation, produced by total sciatic-nerve transection without reinnervation [19, 20]. Likewise, it is quite possible that in some, perhaps many examples of AAM (so-called sarcopenia) of aging animals a neurogenic mechanism may have a major role.

• Ideally, the AAM animals whose muscles are ho-mogenized for biochemical and molecular-genetic studies, should also:

   1 be pre-screened "clinically," including by elec-trophysiology, for identifiable abnormalities that in aging humans are considered to cause muscle-fiber atrophy, especially ones causing type-2 fiber atrophy. These potential abnormalities include: overt or subtle partial or pan-denervation or pan-dysinnervation, hyponutrition/cachexia, and hormone dysregulations. Without this clinical evaluation, it is difficult to be precise about the type of pathogenesis of muscle atrophy in AAM animals;

   2 have the same experimental muscle (or the contralateral one) concurrently studied histochemically to visualize and correlate diag-nostically the morphology and distribution of the presumably abnormal fibers one is homogenizing, with an awareness that different muscles have different mixtures of muscle-fiber types.

• As "disease-controls" for biochemical/molecular-genetic studies of muscle atrophy of aged animals, the same investigative techniques should be utilized to examine in mid-adult-age animals the effects of: (a) induced acute denervation, slow denervation and dysinnervation; and (b) hyponutrition/cachexia.

• Because a relatively greater atrophy of myofibrils characterizes most muscle-fiber atrophies, including type-2 fiber atrophy, denervation atrophy, and atrophic fibers in the several myositides and other myopathies, is there an absolutely unchanging denominator that should be used in studying the various aspects of muscle atrophy in humans and animals? Is use of the "housekeeping" gene/protein actin absolutely reliable?

A critical question

How could one ever prove that there is *not* a neuropathic denervation-dysinnervation component underlying some or many examples of the type-2 fiber atrophy in aged animals, or humans?

Treatment and prevention of human AAM

There is no sure method. Considerations include the following.

Specific treatments

Carefully seek all possibly relevant treatable diseases, and treat any identified correctable causative disorder. e.g. dysimmune neuropathy or primary hyperparathyroidism.

Non-specific treatments

1 Correct any *hyponutrition*, which, in our experience, many undernourished patients deny.
2 Consider available general treatments of "muscle atrophy" discussed below.
3 Monitor the literature for new drugs from animal and human studies.
4 If in a specific situation the type-2 atrophy itself is considered to be actually beneficial – e.g. altruistic

martyring via the survivalistic muscle alanine to liver gluconeogenesis pathway in starvation (see above) – one might not be able to symptomatically stop the type-2 atrophy without correcting its cause.

Results from animal and human studies

There are numerous studies of muscle atrophy in aging animals, but their practical relevance to understanding and treating muscle-fiber weakness and atrophy of aging humans is still being determined. They are disclosing interesting molecular mechanisms, but as yet no successful, enduring prevention or treatment has come from them; no new clinically useful drugs for aging atrophy have emerged [98–102]. Accordingly, myophysiologists and myopharmacologists consider that currently the only somewhat beneficial measure is exercise, preferably resistance exercise, *if it can be performed diligently*.

Exercise

The dictum is "maintain a physically active life" (see [103–105]). Despite a plethora of recent and ongoing pharmacologic research, "exercise is the primary therapy," but that can be difficult. Many of the aged persons with muscle weakness and atrophy have *coexisting exercise-limiting conditions* such as: pain from arthritis, peripheral neuropathy, radiculopathy or another cause; obesity; general fatigue from another disorder such as cardiac, pulmonary, renal, or neoplastic disease; fatigue from various prescription medicines; or even the weakness itself produced by the atrophying muscles. Exercise-wise, the following should be done.

1 Exercise to the extent possible, and active resistance exercise is encouraged. The actual ongoing amount of exercise required to develop and sustain improved strength in aging persons is not known; in actual studies of exercise in aged humans, usually only short-term studies were done.
2 Reduce neuropathic and joint pain: this will also facilitate mobility and exercising. Exercising in a pool can be easier.
3 Reduce obesity: that will facilitate mobility and exercising and, as an extra benefit, perhaps mitigate or prevent a type-2 diabetes status.

Oral leucine, with or without isoleucine and valine (branch-chain amino acids)

These are considered anabolic and utilizable directly by the muscle fibers for their protein synthesis [106]. For patients, the precise salutary amounts and scheduling of these branch-chain amino acids are not established (see Chapter 6 in this volume). They are somewhat difficult to dissolve in liquid.

If these substances actually benefit, possible schedules are: (a) before exercise sessions, as suggested by others; or (b) multiple times during the day is our suggestion, especially for less mobile older persons. However, some investigators consider that these substances are beneficial only when combined with diligent exercise, a difficult assignment for many of the elderly.

Testosterone

Aging men without significant illness typically have a gradual decrease of free and total circulating testosterone after about age 65–70. This can be of testicular origin (associated with elevated circulating follicle-stimulating hormone (FSH) and luteinizing hormone (LH), or of pituitary origin (associated with low circulating FSH and LH). It is not known whether the degree of reduced testosterone correlates with an amount of type-2 fiber atrophy. Both LMNs and muscle fibers have androgen receptors responsive to testosterone/dihydrotesterone; thus, testosterone-therapy benefit could be on LMNs, muscle fibers, or both. Weekly injections of *depo-testosterone*, a known masculinizing anaboloid, in some men with a neuromuscular disease (e.g. ALS, s-IBM, or myotonic dystrophy-1), have increased skeletal muscle endurance and strength for about 4–8 days (Engel, unpublished results). (Probably testosterone is the reason human male muscle is stronger than female muscle.) Castration experiments, in animals, suggest that androgens are not required for peak muscle performance in females but are in males, where they act through the androgen receptor to regulate multiple gene pathways that control muscle mass, strength, and resistance to fatigue [66]. In a clinical use of depo-testosterone, one must be mindful of the patient's ongoing prostate-specific antigen (PSA) status, and also avoid giving it concurrently with a glucocorticoid (a combination that can provoke diabetes-2).

Therapeutically, and potentially prophylactically, the ideal amount, route (intramuscular or transcutaneous), and frequency of testosterone therapy are not known, and must be weighed against its recognized side effects, including but not limited to: (a) short-temper; irritability, and anger; (b) possibly increased chance of prostate cancer; (c) possibly aggravation of an existing diabetes-2 or a genetic- or obesity-based diabetes-2 tendency, especially if the patient is concurrently taking a glucocorticoid or growth hormone; (d) elevation of hematocrit. Cautious ascending-dose titration is important. Oral androgen preparations can engender liver abnormalities. A normal aromatized metabolic product of testosterone is a high level of *estradiol*: its feminizing and/or other possible side effects on the human male neuromuscular system are not established. Some clinicians have considered combining an *aromatase inhibitor*, such as letrozole, anastrozole, or exemestane, to sustain the benefit of testosterone and block estrogenization (but one should note that aromatase inhibitors can have their own side effects). Needed is development of a water-soluble, non-estrogenic androgen preparation that can be safely given subcutaneously or orally.

In general, androgenic anabolic effects involve early downregulation of axin and induction of IGF-1, causing nuclear accumulation of β-catenin (a pro-myogenic, anti-adipogenic stem-cell regulatory factor). This is related to type-2 fiber hypertrophy and atrophy [107]. The androgen receptor is a ligand-dependent transcription factor, containing binding sequences for the Mef2 family of transcription factors, suggesting a functional interaction in skeletal muscle between the androgen receptor and Mef2c [108].

In the future, if surreptitiously developed and used androgens really do enhance athletic performance (more home-runs!), and are safe, perhaps they can be brought to light and tested for counteracting muscle weakness of aging and other enfeebling conditions.

Growth hormone (somatropin)

This drug is US Food and Drug Administration-approved for "HIV associated cachexia," i.e. the HIV muscle atrophy (wasting) that is typically type-2 fiber atrophy. The cause of the muscle weakness and atrophy in HIV patients can be multifactorial, due to: cachexia/hyponutrition; hypoactivity; and virogenic-autoimmune and virotoxic peripheral neuropathies (see above). For AAM, (an imprecise designation, v.s.) growth hormone has not yet been proved effective in a formal trial. Potential side effects of growth hormone therapy must be considered.

Anti-myostatins

Intended for general treatment of muscle-fiber atrophy in aging and in several other settings, anti-myostatins are being developed as a new approach, but they have not yet become established for clinical use in any human muscle atrophy.

• *Follistatin* is a *normal, powerful inhibitor of myostatin action*. Investigatively, it is being given intramuscularly by gene transfer of an alternately spliced cDNA of follistatin, and reportedly it has shown anti-atrophy benefit in mice and monkeys [109, 110]. Very limited human trials are in progress, but apparently none yet for "muscle atrophy of aging".

• *ActRIIB-Fc* is a *myostatin/GDF-8 decoy-receptor*, now in human trials. In animals, ActRIIB-Fc reportedly can reverse cancer cachexia and muscle wasting. In several cancer models, pharmacological blockade of the ActRIIB pathway prevented further muscle wasting and is said to have "completely reversed" prior loss of skeletal muscle (as well as the cancer-induced cardiac atrophy). It also "dramatically prolonged survival" even when the tumor growth was not inhibited. That blockage abolished induction of the ubiquitin ligases and activation of the ubiquitin-proteasome system [31].

• Other potential therapeutic targets in the adverse catabolic pathways of muscle fibers are also being considered.

Potentially salutatory molecular components for future therapeutic consideration

IGF-1

In rats with experimental adjuvant arthritis, systemic IGF-1 reportedly counteracted the muscle atrophy and decreased the atrogen-1 and IGFBP-3 [63] (also, see above).

β-Adrenergic agonists

These are experimental anabolic agents for muscle fibers, causing increased protein synthesis and decreased catabolism. An IGF-1-independent path activates β-adrenoreceptors, enhancing skeletal muscle growth and producing hypertrophy of cultured C2C12 cells (a muscle-derived cell line) [111]. However, clinically significant side effects are of potential concern. β-Adrenergic receptors have been demonstrated autoradiographically in human muscle [112].

JunB

The *JunB transcription factor allegedly maintains skeletal muscle mass and can promote hypertrophy*. JunB is also a major determinant of whether adult muscles grow or atrophy. In adult muscle, decreasing JunB expression by RNA interference causes atrophy, and overexpression of JunB causes independently stimulated protein synthesis and muscle-fiber hypertrophy. JunB transfected into denervated muscle "prevents" fiber atrophy. JunB protects atrophy-targeted proteins by blocking FoxO3 binding to promoters of the ubiquitin ligases atrogin-1 and MuRF-1, and thus reducing protein breakdown in proteasomes. Thus, JunB in adult muscle is required for maintenance of muscle size: it can induce hypertrophy and block atrophy [30]. Autophagy inhibition reportedly can induce "atrophy and myopathy" in adult skeletal muscles, and does not protect skeletal muscles from atrophy during denervation and fasting [113].

Conjugated linoleic acid

Based on treatment of cultured muscle cells, this has been suggested for treatment of cancer cachexia [114].

Pharmacological/biochemical substances without established value for human muscle atrophy of aging

Many substances have been tried, including creatine and DHEA, but none has yet proved effective for AAM, partly because we do not yet understand the essential pathogenesis, or pathogeneses.

Finally, persons should be wary of *nostrums* advertised for "preventing or treating muscle aging."

References

1 Engel WK, Warmolts JR. (1971) Myasthenia gravis: a new hypothesis of the pathogenesis and a new form of treatment. *Ann NY Acad Sci* **18**, 72–87.

2 Engel WK, Warmolts JR. (1973) The motor unit: Diseases affecting it in toto or in portio. In: Desmedt JE (ed.). *New Developments in Electromyography and Clinical Neurophysiology*. Karger, Basel, pp. 141–177.

3 Engel WK, Gold GN, Karpati G. (1968) Type I fiber hypotrophy and central nuclei. A rare congenital muscle abnormality with a possible experimental model. *Arch Neurol* **18**, 435–444.

4 Engel WK. (1962) The essentiality of histo- and cytochemical studies of skeletal muscle in the investigation of neuromuscular disease. *Neurology* **12**, 778–794.

5 Engel WK, Cunningham GG. (1963) Rapid examination of muscle tissue-an improved trichrome method for fresh-frozen biopsy sections. *Neurology* **13**, 919–923.

6 Padykula HA, Herman E. (1955) Factors affecting the activity of adenosine triphosphatase and other phosphatases as measured by histochemical techniques. *J Histochem Cytochem* **3**, 161–169.

7 Drews GA, Engel WK. (1966) Reversal of the ATPase reaction in muscle fiber by EDTA. *Nature* **212**, 1551–1553.

8 Engel WK. (1965) A clinical approach to the myopathies. *Clin Orthop Rel Res* **39**, 6–18.

9 Engel WK. (1965) Muscle biopsy. *Clin Orthop Rel Res* **39**, 80–105.

10 Engel WK. (1965) Diseases of the neuromuscular junction and muscle. In: Adams C (ed.). *Neurohistochemistry*. Elsevier Press, Amsterdam, pp. 622–672.

11 Engel WK. (1970) Selective and nonselective susceptibility of muscle fiber types. A new approach to human neuromuscular diseases. *Arch Neurol* **22**, 97–117.

12 Engel WK. (1967) Focal myopathic changes produced by electromyographic and hypodermic needles. *"Needle myopathy". Arch Neurol* **16**, 509–511.

13 Campa JF, Engel WK. (1970) Histochemistry of motor neurons and interneurons in the cat lumbar spinal cord. *Neurology* **20**, 559–568.

14 Campa JF, Engel WK. (1970) Histochemical classification of anterior horn neurons. *Neurology* **20**, 386.

15 Campa JF, Engel WK. (1971) Histochemical and functional correlations in anterior horn neurons of the cat spinal cord. *Science* **171**, 198–199.

16 Karpati G, Engel WK. (1968) "Type grouping" in skeletal muscles after experimental reinnervation. *Neurology* **18**, 447–455.

17 Hogenhuis LAH, Engel WK. (1965) Histochemistry and cytochemistry of experimentally denervated guinea pig muscle. I. Histochemistry. *Acta Anat* **69**, 39–65.

18 Karpati G, Engel WK. (1967) Transformation of the histochemical profile of skeletal muscle by "foreign innervation". *Nature* **215**, 1509–1510.

19 Karpati G, Engel WK. (1968) Correlative histochemical study of skeletal muscle after a suprasegmental denervation, peripheral nerve section, and skeletal fixation. *Neurology* **18**, 681–692.

20 Karpati G, Engel WK. (1968) Histochemical investigation of fiber type ratios with the myofibrillar ATPase reaction in normal and denervated skeletal muscles in guinea pig. *Am J Anat* **122**, 145–155.

21 Fenichel GM, Engel WK. (1963) Histochemistry of muscle in infantile spinal muscular atrophy. *Neurology* **13**, 1059–1066.

22 Burke RE, Levine DN, Zajac F et al. (1971) Mammalian motor units: physiological-histochemical correlation in 3 types of cat gastrocnemius muscle. *Science* **174**, 709–712.

23 Burke RE, Tsairis P, Levine N et al. (1973) Direct correlation of physiological and histochemical characteristics of motor units of cat triceps surae muscle. In: Desmedt JE (ed.). *New Developments in Electromyography and Clinical Neurophysiology*. Karger, Basel, pp. 23–30.

24 Warmolts JR, Engel WK. (1973) Correlation of motor unit behavior with histochemical and myofiber type in humans by open-biopsy electromyography. In: Desmedt JE (ed.). *New Developments in Electromyography and Clinical Neurophysiology*. Karger, Basel, pp. 35–40.

25 Warmolts JR, Engel WK. (1972) Open biopsy electromyography. I. Correlation of motor unit behavior with histochemical muscle fiber type in human limb muscle. *Arch Neurol* **27**, 512–517.

26 Engel WK, Irwin RL. (1967) A histochemical-physiological correlation of frog skeletal muscle fibers. *Am J Physiol* **213**, 511–518.

27 Brooke MH, Kaiser KK. (1970) Muscle fiber types: how many and what kind? *Arch Neurol* **23**, 369–379.

28 Askanas V, Engel WK. (1975) Distinct subtypes of type I fibers of human skeletal muscle. *Neurology* **25**, 879–887.

29 Raffaello A, Milan G, Masiero E et al. (2010) JunB transcription factor maintains skeletal muscle mass and promotes hypertrophy. *J Cell Biol* **191**, 101–113.

30 Menzies FM, Hourez R, Imarisio S et al. (2010) Puromycin-sensitive aminopeptidase protects against aggregation-prone proteins via autophagy. *Hum Mol Genet* **19**, 4573–4586.

31 Zhou X, Wang JL, Lu J et al. (2010) Reversal of cancer cachexia and muscle wasting by ActRIIB antagonism leads to prolonged survival. *Cell* **142**, 531–543.

32 Brault JJ, Jespersen JG, Goldberg AL. (2010) Peroxisome proliferator-activated receptor gamma coactivator 1alpha or 1beta overexpression inhibits muscle protein degradation, induction of ubiquitin ligases, and disuse atrophy. *J Biol Chem* **285**, 19460–19471.

33 Zhao J, Brault JJ, Schild A et al. (2008) Coordinate activation of autophagy and the proteasome pathway by FoxO transcription factor. *Autophagy* **4**, 378–380.

34 Sandri M, Lin J, Handschin C et al. (2006) PGC-1alpha protects skeletal muscle from atrophy by suppressing FoxO3 action and atrophy-specific gene transcription. *Proc Natl Acad Sci USA* **103**, 16260–16265.

35 Mammucari C, Milan G, Romanello V et al. (2007) FoxO3 controls autophagy in skeletal muscle in vivo. *Cell Metab* **6**, 458–471.

36 Sacheck JM, Hyatt JP, Raffaello A et al. (2007) Rapid disuse and denervation atrophy involve transcriptional changes similar to those of muscle wasting during systemic diseases. *FASEB J* **21**, 140–155.

37 Cohen S, Brault JJ, Gygi SP et al. (2009) During muscle atrophy, thick, but not thin, filament components are degraded by MuRF1-dependent ubiquitylation. *J Cell Biol* **185**, 1083–1095.

38 Engel WK. (2010) Multi-microcramps (MMC) syndrome: a new pathogenic concept of subtle lower motor-neuron (LMN) lability causing very disturbing, continuing muscle pains, sometimes gratifying treatable - but often misinterpreted as mysterious "fibromyalgia" or "psychogenic". *Neurology* **74** (Suppl. 2), A465.

43 Engel WK. (1961) Muscle target fibers - a newly recognized sign of denervation. *Nature* **191**, 389–390.

40 Mendell JR, Engel WK. (1971) The fine structure of type II muscle fiber atrophy. *Neurology* **21**, 358–365.

41 Pleasure DE, Walsh GO, Engel WK. (1970) Atrophy of skeletal muscle in patients with Cushing's syndrome. *Arch Neurol* **22**, 118–125.

42 Engel WK. (1965) Histochemistry of neuromuscular disease-significance of muscle fiber types. "Neuromuscular Diseases". In: *Proceedings of the 8th International Congress of Neurology*. Excerpta Medica Foundation, Amsterdam, vol. **2**, pp. 67–101.

43 Engel WK. (1966) The multiplicity of pathologic reactions of human skeletal muscle. In: Luthy F, Bischoff A (eds). *Proceedings of the 5th International Congress of Neurology*. Excerpta Medica Foundation, Amsterdam, pp. 613–624.

44 Broccolini A, Engel WK, Askanas V. (1999) Localization of survival motor neuron protein in human apoptotic-like and regenerating muscle fibers, and neuromuscular junctions. *Neuroreport* **10**, 1637–1641.

45 Altun M, Besche HC, Overkleeft HS et al. (2010) Muscle wasting in aged, sarcopenic rats is associated with enhanced activity of the ubiquitin proteasome pathway. *J Biol Chem* **285**, 39597–39608.

46 Terracciano C, Gattelli A, Lena E et al. (2010) Differential features of muscle atrophy in patients with osteoporosis and osteoarthritis. *Acta Myologica* **29**, 88.

47 Allen DL, Cleary AS, Hanson AM et al. (2010) CCAAT/enhancer binding factor-delta expression is increased in fast skeletal muscle by food deprivation and regulates myostatin transcription in vitro. *Am J Physiol Regul Integr Comp Physiol* **299**, R1592–R1601.

48 Allen DL, Loh AS. Post-transcriptional mechanisms involving microRNA-27a and b contribute to fast-specific and glucocorticoid-mediated myostatin expression in skeletal muscle. *Am J Physiol Cell Physiol* **300**, C124–C137.

49 Gonzalez-Cadavid NF, Taylor WE, Yarasheski K. et al. (1998) Organization of the human myostatin gene and expression in healthy men and HIV-infected men with muscle wasting. *Proc Natl Acad Sci USA* **95**, 14938–14943.

50 Jespersen JG, Nedergaard A, Andersen LL et al. (2011) Myostatin expression during human muscle hypertrophy and subsequent atrophy: increased myostatin with detraining. *Scand J Med Sci Sports* **21**, 215–223.

51 Kamanga-Sollo E, Pampusch MS, White ME et al. (2003) Role of insulin-like growth factor binding protein (IGFBP)-3 in TGF-beta- and GDF-8 (myostatin)-induced suppression of proliferation in

porcine embryonic myogenic cell cultures. *J Cell Physiol* **197**, 225–231.

52 Ma K, Mallidis C, Bhasin S et al. (2003) Glucocorticoid-induced skeletal muscle atrophy is associated with upregulation of myostatin gene expression. *Am J Physiol Endocrinol Metab* **285**, E363–E371.

53 Trendelenburg AU, Meyer A, Rohner D et al. (2009) Myostatin reduces Akt/TORC1/p70S6K signaling, inhibiting myoblast differentiation and myotube size. *Am J Physiol Cell Physiol* **296**, C1258–C1270.

54 Welle S, Burgess K, Mehta S. (2009) Stimulation of skeletal muscle myofibrillar protein synthesis, p70 S6 kinase phosphorylation, and ribosomal protein S6 phosphorylation by inhibition of myostatin in mature mice. *Am J Physiol Endocrinol Metab* **296**, E567–E572.

55 Wojcik S, Nogalska A, Engel WK et al. (2008) Myostatin and its precursor protein are increased in the skeletal muscle of patients with Type-II muscle fibre atrophy. *Folia Morphol (Warsz)* **67**, 6–12.

56 Garcia PS, Cabbabe A, Kambadur R et al. (2010) Brief-reports: elevated myostatin levels in patients with liver disease: a potential contributor to skeletal muscle wasting. *Anesth Analg* **111**, 707–709.

57 Anderson SB, Goldberg AL, Whitman M. (2008) Identification of a novel pool of extracellular promyostatin in skeletal muscle. *J Biol Chem* **283**, 7027–7035.

58 Lenk K, Schur R, Linke A et al. (2009) Impact of exercise training on myostatin expression in the myocardium and skeletal muscle in a chronic heart failure model. *Eur J Heart Fail* **11**, 342–348.

59 Benny Klimek ME, Aydogdu T, Link M.J et al. (2010) Acute inhibition of myostatin-family proteins preserves skeletal muscle in mouse models of cancer cachexia. *Biochem Biophys Res Commun* **391**, 1548–1554.

60 Gustafsson T, Osterlund T, Flanagan JN et al. (2010) Effects of 3 days unloading on molecular regulators of muscle size in humans. *J Appl Physiol* **109**, 721–727.

61 Murphy KT, Cobani V, Ryall JG et al. (2011) Acute antibody-directed myostatin inhibition attenuates disuse muscle atrophy and weakness in mice. *J Appl Physiol* **110**, 1065–1072.

62 Castillero E, Nieto-Bona MP, Fernandez-Galaz C et al. (2011) Fenofibrate, a PPAR alpha agonist, decreases atrogenes and myostatin expression and improves arthritis-induced skeletal muscle atrophy. *Am J Physiol Endocrinol Metab* **300**, E790–E799.

63 Lopez-Menduina M, Martin AI, Castillero E et al. (2010) Systemic IGF-I administration attenuates the inhibitory effect of chronic arthritis on gastrocnemius mass and decreases atrogin-1 and IGFBP-3. *Am J Physiol Regul Integr Comp Physiol* **299**, R541–R551.

64 Moriscot AS, Baptista IL, Bogomolovas J et al. (2010) MuRF1 is a muscle fiber-type II associated factor and together with MuRF2 regulates type-II fiber trophicity and maintenance. *J Struct Biol* **170**, 344–353.

65 Zhao J, Brault JJ, Schild A et al. (2007) FoxO3 coordinately activates protein degradation by the autophagic/lysosomal and proteasomal pathways in atrophying muscle cells. *Cell Metab* **6**, 472–483.

66 MacLean HE, Chiu WS, Notini AJ et al. (2008) Impaired skeletal muscle development and function in male, but not female, genomic androgen receptor knockout mice. *FASEB J* **22**, 2676–2689.

67 Glass DJ. (2010) Signaling pathways perturbing muscle mass. *Curr Opin Clin Nutr Metab Care* **13**, 225–229.

68 Sandri M. (2011) New findings of lysosomal proteolysis in skeletal muscle. *Curr Opin Clin Nutr Metab Care* **14**, 223–229.

69 Mammucari C, Schiaffino S, Sandri M. (2008) Downstream of Akt: FoxO3 and mTOR in the regulation of autophagy in skeletal muscle. *Autophagy* **4**, 524–526.

70 Wenz T, Rossi SG, Rotundo RL et al. (2009) Increased muscle PGC-1alpha expression protects from sarcopenia and metabolic disease during aging. *Proc Natl Acad Sci USA* **106**, 20405–20410.

71 Menconi MJ, Arany ZP, Alamdari N et al. (2010) Sepsis and glucocorticoids downregulate the expression of the nuclear cofactor PGC-1beta in skeletal muscle. *Am J Physiol Endocrinol Metab* **299**, E533–E543.

72 Bossola M, Pacelli F, Tortorelli A et al. (2008) Skeletal muscle in cancer cachexia: the ideal target of drug therapy. *Curr Cancer Drug Targets* **8**, 285–298.

73 Penna F, Costamagna D, Fanzani A et al. (2010) Muscle wasting and impaired myogenesis in tumor bearing mice are prevented by ERK inhibition. *PLoS One* **5**, e13604.

74 Schakman O, Gilson H, Thissen JP. (2008) Mechanisms of glucocorticoid-induced myopathy. *J Endocrinol* **197**, 1–10.

75 Gilson H, Schakman O, Combaret L et al. (2007) Myostatin gene deletion prevents glucocorticoid-induced muscle atrophy. *Endocrinology* **148**, 452–460.

76 Engel WK, McFarlin DE. (1966) Muscle lesions in myasthenia gravis. *Ann NY Acad Sci* **135**, 68–78.

77 Bender AN, Ringel SP, Engel WK. (1976) The acetylcholine receptor in normal and pathologic states. Immunoperoxidase visualization of alpha-bungarotoxin binding at a light and electron-microscopic level. *Neurology* **26**, 477–483.

78 Ringel SP, Bender AN, Engel WK. (1976) Extrajunctional acetylcholine receptors. Alterations in human and experimental neuromuscular diseases. *Arch Neurol* **33**, 751–758.

79 Engel WK, Trotter JL, McFarlin DE et al. (1977) Thymic epithelial cell contains acetylcholine receptor. *Lancet* **1**, 1310–1311.

80 Oldfors A, Moslemi AR, Jonasson L et al. (2006) Mitochondrial abnormalities in inclusion-body myositis. *Neurology* **66**, S49–55.

81 Chomyn A, Attardi G. (2003) MtDNA mutations in aging and apoptosis. *Biochem Biophys Res Commun* **304**, 519–529.

82 DiMauro S, Hirano M, Schon EA (eds) (2006) *Mitochondrial Medicine*. Informa Healthcare, London.

83 Romanello V, Guadagnin E, Gomes L et al. (2010) Mitochondrial fission and remodelling contributes to muscle atrophy. *EMBO J* **29**, 1774–1785.

84 Hood D. (2010) Mitochondrial dysfunction in aging skeletal muscle: a potential therapeutic focus. *Acta Myologica* **29**, 87.

85 Olson W, Engel WK, Walsh GO et al. (1972) Oculocraniosomatic neuromuscular disease with "ragged-red" fibers. *Arch Neurol* **26**, 193–211.

86 Tsairis P, Engel WK, Kark AP. (1973) Familial myoclonic epilepsy syndrome associated with skeletal muscle mitochondrial abnormalities. *Neurology* **23**, 408.

87 Lombes A, Mendell JR, Nakase H et al. (1989) Myoclonic epilepsy and ragged-red fibers with cytochrome oxidase deficiency: neuropathology, biochemistry, and molecular genetics. *Ann Neurol* **26**, 20–33.

88 Engel WK. (1971) "Ragged-red fibers" in opthamoplegia syndromes and their differential diagnosis. *Excerpta Med Inter Cong Series* **237**, 28.

89 Engel WK, Eyerman EJ, Williams HE. (1963) Late-onset type of skeletal muscle phosphorylase deficiency: a new familial variety of completely and partially affected subjects. *New Engl J Med* **268**, 135–137.

90 Askanas V, Engel WK, Alvarez RB. (1993) Enhanced detection of congo-red-positive amyloid deposits in muscle fibers of inclusion body myositis and brain of Alzheimer's disease using fluorescence technique. *Neurology* **43**, 1265–1267.

91 Kula RW, Engel WK, Line BR. (1977) Scanning for soft-tissue amyloid. *Lancet* **1**, 92–93.

92 Engel WK, Askanas V. (1998) Treatment of inclusion-body myositis and hereditary inclusion-body myopathy with reference to pathogenic mechanisms: personal experience. In: Askanas V, Serratice G, Engel WK (eds), *Inclusion-body Myositis and Myopathies*. Cambridge University Press, Cambridge, pp. 351–382.

93 Engel WK. (1977) Rod (nemaline) disease. In: Goldensohn ES, Appel SH (eds), *Scientific Approaches to Clinical Neurology*. Lea Febiger, Philadelphia, pp. 1667–1691.

94 Engel WK. (2007) Late-onset rod myopathy with monoclonal immunoglobulin can be treatable with IVIG. *Neuromuscul Disord* **17**, 885.

95 Engel WK, Resnick JS. (1966) Late-onset rod myopathy - a newly recognized, aquired and progressive disease. *Neurology* **16**, 308–309.

96 Mahajan S, Engel WK, Luthra I, Gupta V. (2011) Adult-onset rod myopathy syndrome (AORMS): sustained benefit from IVIG plus rituximab. *Ann Neurol*, in press.

97 Engel WK, Brooke MH, Nelson PG. (1966) Histochemical studies of denervated or tenotomized cat muscle. Illustrating difficulties in relating experimental animal conditions to human neuromuscular diseases. *Ann NY Acad Sci* **138**, 160–185.

98 Murphy KT, Lynch GS. (2009) Update on emerging drugs for cancer cachexia. *Expert Opin Emerg Drugs* **14**, 619–632.

99 Cruz-Jentoft AJ, Baeyens JP, Bauer JM et al. (2010) Sarcopenia: European consensus on definition and diagnosis: Report of the European Working Group on Sarcopenia in Older People. *Age Ageing* **39**, 412–423.

100 Kung T, Springer J, Doehner W et al. (2010) Novel treatment approaches to cachexia and sarcopenia: highlights from the 5th Cachexia Conference. *Expert Opin Investig Drugs* **19**, 579–585.

101 Thomas DR. (2010) Sarcopenia. *Clin Geriatr Med* **26**, 331–346.

102 von Haehling S, Stepney R, Anker SD. (2010) Advances in understanding and treating cardiac cachexia: highlights from the 5th Cachexia Conference. *Int J Cardiol* **144**, 347–349.

103 Waters DL, Baumgartner RN, Garry PJ et al. (2010) Advantages of dietary, exercise-related, and therapeutic interventions to prevent and treat sarcopenia

in adult patients: an update. *Clin Interv Aging* **5**, 259–270.

104 Merry TL, Steinberg GR, Lynch GS et al. (2010) Skeletal muscle glucose uptake during contraction is regulated by nitric oxide and ROS independently of AMPK. *Am J Physiol Endocrinol Metab* **298**, E577–E585.

105 Gielen S, Sandri M, Erbs S et al. (2011) Exercise-induced modulation of endothelial nitric oxide production. *Curr Pharm Biotechnol*, in press.

106 D'Antona G, Nisoli E. (2010) mTOR signaling as a target of amino acid treatment of the age-related sarcopenia. *Interdiscip Top Gerontol* **37**, 115–141.

107 Gentile MA, Nantermet PV, Vogel RL et al. (2010) Androgen-mediated improvement of body composition and muscle function involves a novel early transcriptional program including IGF1, mechano growth factor, and induction of beta-catenin. *J Mol Endocrinol* **44**, 55–73.

108 Wyce A, Bai Y, Nagpal S et al. (2010) Research Resource: The androgen receptor modulates expression of genes with critical roles in muscle development and function. *Mol Endocrinol* **24**, 1665–1674.

109 Kota J, Handy CR, Haidet AM et al. (2009) Follistatin gene delivery enhances muscle growth and strength in nonhuman primates. *Sci Transl Med* **1**, 6ra15.

110 Rodino-Klapac LR, Haidet AM, Kota J et al. (2009) Inhibition of myostatin with emphasis on follistatin as a therapy for muscle disease. *Muscle Nerve* **39**, 283–296.

111 Ryall JG, Church JE, Lynch GS. (2010) Novel role for beta-adrenergic signalling in skeletal muscle growth, development and regeneration. *Clin Exp Pharmacol Physiol* **37**, 397–401.

112 Lavenstein B, Engel WK, Reddy NB et al. (1979) Autoradiographic visualization of beta-adrenergic receptors in normal and denervated skeletal muscle. *J Histochem Cytochem* **27**, 1308–1311.

113 Masiero E, Sandri M. (2010) Autophagy inhibition induces atrophy and myopathy in adult skeletal muscles. *Autophagy* **6**, 307–309.

114 Larsen AE, Crowe TC. (2009) Effects of conjugated linoleic acid on myogenic and inflammatory responses in a human primary muscle and tumor coculture model. *Nutr Cancer* **61**, 687–695.

CHAPTER 2

Aging of the human neuromuscular system: clinical considerations

W. King Engel and Valerie Askanas

Departments of Neurology and Pathology, University of Southern California Neuromuscular Center, University of Southern California Keck School of Medicine, Good Samaritan Hospital, Los Angeles, CA, USA

Concepts applicable to various neuromuscular disorders associated with aging

In this chapter we describe our experience and concepts related to clinical and pathogenic aspects of human neuromuscular aging. There is a large literature on the topic, but this chapter is not intended to be a review of that literature: it is a summary of personal experience and opinions, including various therapeutic approaches. Some relevant clinical vignettes are presented in Chapter 3 of this volume.

General principles

When does a person's biological "aging era" begin? Probably about age 40 in both genders, by which time aging-associated disorders, e.g. the female menopause, and perhaps the early phase of the andropause, have begun. Some would emphasize that some slow-downs become evident in the 20s.

"You're just getting old," or "aging," or "just old age" are not diagnoses, and they are not satisfactory explanations for the cause of neuromuscular (or other) symptoms in an aging person. These answers block further inquiry, whereas "I don't know" invites analytical thinking and exploration. But, aging certainly is a *risk factor* for a number of age-related disorders.

A full neuromuscular evaluation is needed to adequately analyze the cause of a neuromuscular problem in an aging patient, as it is in a patient of any age. This includes detailed blood tests, nerve conductions, electromyography (EMG), and a muscle biopsy (performed under local anesthetic, as an out-patient) studied by a battery of histochemical techniques. Often, cerebrospinal fluid (CSF) examination is also needed. Sometimes relevant magnetic resonance imaging is necessary.

Even though fatigue, exercise intolerance, and falling are associated with the *frailties of aging* they are *not* "normal in aging" and each has various possible causes, some treatable. Findings that are considered abnormal in early- and mid-adult life cannot arbitrarily be considered "normal" in aged persons, even if statistically they are more common in the aged; for example, hypertension, shortness of breath, peripheral and central vascular insufficiency, myocardial infarction, osteoarthritic joints, and reduced testosterone or estrogen, as well as imbalance, falling, fatigue, muscle weakness, numbness/tingling/pain of peripheral neuropathy, elevated spinal-fluid protein, slower nerve conductions, and muscle-fiber atrophy. Each of these has pathologic causes, and some are treatable.

We have sometimes found that a *treatable neuromuscular disorder* coexists with another neurologic, or nonneurologic, disorder. In any patient, and especially in an older patient, both conditions might

Muscle Aging, Inclusion-Body Myositis and Myopathies, First Edition. Edited by Valerie Askanas and W. King Engel.
© 2012 Blackwell Publishing Ltd. Published 2012 by Blackwell Publishing Ltd.

be contributing to the clinical picture, and at least one might be treatable: this possibility of concurrently multiple neuromuscular malfunctions is a *non-Oslerian, non-Occam's razor* concept that medical insurance companies can be reluctant to acknowledge (perhaps overly focusing on an untreatable component). However, it is not fair to the patient to deny treatment for a treatable condition simply because it is accompanied by a milder, untreatable one. The physician's duty is to *seek any treatable component* existing in the patient. Examples of combinations we have encountered in our patients include the following.

• *"Double neuropathy"*: chronic, mild, relatively nonprogressive hereditary neuropathy from childhood, with very high arches and steppage gait, namely a form of Charcot-Marie-Tooth (CMT) syndrome, also present in a sibling or parent, plus a *treatable "genetico-diabetoid-2," diabetes-2* (type-2 diabetes), or other dysimmune neuropathy (a concept explained below in the Clinical Comments section). The dysimmune neuropathy can be a cause of significant worsening of the weakness, peripheral sensory loss, and pain beginning at age 50–65 (see vignette 15 in Chapter 3). And, in our experience this *late-onset dysimmune neuropathy* is often very gratifyingly and continuously responsive to ongoing *intravenous immunoglobulin (IVIG)* treatment, upon which the patient is dependent [1–7].

• *Bulbospinal muscular atrophy (BSMA; Kennedy's disease)* plus *treatable genetico-diabetoid-2 or other dysimmune neuropathy*, the latter ones being very treatable with IVIG (as explained below). Although peripheral sensory neuropathy is sometimes considered part of the untreatable androgen-receptor genetic mutation of BSMA, in a BSMA patient we have found that a concurrent treatable dysimmune neuropathy should be sought.

• *Symptomatically treatable muscle cramps* accompanying various disorders, especially neuropathic abnormalities, are often well controlled with clonazepam [8, 9] (see vignette 8 in Chapter 3). Most muscle cramps are neurogenic, a few are myopathic. Cramps can be caused by a neuropathy that might otherwise be mild. If the neuropathy is worse than mild, it might itself be treatable with IVIG or other anti-dysimmune measure (see below).

• *"Pseudo-ALS"* example: cervical-disk myelopathy plus treatable *myasthenia gravis*. Pseudo-ALS is our term for a clinical condition mimicking important aspects of amyotrophic lateral sclerosis (ALS), but due to a non-ALS condition that is sometimes treatable. In this example, the myasthenia gravis mimicked (a) the bulbar aspects of ALS by producing severe dysphonia and dysphagia (necessitating a gastrotomy tube), and (b) the limb weakness. All of these aspects were well treatable to essentially normal status with high-single-dose alternate-day prednisone (and intentionally *not* using pyridostigmine/mestinon along with the prednisone) [10–13]. The concurrent cervical-disk myelopathy caused Babinski responses and slight ALS-like hyperreflexia of the lower limbs, but in retrospect those aspects were considered not progressive and not clinically important. (Myasthenia gravis itself can cause slightly brisk tendon reflexes, but not a Babinski response.)

• *Pseudo-ALS* example: *fasciculating dysimmune neuropathy*. treatable with IVIG, plus unilateral cerebral arteriovenous malformation in the motor area causing hyperreflexic hemiparesis, treated with focal microembolization. The ipsilaterality was postulated to be due to a vascular *steal* from the contralateral brain motor area.)

• Sporadic inclusion-body myositis (s-IBM) plus *genetico-diabetoid-2 dysimmune peripheral neuropathy*, the latter very treatable with IVIG (see below).

• Chronic, very slowly progressive autosomal dominant hereditary *oculopharyngeal* (but anatomically more correctly called *palpebro-pharyngeal* because there is prominent eyelid ptosis *without* impaired eye movements) *muscular dystrophy (OPMD)*, evident from teen-age in a woman and, beginning at age 61, additional moderately progressive proximal limb-muscle weakness for the last 2 years due to treatable *polymyositis*. The later, rather aggressive weakness, was previously misinterpreted as a "late progressive phase of OPMD" (which does not occur). We identified, by high serum creatine kinase (CK) and muscle-biopsy histochemistry, that the newly progressive weakness was caused by newly coexisting polymyositis. That polymyositis initially was very responsive to prednisone, but death ensued 18 months later due to a previously undetectable *metastatic cancer* of undetermined primary site; the *polymyositis* was probably a *dysimmune remote effect*.

• *Ophthalmoparesis*, presumably from *mitochondrial myopathy* diagnosed by a biceps-muscle biopsy, plus a *dysimmune neuropathy* associated with elevated CSF protein 120 mg/dL (upper normal is 45 mg/dL), which was treatable with IVIG. One should not assume that all neuromuscular aspects of a mitochondrial myopathy patient are due to an untreatable mitochondrial or nuclear DNA mutation.

• Progressive brain and spinal-cord *multiple sclerosis (MS)* plus *dysimmune peripheral neuropathy*, probably sharing with the MS a dysimmune etiologic commonality and treatability, in a woman. With IVIG treatment for >13 years, both aspects have not only stopped progressing, but have also been definitely improved. We had a similar clinical combination in a man who regained the ability to walk easily and energetically without the cane he previously needed for his imbalance and legs spasticity. His benefit from continuing IVIG lasted for more than a year, until his insurance stopped the treatments.

Clinical comments on selected neuromuscular phenomena and diseases

Every normal motor and sensory peripheral nerve fiber is, individually, an integrated "teamlet" composed of tightly apposed, very interdependent players. The normal nerve fibers (axons) transmit the electrical signal as either (a) *motor commands*, from their neuronal cell bodies situated in the spinal cord, each to about 200 muscle fibers, or (b) *sensory information* from the distal axonal endings and sensory transducers back to their neuronal cell body in the dorsal-root ganglia, near the spinal cord and thence, by cellular relay, up to brain. Tightly encircling, and arranged along each nerve fiber, like long beads on a string, are the myelin-containing *Schwann cells*. The Schwann cells supply absolutely essential trophic factors to the axon: without those factors the axon does not function normally, resulting in a "dysschwannian neuropathy." Conversely, the Schwann cells are themselves totally dependent on essential trophic factors from the neuronal axon for maintaining their normal maturity and health; impairment of that normal influence originating from the nerve fiber occurs in a primary "dysneuronal neuropathy" and results in secondary Schwann-cell damage. Note that from a motor or sensory neuropathy, *all* symptoms are directly attributable to the neuronal dysfunction, which may or may not be secondary to a Schwann-cell dysfunction.

"Diabetic neuropathy"

A patient with peripheral neuropathy and diabetes is still too often simply diagnosed as "diabetic neuropathy" and told there is no successful treatment (this is, unfortunately, sometimes still being stated in books and published articles). However, since 1992 we have been successfully treating diabetes-2-associated dysimmune neuropathies with anti-dysimmune measures [1, 3, 4, 14]. It is now increasingly accepted that in diabetes-2 there is often a *dysimmune neuropathy*, commonly with elevated CSF protein, that frequently is very well treatable with IVIG (see vignette 12 in Chapter 3, and [1, 14]) or sometimes with other less-effective anti-dysimmune measures. We have proposed that: (a) the *genetic milieu of diabetes-2 predisposes to dysimmune neuropathy* (in a cause–effect relationship [4], by a mechanism possibly *not* related directly to glucose dysmetabolism); and (b) this same mechanism can produce a *"genetico-diabetoid-2 dysimmune polyneuropathy"* (see below).

"Genetico-diabetoid-2 dysimmune polyneuropathy"

Genetico-diabetoid-2 dysimmune polyneuropathy is our term, which we have been using for 15 years to describe the same clinical and laboratory features in patients as in the above-mentioned "diabetes-2 dysimmune neuropathy," who themselves do not yet have detectable glucose dysmetabolism parameters that would be considered indicative of actual diabetes-2, but have a close family history of diabetes-2 [4] (and Engel, unpublished work). In such patients, we have found that their polyneuropathy can be manifest as long as 10 years before their diabetes-2 becomes clinically evident. This genetico-diabetoid-2 dysimmune polyneuropathy is often very treatable with IVIG [4].

In a patient who does have a close family history of diabetes-2, a glucocorticoid should be avoided if possible, because it can increase insulin resistance and make manifest diabetes-2 glucose dysmetabolism. Accordingly, asking about a close family history of diabetes-2 is very important in managing a chronic immune dysschwannian polyneuropathy (CIDP) (sometimes less precisely called chronic inflammatory demyelinating polyneuropathy), or other dysimmune patient.

Sporadic ALS and putative putative retrovirogenic-dysmetabolic mechanism involving "neuronal-nurturing cells:" an X-Y-Z hypothesis regarding this devastating and still-enigmatic disease

There is no successful treatment for sporadic ALS (sALS). Without artificial ventilation and feeding, typical patients are still dying within 1–5 years, despite a prodigious amount of time and money spent on possibly related human and tenuously related mouse research. sALS is considered an aging-evoked degeneration especially, but not exclusively, of motor-neuron systems (targeted "Cells-Z") [15, 16]. Anatomically, the sALS spinal-cord involvement has a monotonously characteristic topography. Interestingly, hereditary forms of ALS (hALS), which are similar but not identical to sALS, are typically first clinically manifest in aging, even though the gene mutation had been present throughout life, from conception. Two questions in ALS are: (a) what triggers that late-onset catastrophic neuronal cell death, clinically evident and fatal in 1–5 years; and (b) what kept the clinical disease suppressed for three to six decades? If the latter is one "factor," it should, speculatively, be an excellent treatment for hALS, and possibly for sALS.

Because the pathogenesis and treatment of sALS are still unknown, new approaches are desperately needed. The sALS myelopathic pattern suggests a *generalized dysmetabolism*, as does the posterior-column *middle-root-zone pattern* in some hALS families [17]. A dysmetabolic mechanism, if identi-fied, might be treatable by simple replacement with a "*factor-Y*," even if the putatively impaired *neuronal nurturing cells (NNCs)*/cells-X have expired long before the clinical onset of sALS.

The abundant accumulation in the sALS spinal cord of a) PAS-positive corpora amylacea within astrocytes and b) lipofuscin within motor neurons is of unknown significance [74].

We previously suggested that sALS is of *retroviral origin* [16, 18]. More recently, McCormick et al. [19], using a qPERT technique, detected retroviral reverse transcriptase in sALS sera but not in CSF. If a pathogenic ALS virus would be identified, we hypothesized that, by a *virogenic-dysmetabolic mechanism*, the proposed ALS virus might be acting (a) directly on neurons, especially lower and upper motor neurons; or (b), more intriguingly and potentially more amenable to simple treatment, the virus might be acting directly, or indirectly, on hypothetical *NNCs/cells-X* that normally a) produce, or facilitate delivery of, a metabolic *factor-Y vital* to motor neurons ("cells-Z") [15, 16], or b) inactivate a "*toxin-Y*" that preferentially *damages* motor neurons. The NNCs could be located (a) *near to or remote from* the motor-neuron somas and tracts. "Near-NNCs" (*paracrine effect*) could be the hypothetical "*para-motor-neuron astrocytes*" [16] which, like other astrocytes in ALS, manifest oxidative stress [16]; these hypothesized para-motor-neuron astrocytes are situated close to, and embryologically are putatively induced by, motor neuron somas and long tracts. Or, "remote NNCs" (*endocrine effect*) could be analogous, in principle, to gastric parietal cells that normally produce intrinsic factor required for cobalamin/B_{12} absorption in the distal ileum; deficiency and permanent loss of intrinsic factor causes its own topographically characteristic B_{12}-*deficiency myelopathy*. In ALS, disturbance of NNCs could be: (a) *indirect*, for example dysimmune, as in anti-parietal-cell antibody-induced metabolically treatable cobalamin/B_{12} deficiency; or (b) by *direct infection*, e.g. as speculated for ALS hepatocytes [15, 20]. Similarly, *indirect dysmetabolic mechanisms* were hypothesized for some forms of hALS [17].

Note: the undetectability of *reverse transcriptase* in ALS CSF, does not exclude a retrovirus in sALS; it suggests active virus may be outside the central nervous system (CNS) in remote cells, such as the NNCs/cells-X, where it could be morphologically undetectable but deranging cellular function by being integrated into the NNC molecular machinery. Accordingly, it seems appropriate to seek, by multi-tissue screening, evidence for a retroviral reverse-transcriptase and for tracks of another occult virus. We also suggest therapeutic antiviral trials, e.g. with the anti-HIV highly active antiretroviral therapy (HAART) agents, and others.

Interestingly, one of our ALS patients had the retrovirus HTLV1 [21]. Two current ALS patients have a very high serum hepatitis C viral RNA load, e.g. 291,000 IU (normal <615 IU) and PCR HCV RNA 5.52 (normal <1.63) but with repeatedly-normal liver-function tests (γ-glutamyl transpepti-dase (GGTP), aspartate aminotransferase (AST), ala-nine aminotransferase (ALT), lactate dehydrogenase (LDH)).

In a few sALS patients we found that two types of treatment have produced *transient* symptom-atic improvements of strength, but neither was able to stop the *insistent progression* of the under-lying "degenerative" ALS disease. (a) In four of our carefully followed typical sALS patients we observed, repeatedly, a slight but definite benefit for about 3–5 days following each 5-day course of IVIG, 0.4 g/kg/day (Engel, unpublished obser-vations) [22]. (b) With initial TRH (thyrotropin releasing hormone) treatment of 12 sALS pa-tients [23], transient improvements, each lasting for hours to 1–2 days, also occurred repeatedly. These responses suggest temporary re-awakening of "comatose" motor neurons, which can be interpreted as demonstrating our concept that *in every ALS patient there are some potentially revivable/ recoverable motor neurons*, and consequently a truly beneficial treatment should not only stop progression but should produce some *actual sum-mating improvements*. The TRH mechanism may have been a neurotransmitter effect stimulating partially impaired but still-alive lower motor neurons, analogous in principle to pyridostig-mine action in myasthenia gravis, and also had a confounding autorefractoriness [22]). Unfortu-nately, TRH apparently did not produce a neu-rotrophic effect able to reverse the degenerative

ALS process. The beneficial mechanism of IVIG in the ALS patients is not known, but could be based on its known anti-dysimmune or antiviral properties, or on another action. Perhaps it is an undeciphered clue to one aspect of the sALS pathogenesis.

We have also hypothesized that a metabolic defect impairing the *normally high phosphorylase* in lower motor neurons [24, 25] might play a role in ALS pathogenesis.

hALS

About 10% of all ALS patients are hereditary, asso-ciated with a mutation of *SOD1*, *TDP43*, *FUS* [26], or a newly-discovered mutution of gene *C9ORF72* at chromosome 9p21 [75]. From this latter was sug-gested a defective RNA metabolism in some cases of both hALS and sALS. An RNA hypothesis for ALS was also previously suggested [15]. Whether any of the hALS patients will have the same ultimate molecular pathogenesis as sALS is uncertain.

"Pseudo-ALS"

"Pseudo-ALS" is a *most desirable alternative* to a diag-nosis of ALS, and should always be sought. See also examples of *ALS mimics* (above) and see in Chapter 3, vignette 21 about pseudo-ALS, and vignettes 8 and 10. Several conditions sometimes mistakenly diag-nosed as regular ALS are:

• *Multifocal motor neuropathy* (Chapter 3, vignette 8).

• *Multi-microcramps* (Chapter 3, vignette 10) [8, 9].

• Dysimmune "*Fasciculating progressive muscular atrophy*" (DF-PMA), probably a motor-predominant form of CIDP, which can be remarkably responsive to anti-dysimmune treatment [27]. A 47-year-old man had treatable upper-limb DF-PMA evolving into a "*hanging arms*" or "*man-in-a-barrel*" appear-ance, which had developed slowly and asymmetri-cally during 19 years. We initiated IVIG treatment, which produced rapid (beginning the next day following the initial 5 days of IVIG), cumulatively dramatic improvement (he can raise and hold both arms fully overhead), enduring 14 years from continuing, but now less-frequent, IVIG [28].

• "*Benign focal amyotrophy*" is ("benign" in the sense that it is not fatal like ALS, but it can be quite crippling). It has a gradual onset with weakness,

Table 2.1 Manifestations of disturbed activity of lower motor and sensory neurons.

Abnormal	Nonfunction	Labile, hyperfunction
Motor nerve		
Muscle action	Weakness, atrophy	Fasciculations, cramps, microcramps, brisk reflexes
Muscle fibers: denervated, de-inhibited, labilized	Fibrillations, positive waves	
Sensory nerve: small fiber		
Pain sensation	Numbness	Pain, tingling, burning, walking on stones, glass, tightness, electric shocks
Sensory nerve: large fiber		
Vibration, position sense	Numbness, imbalance	Tingling, tightness, electric shocks

atrophy, and fasciculations, usually asymmetric, in the shoulder and proximal upper limbs (Engel, unpublished observations) [29]. It can have a benign course, but we consider anti-dysimmune treatment appropriate, using IVIG or another agent to halt the progressive crippling, enhance the amount of recoverable strength, and facilitate the speed of improvement (Engel, unpublished observations) [29]. We have had one 50-year-old man from Australia who had been left with a chronically absolutely limp arm, which he implored us to surgically remove because it was getting in the way and being painfully injured. Instead, we offered anti-dysimmune treatment, which he declined. Another man, age 68, developed an acute hanging arm within a few days following a "horse serum" injection after a mild scorpion sting in northern Mexico; although his arm had been hanging untreated for a year, it gradually and, to everyone's pleasant surprise, nearly completely recovered with anti-dysimmune prednisone, oral cyclophosphamide, and plasmaphereses (before IVIG was available). s-IBM is often misdiagnosed as ALS (see Chapters 1 and 3).

"Benign fasciculations"

These can occur in normal, younger or aged persons after vigorous exercise and/or *"excessive" caffeine* (excessive for that individual), and they also can occur at rest and during sleep. (Caffeine in an older person might also precipitate sometimes very serious cardiac atrial fibrillation. Note that a person's *caffeine intolerance* gradually increases as one progresses through ages 40, 50, 60, and beyond. Sometimes fasciculations are also associated with painful muscle macro-cramps. Fasciculations and cramps are both caused by excess lability of lower motor neurons (Table 2.1) and can often be well treated with small doses of clonazepam (see below). One should not over-diagnose benign fasciculations with or without cramps as "possibly" the frighteningly-fatal ALS.

Therapeutically, the first step to stop fasciculations and cramps is to eliminate provocative substances, for example, all caffeine and other stimulants, including decongestant adrenergic agents in allergy medicines, β2-agonist bronchodilators, and CNS-stimulant drugs, including donepezil. Unfortunately, the stimulant caffeine is not forbidden to children, nor in the Olympics, nor in high-school and other sports performances, even though most consider caffeine a *performance enhancer*. Remarkably, highly caffeinated "energy drinks" are widely promoted as performance enhancers by their purveyors, even to minors, and those purveyors enthusiastically sponsor and put their name on major sports events, performance venues, and teams. Generally unrecognized is the possibility that some of the disabling muscle cramps of athletes might be related to their intake of caffeine (or perhaps other stimulants).

Fasciculations associated with progressive weakness are not benign – the underlying disease might be mild or, infrequently, serious, for example, if there is progressive weakness evolving into ALS. When abnormal, fasciculations and cramps more commonly signal treatable CIDP than ALS.

Amyloidoses

Amyloid diseases are typically associated with aging, although some genetic neuropathy forms can begin earlier. Not yet clarified are two questions: (a) what starts the accumulation of misfolded proteins that lead to the amyloidic process and (b) how do the amyloidic processes impair function of normal cells, i.e. what is the molecular mechanism of amyloid-associated cellular toxicity?

"Amyloid" is the general term designating the homo-aggregation of the same misfolded protein molecules, binding to each other to initially form the "primary protein" monomers and oligomers. These can aggrandize to become polymeric fibrils. Then the fibrils can co-aggregate into a β-pleated sheet configuration, which is the visible amyloid, stainable with crystal violet [30] or the Askanas fluorescent Congo red technique ([31] and see Chapters 7 and 10). The accumulated amyloid can be extracellular or intracellular. The extracellular amyloid in soft tissues can be clinically imaged by MiBi nuclear scans [32].

As a basis of various pathologic conditions, about 40 or more different proteins each can self-aggregate to form the "primary protein" of an amyloid. For example, in amyloid peripheral neuropathies the deposited extracellular amyloid often contains: (a) the variable portion of immunoglobulin light chain in some B-lymphocyte dyscrasias, or (b) mutant transthyretin in some autosomal dominant hereditary amyloid neuropathies.

A number of "secondary proteins" have been detected bound to the amyloid deposits, as evident extracellularly in various amyloid disorders, and within muscle fibers of s-IBM patients and paralleled by immunoprecipitation studies (Chapters 7 and 10).

In *amyloid peripheral neuropathy*, two mechanisms of amyloid-associated toxicity have been proposed: (a) the electron-microscopically invisible amyloid molecular precursors (now thought to be monomeric or oligomeric misfolded protein molecule precursors of the amyloid fibril) may be the molecular cytotoxic agents damaging the neural tissue by a yet-unknown biochemical *"toxic affinity"* mechanism [33]; (b) much less important are the summating effects of small deposits of aggregated amyloid exerting damaging physical pressure. We favor (a) as the major damaging pathogenic mechanism. Perhaps the electron-microscopically invisible pre-amyloid toxic molecules have a selective affinity/stickiness for certain exposed surface plasmalemmal receptors of various inadvertently targeted cells in peripheral nerves (such as small-fiber and large-fiber sensory neurons, and motor neurons, with or without their Schwann cells); by binding there they may damage cellular function.

This cyto-erosive mechanism of molecular toxic affinity, a *"misintended adhesion,"* can be considered for: (a) the toxicity of misfolded amyloid-β, prion, α-synuclein; (b) possibly for hyperphosphorylated tau in s-IBM and Alzheimer disease; and (c) very speculatively, as a cause of ALS (regarding a putative yet-to be-identified toxic molecule generated within the CNS or possibly in a remote tissue). But the underlying reason for many molecules of a given protein to start being misfolded is not known. Regarding *"aging phenomena,"* possibly there are *post-translationally malfolded toxic*, but not necessarily amyloidogenic, *proteins* producing *"aging changes"* in muscle, neurons nerve, Schwann cells, and other cells of the body: this is our current musing. To understand the cause and treatment of *putatively toxic aging-associated malfolding mechanisms* is an important research challenge.

In s-IBM the amyloid is accumulated intracellularly in two major types of *inclusions*, especially containing, as the presumed *primary protein*, either (a) amyloid-β42 plus co-deposited other proteins, or (b) hyperphosphorylated tau, plus co-deposited other proteins (see Chapters 7 and 10). It is possible that one or more of the other *co-accumulated proteins* might actually have a pathogenic role in initiating or continuing the multi-focal protein accumulations. But probably more relevant to the cyto-destruction in s-IBM is our proposal that an *invisible pre-amyloid* (pre-inclusion) *monomers or oligomers* having cytotoxic molecularly-destructive affinities for crucial intracellular components. Whether any of the proteins bound to the aggregated proteins becomes deficient enough within the cell to cause harm is not known.

In the Alzheimer brain, although the amyloid-β-containing extracellular plaques are an eye-catching finding (and are structures being imaged clinically), years ago we proposed that, like we postulated in s-IBM, there is a similarly *invisible intracellular toxicity* occurring *within Alzheimer brain neurons* (a concept that is now becoming more widely accepted (see Chapters 7 and 10, and below).

Neuromuscular fatigue and exercise intolerance

Neuromuscular fatigue and exercise intolerance should never be quickly dismissed as being caused by inexplicable and untreatable "*aging.*" They might actually be due identifiable problems, such as neuromuscular, cardiac, respiratory, or other disorders. In the usual clinical neuromuscular exam, *fatigue is not evaluated*, and sometimes it is not quantitated in therapeutic trials. With an *effective treatment* of a neuromuscular disorder, *subjectively lessened fatigue* is often the first and must pervasive symptom to improve, and to reappear upon reduction or withdrawal of an effective treatment. An observant patient can give a reliable report of any *change of the fatigue component of daily activities*, such as individually standardized walking (according to minutes or blocks), stair-climbing, arising from a chair, lifting, and gripping. These valid indicators of treatment efficacy must not be rejected by insurance company reviewers.

Deconstructing "chronic fatigue syndrome"

Based on patients we have seen, the "diagnosis" of untreatable *chronic fatigue syndrome (CFS)* has often been made hastily and nebulously, sometimes dismissively, without detailed investigations of the patient that could disclose a clearly identifiable cause and possibly a treatable one, such as we have found, for example: a subtle CIDP or other neuropathy; myasthenia gravis, periodic paralysis, muscle carnitine deficiency (see below), or hyperparathyroidism [8, 34]. The fairly recent and contradictory reports of the "XMRV retrovirus" allegedly associated with CFS, recently have not been confirmed. In the meantime, the US Food and Drug Administration (FDA) has banned "CFS patients" from donating blood. A number of patients labeled as "CFS" have malaise and depression, but whether

that is primary or is secondary to an occult debilitating neuromuscular disorder, such as a neuropathy, can be difficult to determine in the individual patient. In each CFS-like patient, we recommend performing: (a) a full battery of blood tests, including dysimmune and viral parameters; (b) a histochemically analyzed diagnostic muscle biopsy; (c) nerve conductions and EMG; (d) a spinal fluid analysis including an "m.s. panel" for dysimmune parameters.

What is treatable "neural-labile pseudo-fibromyalgia"?

In our opinion, the diagnosis of "*fibromyalgia*" is often used to describe various unexplained pain symptoms, not a distinct disease. The classic tender points are often sites of neurogenic muscle *macrocramps* or *microcramps*, caused by pathologic neural lability originating in some region of unhappy lower motor neurons. The small painful and tender cramps or microcramps can sometime feel like a "sausage," according to palpation by the patient and physician. Not uncommonly, fibromyalgia is used as a *dismissive diagnosis* for muscle aches and pains. Sometimes incorrectly called fibromyalgia are five manifestations that we consider to be based on proven neuropathic pathogeneses, and which are often directly treatable.

1 *Mechanical cervical radiculopathy*, involving one, or sometimes a few, nerve roots, causing pain, muscle tenderness, and "muscle tightness," which are actually focal crampings, in the neck, upper shoulders or arms [35]. A positive result in a carefully done "neck-stretch test" [35], using the physician's hands can produce some degree of immediate relief, usually transiently, but nevertheless it can be diagnostic; even a transient worsening of the pain typically indicates a focal mechanical radiculopathy. Longer-term improvement is often achieved by properly instructed, repeated neck stretchings utilizing a home neck-stretch apparatus (begun after magnetic resonance imaging excludes serious neck pathology). "*Ponderous purse disease*" (PPD) [36], much more often in women, is caused by a heavy shoulder purse (or a shoulder computer bag, or a shoulder bag of baby paraphernalia), which can aggravate or bring out cervical radiculopathy symptoms and simulate "fibromyalgia." PPD can usually be mitigated or eliminated by the apparently abhorrent concept of carrying a much lighter hand purse to eliminate or markedly lighten the shouldered "beast of burden."

2 *Mechanical lumbosacral radiculopathy* can produce a focal painful and tender persisting tightness cramp – a "sausage" – in the low-back or gluteal musculature, or sometimes lower in the thigh or leg.

3 *Hyperparathyroidism* sometimes is overlooked, especially when normocalcemic (see below [34]; Engel, unpublished observations).

4 Persistingly migrating *"multi-microcramps"* syndrome, with occasional macrocramps (see below) [8].

5 A *predominately motor CIDP*.

Falling

Falling of older patients is more than "just getting old." It is often, but not always, the result of enfeeblement of lower-limb muscles affected by a neuromuscular disorder, or sometimes from a sensory-neuropathy ataxia. The patient who falls may have (a) certain common, relatively easily correctible causes of falling, such as: medication effects; dysregulations of blood pressure, cardiac function, and plasma glucose; and other disorders in the general physician's purview; or (b) a sometimes overlooked (especially in today's hurried clinical atmosphere), a gradually incapacitating but possibly treatable neuromuscular/neurologic condition. Each falling patient deserves careful neurological and neuromuscular analysis (see above). Some work-around *assistive devices* can be tried – e.g. canes, crutches, braces, walkers, and wheelchairs – but they are often disdained by *perilously proud seniors*. Also very important: seniors should have, and wear, the best possible *corrective eye-glasses*.

Some disorders causing treatable weakness, sensory imbalance, and/or disabling spasticity are discussed in the Chapter 3 vignettes, and below.

• *Peripheral neuropathies* can cause falling due to both weakness from motor-nerve involvement and impaired balance from sensory-nerve deficits: these defects are often concurrent.

• *Motor neuron disorders*, such as ALS and PMA, can cause lower-limb weakness, floppy feet, and falling.

• *Sudden automatic reaction to sudden pain*, as from a painful neuropathy or arthritic conditions, including back pain, can throw the patient off balance and produce a fall.

• *Painful muscle "macrocramps" and "microcramps"* can impair gait and cause falling. They are typically neurogenic, more often produced by peripheral neuropathy or mechanical radiculopathy. The pathogenic aspects of these are often treatable (see above and below), and symptomatically we have found that low-dose clonazepam often provides gratifying relief [8, 9]. Much less commonly, the cause of the cramps is ALS, a feared but uncommon diagnosis.

• *Generalized type-2 muscle fiber atrophy* can result from visible, or sometimes occult, undernourishment (cachexia), remote effect of a neoplasm (e.g. via undernourishment or a tumorogenous "neuromuscular toxicant"), inactivity (disuse), or glucocorticoid toxicity. Treating the underlying condition sometimes improves the atrophy and weakness (see Chapter 1 in this volume). To conditions causing type-2 fiber atrophy in an elderly animal, or human, the imprecise and intellectually misleading general term "sarcopenia" is sometimes applied. It is often misinterpreted as a "diagnosis," but it only means *atrophy of aging muscle*, for which *AAM* is our more direct designation (see Chapter 1). To say that an aging animal or patient with muscle atrophy and weakness has "sarcopenia" only obfuscates the problem.

• *Occult hyperparathyroidism*, associated with an elevated, or normal, level of ionized calcium, can present as fatigue, weakness, and falling due to muscle denervation atrophy plus type-2 fiber atrophy [8]. It is often easily treatable by surgical excision of a *parathyroid hormone (PTH) adenoma* (see Chapter 3, vignette 9; Engel, unpublished observations). A PTH adenoma is sought by ultrasound scan, CT or radioisotope scan. If the cells overproducing PTH are not grouped in an adenomatous lump, but are more diffuse, the scans can be negative, but that does not exclude the presence of overproducing PTH cells that require surgical removal. In that situation it seems to us that exploratory surgery utilizing real-time measurements of PTH in the several veins draining the parathyroid gland regions might identify the general locus of the over-producing cells requiring removal.

- *Cervical spinal problems* impairing gait are increasingly common in seniors. They include mechanical pressures. *Spondylotic myelopathy*, from pressure on the cervical spinal cord, can cause spasticity of gait and/or focal pressure on roots of nerves in one or both upper limbs. *Lumbosacral spondylotic radiculopathy*, can cause impairment of motor and sensory nerve-roots to the lower limbs. Those mechanical pressures are sometimes treatable by surgery, which must be done extremely carefully so as to not impair the delicate blood supply of the spinal cord and roots. However surgery is not always needed, and if done is not always successful.
- *Brain disorders* that cause imbalance and/or spasticity might be overlooked, for example, potentially treatable ones such as normal-pressure hydrocephalus, subdural hematoma (e.g. in a patient on anticoagulant therapy who has recently fallen), and early abscess or tumor. Other brain disorders affecting balance and gait are various.

Special vasculopathic aspects of neuromuscular diseases

These raise the consideration of vasodilative and/or anticoagulative concurrent treatment.

Immunoglobulin and complement deposition in venules and arterioles is characteristic of dermatomyositis [37, 38].

Arterioles, or perhaps more proximal vessels: ischemia, intermittent or prolonged:

- *Duchenne muscular dystrophy*: small foci of same-stage necrotic muscle fibers or regenerating muscle fibers (with high serum CK), plus excessive fibrosis, were identified in patients. These (and elevated serum CK) were reproduced in our rat model that combined aorta ligation below the level of the renal arteries with a vasoconstrictor, serotonin or norepinepherine [39–43]. These findings in Duchenne dystrophy, studied before the dystrophin gene mutations were found, may indicate a co-pathogenic mechanism.
- *Ischemic leg necessitating amputation, in an elderly patient*: this had the same same-stage multifocal myopathic lesions [39–43], thereby supporting the ischemia hypothesis of a vascular co-component of the Duchenne dystrophy pathogenesis.

Capillaries: *calcium deposits*, when seen in patients with normal renal function, normal PTH, and normal calcium levels, are virtually diagnostic of *diabetes-2* (Engel, unpublished observations since 1981).

Boxing

In the "sport" of boxing, the main aim is brain maim. The boxer's intent is to produce unconsciousness by concussing another person's brain. Numerous repetitions of these often eventuate in *dementia pugilistica* or other crippling brain abnormalities, including "premature aging changes." In the media there is more concern expressed regarding accidental concussions in hockey and football than intentional boxing concussions, public displays of which are enjoyed often by thousands of attendees and by millions via television. Enthusiasts focus on the victor, neurologists on the vanquished. Formal recommendations of the American Academy of Neurology and the American Medical Association to ban boxing have not been influential. (Interestingly, in some states, being involved in the activity of cock fights can engender incarceration.)

Clinical exam suggestions

- *Simple vital capacity*: we measure this on every patient at every clinic visit, and daily for in-patients, employing an easy-to-use hand-held respirometer.
- In a *spastic or rigid patient*, one should test muscle strength by the *power to resist force*, not by ability to actively move the muscle being tested. In fact, this should be done when testing all neuromuscular patients.
- When testing patellar and biceps *tendon reflexes*, in order to focus the tap, the examiner's finger should be put across the tendon and very firmly hit with a "Queen Square" reflex hammer.
- The *Babinski test* can be done correctly only if flexion and extension strength of the toes is normal. Also, distal reduction of pain sensation in the soles can produce a nonresponsive result.
- In a peripheral neuropathy with sensory-nerve involvement: (a) *distally reduced pain sensation* is tested by carefully testing distally to proximally up a limb with a disposable toothpick, but (b) to detect *distal pain hypersensitivity*, we carefully test proximally to distally down a limb. Hypersensitivity is produced by exces-

sive lability of dysfunctional small-diameter pain fibers in a peripheral neuropathy.

• Looking and palpating for *enlarged sural nerves* should always be done in a clinical neuromuscular exam. They can be brought into prominence by the examiner holding the foot fully inverted and flexed.

• The neurologic examiner should always *personally check the pulse* (it only takes a minute). Aging patients can have an *unrecognized tachycardia* or *arrhythmia*, potentially dangerous, potentially quite treatable. A number of times we have found a previously undetected atrial fibrillation or other arrhythmia, or a pulse >90 BPM, and even >110 BPM.

• Always ask about a *family history of diabetes-2*. A close family history can predispose to (a) manifestation of diabetes-2 by glucocorticoid/prednisone treatment, and (b) genetico-diabetoid-2 dysimmune polyneuropathy.

• Always test for *jaw hyperreflexia* and *Chvostek facial neuromuscular hypersensitivity*.

• When *examining strength* of patients with *sensory peripheral neuropathy*, having them *look at the area being tested* often elicits their improved, maximal response.

Laboratory testing and interpretation

• In an aging person, *a laboratory result that would be abnormal in a young adult* should not be summarily dismissed as "normal in aging."

• Every *circulating antibody* is member of a "nano-family" composed of identical "monoclonal antibodies" produced from one B-lymphocyte clone. In clinical parlance, when there is increased size of a quantitated peak or band representing one such nano-family, that nano-family is designated a "*monoclonal antibody*."

• "Monoclonal gammopathy of unknown significance" (MGUS) is an *oxymoronic misunderstanding* when used in reference to a neurologic patient in whom the serum or urine monoclonal antibody is suspected to be having a pathogenic role. Historically, the term "MGUS" was initiated by R.A. Kyle, a myeloma expert [44], simply in reference to a monoclonal antibody that was not associated with a de-

tectable myeloma or other serious B-lymphocyte dyscrasia after careful searching. However, instead of MGUS, a more correct name is "*nonmyeloma monoclonal gammopathy*" (NMMG). In a book by concerned clinicians, the commonly misused, literally illogical and confusing expression of "undetermined significance" is exemplified in their table entitled "Proposal for criteria for demyelinating polyneuropathy *associated with MGUS*". It includes categories of "The relationship is *definite* when ...," and "The relationship is *probable* when ...." But logically, if the relationship is *definite* or *probable* the monoclonal gammopathy cannot be of *unknown* pathogenic significance. We agree with the authors' general emphasis in that table but not with perpetuating that illogical and misleading use of "MGUS". In our group of over 1000 patients presenting, over the years, to our tertiary referral center with peripheral neuropathy and a discoverable monoclonal gammopathy, none has had evidence of myeloma, in 3–10 year clinical follow-ups (although not all had initial bone-marrow, radiologic, and radionuclide imaging).

• A *monoclonal band*, or *free light chains*, or *free heavy chains* in serum, urine, or CSF should not be dismissed as "normal in aging." Rather, those immunoglobulins and fragments are indicative of dysimmunity and of possible pathogenic significance in that patient. *Immunofixation electropheresis* (IFEP) is very sensitive for detecting monoclonal bands and free light- or heavy-chains. Decades ago the IFEP technique made obsolete serum protein electropheresis and immunoelectropheresis but, unfortunately, those two inferior techniques are still being ordered instead of IFEP, sometimes at the insistence of insurance and Health Maintenance Organization (HMO) companies.

• If a monoclonal band, or free light chains or heavy chains, are detected by IFEP, are they the pathogenic ones? These abnormalities demonstrate a *dysimmune milieu* within the patient and a suspicion that the detected abnormality might be the cytotoxic one. However, conceptually the actual dysimmune cytotoxicity could be, qualitatively, due to a different monoclonal nano-family that is not quantitatively high enough above the detection threshold to be identified as "monoclonal."

- The *white blood cell count (WBC)* and *"leucopenia"* are illogical and misleading archaisms from ancient times when blood cells were first seen microscopically and the best that could be done was to categorize them as "red" or "white" cells. Astonishingly, "WBC" and "leucopenia" are still being used in prestigious medical journals (such as the *New England Journal of Medicine*), the Physicians' Desk Reference, and Epocrates, and that illogicality is still being used by medical-school professors, even hermatologists and being taught to our students. Those two terms and that concept *should be banished from medicine*. Reason: the WBC is composed mainly of two disparate cell types, neutrophils and lymphocytes. Its use is worse than nonsensical because it can distort clinical management, especially when used as guidance in anti-dysimmune treatment. Every laboratory computer should always automatically produce *absolute values* in the differential blood count. In our anti-dysimmune treatments: (a) a worry factor is to *keep the absolute neutrophil count up* in the safe range; and (b) therapeutically we like to *push the total lymphocytes down* to a very low level, even though only a small percent of the lymphocytes are thought to be the undesirable pathogenic ones in an autoimmune disease. We cannot yet target *only* the actual trouble-making B- and T-lymphocytes. A step in that direction is the recently popular rituximab, which targets mainly CD20 B-lymphocytes (but it can also produce an undesired neutropenia). A desirable combination of normal neutrophils and low lymphocytes can produce a "low WBC," a "leucopenia," which misleadingly suggests to some clinicians an erroneous need to interrupt the anti-dysimmune treatment. Thus, safety and efficacy monitoring only with a WBC can confuse a desirable therapeutic lymphopenia with a potentially worrisome neutropenia. To help keep the neutrophil count up, we sometimes use a small dose of prednisone, such as 5–15 mg single-dose on alternate days, if the patient does not have diabetes-2 or a close-family history of diabetes-2, or another contraindication for prednisone.

- *Examination of CSF* is important in many neuromuscular disease patients, such as ones in whom an aspect of peripheral neuropathy, a motor neuron disorder, or a CNS component is suspected. Wrong is the sometimes-stated idea that a protein value above the listed "normal" of 45 mg/dL can be "normal in elderly persons." To us, elevated CSF protein *always* means (a) impairment of the blood–nerve or blood–brain barrier, or (b) abnormal production of protein by the CNS (if that protein was not due to a "bloody spinal tap"). For example, a CSF protein elevation can be an aspect of a dysimmune neuropathy, which is more common among the elderly, and protein elevation is especially common in diabetes-2 dysimmune neuropathy. Regarding CSF immunoglobulin bands, we consider even one band abnormal and significant, contrary to certain long-ago-established and possibly erroneous guidelines that require two, or sometimes three, bands to be considered abnormal. CSF immunoglobulin bands due to pathologic inward leakage of the blood–nerve or blood–brain barrier would also be found in the concurrent serum, if they are above the threshold of detectability.

- *Elevation of serum AST, ALT, and LDH* indicates abnormal leakage from either skeletal muscle or liver. These parameters are not solely "liver-function tests", but that is still sometimes being thought and taught. Distinguishing the source requires analysis of GGTP and CK (CPK). Serum GGTP is increased only in some liver disorders, and serum CK (MM type) is increased only in some skeletal-muscle disorders, especially in myopathies, but it also can be slightly elevated in some disorders causing muscle denervation. Serum CK MB type is increased in some cardiac disorders, and can also be somewhat increased if there are a number of regenerating skeletal muscle fibers in a neuromuscular disorder [45]. Neuromuscular evaluations and liver evaluations should always include both CK and GGTP measurements.

Clinical electrophysiology considerations

EMG

Routine clinical EMG done during slight voluntary contraction of a muscle allows *quantitation only of the early-activated type-1 slow-twitch motor units*. It does not see the fast-twitch type-2 motor-units, which are activated only by a vigorous contraction [10, 46, 47]. Thus, size abnormalities of type-2 motor units are presumably not detected.

Electrically enlargement of a motor-unit amplitude and duration probably initially represent "densification" of the distribution of its muscle fibers, which are not normally densely distributed within the overall territory of an individual motor unit. Thus, at first there is probably not a widened geographic territory [25, 48].

It is imprecise and simplistic to consider the EMG pattern of voluntary *"brief-duration, small-amplitude, overly-abundant motor-unit potentials" (BSAPs)* as diagnostic only of "myopathy" or as a "myopathic EMG" [49, 50]. The BSAP pattern basically means there are *fewer than the normal number of activated muscle fibers per motor unit*. Consequently the patient activates more than the usual number of motor units to achieve a certain amount of force. Yes, this can occur in a myopathic process due to a relatively random loss of a portion of the activatable muscle fibers within numerous individual motor units. However, the BSAP pattern can also occur if the loss of muscle-fiber activation is due to (a) impaired transmission at randomly affected neuromuscular junctions (as in myasthenia gravis or botulinum toxicity), or (b) impaired transmission in randomly affected distal motor nerve twigs in a "distal neuropathy," such as the multi-microcramps syndrome and some other peripheral neuropathies. If polyphasic potentials are also an aspect of a BSAP pattern, it is called a BSAPP pattern.

Thus, the BSAP and BSAPP patterns indicate *fractionated motor units*, meaning the patient is activating fewer than the normal number of muscle fibers within many individual motor units; they do not delineate just one diagnostic category, i.e. not exclusively a myopathy.

Nerve conduction velocities

Denervation and dysinnervation abnormalities are usually *neurogenous* (but, atypically, sometimes can be myogenous; see Chapter 1). Conceptually, denervation is a complete loss of neural influence on the muscle fiber (which initially can be reversible by reinnervation and repair, but often progresses to become irreversible). Dysinnervation is only a partial loss of neural influence, which can either (a) remain partial, or (b) worsen to become a completed denervation (details in Chapter 1). In general, a dysinnervation probably would be more easily treatable and reversible, and thereby able to provide short- or long-term benefit.

Routinely tested clinical nerve conduction velocities are *unable to measure the slow-conducting small-diameter nerve fibers*; these (a) normally convey pain sensation, and (b) when they are abnormal, as in injury or disease (such as peripheral neuropathy), they can be excessively labile and emit spontaneous signals of pain. Accordingly, in a predominantly painful sensory-neuropathy form of CIDP or another neuropathy, the measurable nerve conduction velocities of the large-diameter fast-conduction nerve fibers can be normal or abnormal. Therefore, one must not require conduction-slowing of those measurable, but not symptom-producing, fast-conducting fibers as a requirement for the clinical diagnosis of CIDP. Nor should they be a required parameter to be monitored for documenting improvement in a predominantly painful neuropathy.

For monitoring potential improvement of a patient's mixed large- and small-diameter nerve fiberneuropathy, as in CIDP or another disorder, an improvement of nerve-conduction parameters cannot be required. A patient can show good to excellent benefit clinically without any improvement of conduction velocities (Engel, unpublished observations).

We propose that in nerve conduction velocity studies, a ratio between relative slowness of conduction velocity and relatively good or excellent amplitude (our "V/A ratio") could potentially be useful for determining *early slowing* of conduction. However, we have not yet formalized this proposed ratio and the relevant normal values thereof.

Diagnostic muscle biopsy interpretations

Diagnostic muscle biopsies are very important (these are also discussed extensively in Chapter 1). A few general principles are as follows.

• *Denervation/neuropathic aspects*: "*denervation*" can be: (a) an anatomic disconnection; or (b) only a dysfunctional, partial loss of neuronal trophic influence of the lower motor neuron axon to the denervated muscle fiber, i.e. a *dysinnervation* (see above).

1 *Recent denervation not followed by reinnervation* is evident as atrophic small angular muscle fibers.

2 *Early reinnervation following recent denervation* is evident as intermediate-staining fibers on the reverse ATPase reaction, if the reinnervation is by a foreign (opposite type) of motor neuron (see Chapter 1).

3 *Established reinnervation following previous denervation* is manifest as type-grouping.

4 *Nonreinnervation following previous denervation* is evident as very atrophic pyknotic nuclear clumps.

5 *Paucity* of one of the muscle-fiber types: this is usually an aspect of a type-grouping phenomenon (a hypothetical, much less likely alternative is that it might be reflecting a neuropathic or myopathic preferential loss of one type of lower motor neuron or type of one muscle-fiber).

• *Ordinary myopathic aspects*: these include necrosis, phagocytosis, regeneration, and vacuolation of muscle fibers. *Dysimmune "inflammatory" myopathies* typically have accumulated lymphocytes and macrophages in relation to abnormal muscle fibers and/or around blood vessels. Sometimes deposition of immunoglobulins in blood vessels is a major pathogenic mechanism, as in dermatomyositis [37, 38].

• *Type-2 muscle fiber atrophy* can be caused by various abnormalities, such as cachexia, hypoactivity (disuse), glucocorticoid excess, hyperparathyroidism, a manifestation of recent pan-deinnervation [51, 52] or pan-dysinnervation, or upper-motor-neuron abnormality (for extensive discussion, see Chapter 1).

Manifestations of disturbed activity of lower motor and sensory neurons

See Table 2.1.

Therapeutic principles

N-of-1 + 1 + 1 studies

In our opinion, controlled trials involving many patients, seeking a subtle or miniscule beneficial effect, are occasionally helpful but are not the *sine qua non* of providing all the information useful for clinical management. Also, they can be very expensive, often seeming to be satisfied with only an infinitesimally small benefit that requires special statistics to be demonstrated. We believe that a number of "N-of-1" therapeutic experiences involving carefully monitored individual patients often can be very informative and clinically relevant.

To emphasize this principle, a few of our lucky and enduring therapeutic successes may be mentioned:

• *Hypokalemic periodic paralysis*: *acetazolamide* [53, 54]. *Hypo- and hyperkalemic periodic paralyses*: *dichlorphenamide* (another carbonic anhydrase inhibitor) [55]. These prominently reduced paralyzing-attack frequency and severity, and increased interictal strength. They have become standard treatment.

• Two *muscle carnitine deficiency disorders* having increased triglyceride, within muscle fiber, treated differently with:

1 *Diet nearly devoid of long-chain fatty acids*: severe muscle weakness of proximal limbs, swallowing, and breathing, which evolved to respiratory- and gastric-feeding-tube dependency by age 17. The boy was slightly obese, very intelligent, and highly motivated. He had failed carnitine treatment. (Carnitine is needed for transporting long-chain fatty acids into mitochondria for ATP production (but it is not needed for short- and medium-chain fatty acid utilization.) Our new hypothesis [56, 57] was that the accumulating long-chain fatty acids were toxic, by forming micelles with sodium and these have a detergent action solubilizing cellular membranes, a form of "*endodissolution*" (not an "*afuelia*"). Our unique treatment, begun in 1981, was to de-fat him by eliminating long-chain fatty acids from the diet, replace nutrition with multi-component Portagen (Mead-Johnson Co.), containing only short- and medium-chain fatty acids (from coconut oil), and eliminate obesity (initially only 700 calories/day). Within 3 weeks he was off the respirator and feeding tube, and walking a few steps, at 2.5 months he was walking 2.5 km/day, and in 1 year he was playing golf. Now, 30 years later, he maintains normal strength, is a busy international professional, and remains on the unique diet.

2 That same *long-chain fatty-acid-free diet* was used very successfully to treat a three family members who had lifelong weakness and fatty-food intolerance due to autosomal dominant lipid neuromyopathy (with excess lipid within muscle fibers and Schwann cells) and normal levels of muscle carnitine [58].

3 *Emergency use of D,L-carnitine directly from a chemical company, 4 g/day,* for a virtually lifelong-afflicted, diffusely weak 23-year-old woman, on a respirator, who was so near death that her autopsy was being planned. This treatment resulted in dramatic improvement within 10 days. At 8 months muscle function was normal and remained so on 3 g of L-carnitine/day, eventuating 1 year later in her planning her own wedding. The lucky-guess desperation treatment [59] was based on our identifying excess lipid within the antemortem biopsied muscle fibers of her sister, deceased at age 10 (linked in our laboratory by having the same family name of the biopsy specimen submitted from a different state).

• *HTLV1 subacute severe spastic paraparesis*, with some muscle fasciculations and cramps: anti-dysimmune therapy (*prednisone plus oral cyclophosphamide* 2 mg/kg/day in one, and *prednisone plus total-body irradiation* (see below) in the other) in two men, 68 and 70. Those produced remarkably improved walking (no longer wheelchair-dependent) [60]. Treatment was initiated because the culture-negative CSF had 28 and 111 lymphocytes, protein of 86 and 254 mg/dL (normal < 46), and elevated IgG synthesis. All was done before their diagnosis of HTLV1 became known as per the American Red Cross careful lookback-monitoring and before routine testing of surgical donor blood for HTLV1, which was the retrospectively documented source of infection of these men who had had coronary-bypass procedures, each involving many units of transfused blood. This is an example of *virogenic*

dysimmune myelopathy. Knowing of the HTLV1 viremia would have made us hesitate before this treatment. This successful experience encourages consideration for similar HTLV1 myelopathy treatment in the future, and it re-emphasizes the virogenic aspect of dysimmune diseases (see the section on Interferon-α2A below).

• Syndrome of *continuous motor-unit activity* (also called neuromyotonia or multi-microcramps): immunosuppression (*prednisone, oral cyclophosphamide, plasmaphereses*, before IVIG was available) produced an excellent, essentially full response—(regained ability to walk, write, and drive)—in a severely disabled elderly woman. This response provided the first indication that this disorder is an autoimmune disease [61].

Intelligent and observant patients

Clinicians understand that an intelligent and observant patient can detect significant *good or bad changes* in sensory and motor phenomena, and especially *fatigue* aspects, before the clinical exam can, or use of special machines can. Not reliable for monitoring results of treatment are repeated nerve conductions, EMG, and muscle biopsies, although sometimes a repeat study is necessary to help clarify the pathologic process. Sometimes general "clinical guidelines" that are intended to be helpful for patient management are too restrictive. Accordingly, *absence of a guidelines-designated benefit is not absence of relevant benefit*.

Our principles of anti-dysimmune treatment

Always within the limits of safety and side effects:

1 Stop pathogenic damaging, and permit maximal endogenous repair and regeneration.

2 The longer time that cells remain *malfunctioning*, the greater likelihood they will *die* (*normal↔ malfunctioning but alive → dead*).

3 *Individualize* anti-dysimmune treatments.

4 *Maximally reduce cellular malfunction* for as long as possible, *to prevent gradual irreversibility* and cell death.

5 It is *medically inappropriate* for a physician to choose to intentionally provide less than optimal anti-pathogenic therapy of dysimmune disease, or be satisfied with clearly less than optimal improvement—and for insurance companies, HMOs, or a government to do so is contrary to good medical care. That would be similar to providing intentionally suboptimal treatment of infectious diseases, which is clearly inappropriate.

6 Achieve *maximally summated improvement*, based on clinical expectation. For example, when using IVIG, be not content with a less-than-optimal plateau of blunted improvement, nor with some repeatedly unsustained, unsummating little improvements. One should *treat maximally* and *often enough* to prevent a "*Sisyphus phenomenon.*" In Greek mythology, Sisyphus was a misbehaving character, punished by the gods by being compelled to roll an immense boulder up a steep hill, but each time, before he could keep it at the top of the hill, the huge rock would always roll back down, forcing him to begin again, and again, and again, repeating this endless toil throughout eternity. IVIG treatments, if given in suboptimal dosage and frequency, if fail to summate for optimal benefit, resulting in *Sisyphusian futility* for the patient and physician. This should be avoided if at all possible. In our experience with IVIG, optimal benefit usually lasts only 1–2 weeks after the last infusion, sometimes even shorter. Thus, reappearance of symptoms before the next dose suggests a Sisyphusian inadequate frequency, a major hindrance to long-term summation of benefit, and possibly ingravescently adding to aspects of *irreversibility of the cellular damage* the physician is attempting to repair. But we also emphasize that individual IVIG doses given in too-large amount and/or too rapidly in one infusion session can be risky, occasionally producing generally unwell feeling, hypertension, headache, or blood-vessel blockage. Infused IVIG thickens the blood, and so we always give *aspirin* to patients being treated with IVIG, unless they are already taking coumadin or plavix.

7 Try to *develop new drugs* that enhance regeneration in the central and peripheral nervous system, to be given concurrently with anti-pathogenic (e.g. anti-dysimmune) drugs.

Proposed overlapping phases of anti-dysimmune improvement

These are the *timings* that seem to occur regarding *IVIG benefit* [3–6, 28]:

- *Rapid*: 1–14 days=reversing of "*moment-to-moment molecular inhibiton,*" such as cytotoxic action (e.g. cytotoxic affinity of immunoglobulins, cytokines, or other damaging molecules—including putatively pathogenic misfolded proteins.
- *Slow*: incrementing during weeks to months= *repair/regrowth mechanisms* of neurons, Schwann cells, and muscle fibers.

Comments on individual anti-dysimmune treatments

IVIG

An IVIG dosage and schedule *individualized* for each patient is very important. The usual dose per infusion day is 0.4 g/kg on five consecutive days every third week [4, 6]. Although some physicians give 2–2.5 times this daily amount on one day, or on two consecutive days, we consider that this increases risk of *thromboembolic vessel blockage* by the blood-thickening effect of the IgG infusate. We infuse slowly, generally not over 100 mL/hour, and slower for *worrisome patients* who are considered susceptible to hypertension, headache, or vascular occlusion, and for small patients or ones with a general frailty of aging. This is in contrast to some IVIG package inserts that allow up to 250–340 mL/hour for a 70 kg patient. For worrisome patients, we invented, 17 years ago, an infusion schedule of 0.4 g/kg on *two nonconsecutive days every week* [4, 6]. This provides a more even elevation of IgG blood levels and fewer side effects. More recently, we have sometimes utilized a schedule of 3-week cycles, namely 3–3–0 or 3–2–1 infusions per week on alternate or consecutive days: of these two schedules, the former is more days effective for some patients.

Note: the supposed quantitative half-life of the administered IgG circulating in the blood is not a measure of the *biological therapeutic half-life* for the individual patient, nor does it consider the blood level that must be maintained to achieve persisting benefit. In one of our patients, we repeatedly documented that the necessary therapeutic blood level was above 2200 mg/dL (the laboratory-stated normal blood level of IgG is 650–1650 mg/dL); below that level, symptoms began to reappear.

For diabetics, one should use IVIG brands without sucrose. Such as Gammagard-Liquid or Gamunex (the latter requires brief flushing of the intravenous line with 10 mL 5% dextrose in water).

There can be a number of *apparently-benign "pseudo-lupus" laboratory-parameter side-effects from IVIG*, including: high sedimentation rate, elevated immune complexes, rheumatoid factor, and anti-thyroid antibody positivity, some positive lupus-panel tests, and various rashes. Because of these, several of our patients were erroneously told by a local physician "you have lupus."

A possible future for IVIG therapy is to identify the active region of the IgG molecule and synthesize it for simpler, quicker, and cheaper treatments.

Repeated plasmaphereses

Plasmapheresis is an out-patient procedure for acutely removing from the blood putatively-toxic antibodies (and other detrimental molecules such as cytokines and misfolded proteins). The whole blood is flowed from a vein into a centrifuge machine, and a portion of the liquid part (containing noxious antibodies and all other circulating soluble substances and factors) is removed. The patient's own red blood cells are then returned to him or her. The outflow and return flow to the patient must be carefully monitored by an experienced technician to prevent hypotension or hypertension. Although plasmaphereses are sometimes very beneficial, they *do not stop* the ongoing production of toxic antibodies or other toxic molecules, which immunosuppression drugs and radiation treatments are intended to do. Note: the patient's oral and parenteral medications must be given *after* a plasmapheresis treatment—if given before, they would be removed from the blood by the pheresis.

Glucocorticoid

In diabetics or patients with a close family history of diabetes-2, we try to avoid glucocorticoid treatment, which can aggravate or bring out diabetes-2 in such patients. In nondiabetic patients, when we do use a glucocorticoid, usually prednisone, we prefer the schedule of single-dose on alternate days (before 8 am, to avoid insomnia from a caffeine-like side effect) [62, 63]. For a more severely involved pa-

tient, we often start with daily glucocorticoid, sometimes with high–low daily alternating doses, and then gradually convert to the alternate-day schedule.

In the future, perhaps the prednisone molecule can be modified to keep the beneficial motif and eliminate the side-effects motif.

Imuran (azathioprine)

For Imuran, a daily divided, or single, oral dose of about 3 mg/kg (with food) can be planned, but we start at about 2 mg/kg and increase it as tolerated. As a safety aspect, we monitor *absolute neutrophils* every 1–2 weeks, and for the first 3 months monitor liver functions (GGTP, AST, ALT) plus CK monthly. We often use concurrently a small-single-dose alternate-day glucocorticoid (prednisone) to increase the circulating neutrophils, trying to avoid a potentially worrisome drug-induced neutropenia. Over time, the Imuran dose often needs to be gradually reduced to maintain neutrophils in a safe range. *Caution*: generic azathioprine, imposed by insurance companies, can be toxic. We have recently seen an intolerable febrile, malaise, flu-like syndrome in two geographically separate patients, which did not recur when we switched them to the brand Imuran, with resultant excellent and sustained clinical benefit. In another patient there was a prominent generalized pruritic rash with generic azathioprine which was not seen subsequently in that patient with Imuran. An occasional patient can be intolerant to both forms of the drug.

Rituximab

This is a rapidly acting immunosuppressant *toxic to CD20 B-lymphocytes*, a small subset of which is the main pathogenic element in some autoimmune diseases. Rituximab is typically given and closely supervised by a physician experienced in immunotherapy. Not yet established is whether or not there will be a long-term toxicity of chronic rituximab treatment of severely affected dysimmune neuromuscular patients, whose disease itself is not life-shortening. Until now, rituximab has only rarely caused progressive multifocal leucoencephalopathy, a severe JC-polyomavirus disease of the brain.

Often, each intravenous rituximab dose is 375 mg/m^2, initially given weekly for three or four doses. Then the 4-week-cycle is repeated every 6 months. However, we are following one sensory >motor CIDP patient, with a serum IgM-monoclonal, quantitatively elevated IgM, and myelin-associated glycoprotein (MAG) antibody. He has shown a good rituximab response for 5 years, but his symptoms begin to return about 2 months before his next dosage is due. Too-infrequent dosing probably invites Sisyphus relapses, whereas too-frequent dosing might jeopardize the bone marrow. Intuitively, we have recently developed (for a patient with dysimmune adult-onset rod-myopathy syndrome, including CIDP and monoclonal gammopathy) [64–67] what seems to be a better rituximab schedule to follow after the induction course of four-weekly doses: it consists of a once-monthly maintenance-dose every 6 weeks and then every 4 weeks (developed with Dr N. Gupta and I. Luthra).

In the future, perhaps, a lower standard dosage, and/or a less frequent schedule of rituximab, can become established for longer-term use, especially for older dysimmune patients.

Total-body irradiation (TBI)

This has been extremely beneficial for three of our later-adult-onset dermatomyositis-polymyositis patients who were totally weak, totally limp, on a ventilator and gastric feeding tube, and previously unresponsive to all other immunosuppression treatments [68]. Their individual cumulatively dramatic and long-term improvement was achieved, resulting in being off supportive tubes, walking well, and for one, being able to drive farm equipment. For those patients, the total-body irradiation treatments were suggested, and supervised very carefully, by Dr Alan Lichter, MD, radiation therapist. They were *15 rads twice weekly given for 5 weeks, a total course of 150 rads.* Lymphocytes are pathogenic and they are the circulating cells most damaged by TBI.

For the immediate future, total-body irradiation treatment deserves further reconsideration. It must be done with careful cooperation between a knowledgeable radiotherapist and the neuromuscular physician.

Interferon α2A

Can this treatment sometimes result in an actual "cure"? The subject is not an elderly patient, but his N-of-1 story evokes a principle potentially applicable to patients of any age. Previously, *Poly ICLC*, an interferon inducer, each dose of which causes a 12-hour fever as a side-effect, was extremely beneficial in an unusual disorder we call "*fever-responsive dysimmune neuropathy*", in a patient who had had 1–3 week slight improvements following spontaneous fevers [69]. The subsequent patient with fever-responsive neuropathy was a 16-year-old boy (in November 1989) who had a previously-untreatable motor dysschwannian polyneuropathy, gradually progressing into severe, totally quadriplegic areflexic paralysis for 2 years, and low vital capacity 1.5 L. CSF protein was 56 mg/dL (upper normal is 45 mg/dL). Our solo treatment [70–72] was with interferon α2A 12×10^6 units subcutaneously twice a week, which by then had become available, chosen because it also produces a 12-hour fever after each dose. This was given for 14 years and slowly produced cumulatively dramatic improvement (beginning barely detectably, the day after the first treatment). That benefit has now been persisting undiminished for 8 years after stopping the interferon α2A [72]. Currently, he vigorously mountain bikes, ocean-kayaks, and river-canoes, with only some residual distal weakness. We *propose* that the *putatively pathogenic lymphocytes* have been *irrevocably destroyed*. If so, this may be a "*cure*" of his dysimmune disease.

Formulation: interferon has anti-dysimmune and anti-viral actions. Some dysimmune diseases are known to be caused by a persistent immune reaction to a viral, bacterial, or other infection, and most or all of them are suspected to be of that pathogenesis.

The excellent improvement of this fever-responsive dysimmune neuropathy patient suggests that perhaps we should always treat dysimmune patients by combining anti-dysimmune and antiviral (or other antimicrobial) drugs, or one drug that does both. This concept is a putative model for future "combined anti-dysimmune plus anti-microbial therapy." And in each dysimmune patient we should always be searching for tracks of a "*relevant microbe.*"

Possibly relevant: (a) HTLV1 viral myelopathy is at least partly dysimmune [60] (see above); and (b) previously occult oncornavirus manifested morphologically as definite viral-type particles in "normal" chick embryo tissue-cultured muscle [73], probably Rous sarcoma virus, is possibly present in chickens worldwide. In general, we all probably have more exposure to viruses than we realize, and carry more within our tissues.

Oral cyclophosphamide

Up to 2 mg/kg/day of oral cyclophosphamide (plus >10 glasses of liquid/day) has been very beneficial in some patients (as noted above), but the potential side effects of repeated hemorrhagic cystitis leading to bladder cancer have made it less attractive.

Thalidomide and lenalidomide

Thalidomide, and its possibly better analog *lenalidomide*, have immunosuppressant effectiveness. In our experience, sometimes thalidomide can improve on benefit produced by IVIG. However, both drugs can be rather slow to show effectiveness. As a side effect, they can produce a toxic sensory peripheral neuropathy, which is especially confusing and deleterious when treating a patient having, or potentially developing, a dysimmune sensory neuropathy. (Regarding, thalidomide and lenalidomide, we appreciate the drug background information and patient management collaboration of Dr Leo Orr.)

Caution

Be aware that a *generic drug* is *not necessarily identical* in *clinical benefit and side effects to the brand-name drug*. If with a generic version there is (a) lack of the expected efficacy, or (b) undesirable side effects, one should try a course of the original brand-name drug (see our disappointing experience with azathioprine, above). Apparently, the FDA requires physical-chemical equivalence, but not proof of clinical equivalence for approving a generic drug.

Some concepts discussed above are illustrated in clinical vignettes presented in Chapter 3.

References

1 Engel WK, Prentice AF. (1993) Some polyneuropathies (PNs) in insulin-requiring adult-onset diabetes (IRAOD) can benefit remarkably from anti-dysimmune treatments. *Neurology* **43**, 255–256.

2 Engel, WK. (2002) In type-2 diabetes, diabetic neuropathy is usually responsive to intravenous IgG (IVIG) treatment, ergo presumably dysimmune. *Acta Myologica* **21**, A79.

3 Engel WK. (1997) Intravenous immunoglobulin (IVIG) - an often-overlooked treatment - produces rapid, remarkable, sustained benefit in "diabetic neuropathy complex", suggesting a dysimmune mechanism. *Ann Neurol* **42**, 414.

4 Engel WK. (2003) Intravenous immunoglobulin G is remarkably beneficial in chronic immune dysschwannian/dysneuronal polyneuropathy, diabetes-2 neuropathy, and potentially in severe acute respiratory syndrome. *Acta Myologica* **22**, 97–103.

5 Engel WK. (2006) "Pseudo-lupus", benign neutropenia, and other probable non-worrisome blood-component changes due to IVIG treatment. *Neuromuscul Disord* **16**, 647–648.

6 Engel WK. (2006) Longer-term (>3 months), IVIG treatment to optimize clinical benefit and cellular protection usually requires an individualized adjustable schedule - not fixed regimentation. *Neuromuscul Disord* **16**, 703–704.

7 Engel WK. (2009) Intravenous immunoglobulin in relapsing-remittin multiple sclerosis: a dose-finding trial. *Neurology* **73**, 1077–1078.

8 Engel WK. (2010) Multi-microcramps (MMC) syndrome: a new pathogenic concept of subtle lower motor-neuron (LMN) lability causing very disturbing, continuing muscle pains, sometimes gratifying treatable - but often misinterpreted as mysterious "fibromyalgia" or "psychogenic". *Neurology* **74**, A465.

9 Mahajan S, Engel WK. (2010) Symptomatic treatment for muscle cramps (an evidence-based review). Letter to the Editor. *Neurology* **75**, 1397–1398.

10 Engel WK, Warmolts JR. (1971) Myasthenia gravis: a new hypothesis of the pathogenesis and a new form of treatment. *Ann N Y Acad Sci* **183**, 72–87.

11 Warmolts JR, Engel WK. (1972) Benefit from alternate-day prednisone in myasthenia gravis. *N Engl J Med* **286**, 17–20.

12 Warmolts JR, Engel WK, Whitaker JN. (1970) Alternate-day prednisone in a patient with myasthenia gravis. *Lancet* **2**, 1198–1199.

13 Engel WK. (1976) Myasthenia gravis, corticosteroids, anticholinesterases. *Ann NY Acad Sci* **274**, 623–630.

14 Engel WK. (2001) Polyneuropathy in type 2 diabetes mellitus. *Lancet* **358**, 2086.

15 Engel WK. (1991) RNA metabolism in relation to amyotrophic lateral sclerosis. *Adv Neurol* **56**, 125–153.

16 Engel WK. (1991) Does a retrovirus cause amyotrophic lateral sclerosis? *Ann Neurol* **30**, 431–433.

17 Engel WK, Kurland LT, Klatzo I. (1959) An inherited disease similar to amyotrophic lateral sclerosis with a pattern of posterior column involvement. An intermediate form? *Brain* **82**, 203–220.

18 Engel WK. (2008) In ALS, viral-dysmetabolic mechanisms acting via neuronal-nurturing cells (NNCs) could portend replacement therapy and should be sought by multi-tissue screening for rev-transcriptase (RT) and viral tracks. *Neuromuscul Disord* **18**, 764.

19 McCormick AL, Brown RH, Cudkowicz ME et al. (2008) Quantification of reverse transcriptase in ALS and elimination of a novel retroviral candidate. *Neurology* **70**: 278–283.

20 Engel WK, Patterson JM, Tauzin MR et al. (1988) Liver-biopsy abnormalities in amyotropic lateral sclerosis. *Ann Neurol* **24**, 163.

21 Prentice A, Engel WK, Rasheed S. (1992) Amyotrophic lateral sclerosis (ALS) associated with HTLV-I infection. *Neurology* **42**, 454–455.

22 Engel WK. (1989) High-dose TRH treatment of neuromuscular diseases: summary of Mechanisms and critique of clinical studies. *Ann NY Acad Sci* **553**, 462–472.

23 Engel WK, Siddique T, Nicoloff JT. (1983) Effect on weakness and spasticity in amyotrophic lateral sclerosis of thyrotropin-releasing hormone. *Lancet* **2**. 73–75.

24 Engel WK, Beydoun SR. (1985) Myophosphorylase deficiency (MPD) probably also involves lower motor neurons (LMNs) in some cases. *Neurology* **35**, 304.

25 Engel WK. (1977) Introduction to disorders of the motor neuron, nerves and related abnormalities. In: Goldensohn ES, Appel SH (eds), *Scientific Approaches to Clinical Neurology*. Lea Febiger, Philadelphia, pp. 1250–1321.

26 Yan J, Deng HX, Siddique N et al. (2010) Frameshift and novel mutations in FUS in familial amyotrophic lateral sclerosis and ALS/dementia. *Neurology* **75**, 807–814.

27 Engel WK, Hopkins LC, Rosenberg BJ. (1985) Fasciculating progressive muscular atrophy (F-PMA) remarkably responsive to anti-dysimmune treatment (ADIT)-a possible clue to more ordinary ALS? *Neurology* **35**, 72.

28 Engel WK. (1995) Rapid and continued improvement from intravenous immunoglobulin treatment of asymmetrical chronic progressive muscular atrophy after 19 years of disease progression. *Ann Neurol* **38**, 333–334.

29 Adornato BT, Engel WK, Kucera J et al. (1978) Benign focal amyotrophy. *Neurology* **28**, 399.

30 Engel WK, Askanas V. (2006) Inclusion-body myositis: clinical, diagnostic, and pathologic aspects. *Neurology* **66**, S20–29.

31 Askanas V, Engel WK, Alvarez RB. (1993) Enhanced detection of congo-red-positive amyloid deposits in muscle fibers of inclusion body myositis and brain of Alzheimer's disease using fluorescence technique. *Neurology* **43**, 1265–1267.

32 Kula RW, Engel WK, Line BR. (1977) Scanning for soft-tissue amyloid. *Lancet* **1**, 92–93.

33 Engel WK, Trotter JL. (1979) Plasma-cell dyscrasic amyloid neuropathy: a parasparafucile phenomenon? In: Serratrice G, Roux H (eds), *Peroneal Atrophies and Related Disorders*. Masson Publishing Co, New York, pp. 339–347.

34 Patten BM, Bilezikian JP, Mallette LE et al. (1973) Neuromuscular disease in primary hyperparathyroidism. *Ann Intern Med* **80**, 182–193.

35 Engel WK. (1987) A simple, low-tech clinical test and treatment for cervical root compression. *Ann Neurol* **22**, 165.

36 Engel WK. (1978) Ponderous-purse disease. Letter to the Editor. *New Engl J Med* **299**, 557.

37 Whitaker JN, Engel WK. (1972) Vascular deposits of immunoglobin and complement in idiopathic inflammatory myopathy. *New Engl J Med* **286**, 333–338.

38 Whitaker JN, Engel WK. (1973) Mechanisms of muscle injury in idiopathic inflammatory myopathy. *New Engl J Med* **289**, 107–108.

39 Mendell JR, Engel WK, Derrer EC. (1970) Duchenne muscular dystrophy: functional ischemia reproduces its characteristic lesions. *Science* **172**, 1143–1145.

40 Mendell JR, Engel WK, Derrer EC. (1972) Increased plasma enzyme concentrations in rats with functional ischemia of muscle provide a possible model of Duchenne muscular dystrophy. *Nature* **239**, 522–524.

41 Engel WK. (1973) Duchenne muscular dystrophy: a histologically based ischemia hypothesis and comparison with experimental ischemia myopathy. In: Pearson CM, Mostofi FK (eds), *The Striated Muscle*. Williams & Wilkins Co, Baltimore, vol. **12**, pp. 453–472.

42 Engel WK. (1977) Integrative histochemical approach to the defect of Duchenne muscular dystrophy. In: Rowland LP (ed.), *Pathogenesis of the Human Muscular Dystrophies*, American Elsevier Publishing Co, New York, Excerpta Medica, pp. 277–309.

43 Engel WK, Derrer EC. (1975) Drugs blocking the muscle-damaging effects of 5-HT and nonadrenaline in aorta-ligated rats. *Nature* **254**, 151–152.

44 Kyle RA. (1978) Monoclonal gammopathy of undetermined significance. Natural history in 241 cases. *Am J Med* **64**, 814–826.

45 Adornato BT, Engel WK. (1977) MB-creatine phosphokinase isoenzyme elevation not diagnostic of myocardial infarction. *Arch Intern Med* **137**, 1089–1090.

46 Warmolts JR, Engel WK. (1973) Correlation of motor unit behavior with histochemical and myofiber type in humans by open-biopsy electromyography. In: Desmedt JE (ed.), *New Developments in Electromyography and Clinical Neurophysiology*, Karger, Basel, pp. 35–40.

47 Warmolts JR, Engel WK. (1972) Open biopsy electromyography. I. Correlation of motor unit behavior with histochemical muscle fiber type in human limb muscle. *Arch Neurol* **27**, 512–517.

48 Engel WK. (1977) Introduction to the myopathies. In: Goldensohn ES, Appel SH (eds), *Scientific Approaches to Clinical Neurology*, Lea Febiger, Philadelphia, pp. 1602–1632.

49 Engel WK. (1973) "Myopathic EMG" - nonesuch animal. *New Engl J Med* **289**, 485–486.

50 Engel WK. (1975) Brief, small, abundant motor-unit action potentials. *Neurology* **25**, 173–176.

51 Karpati G, Engel WK. (1968) Correlative histochemical study of skeletal muscle after a suprasegmental denervation, peripheral nerve section, and skeletal fixation. *Neurology* **18**, 681–692.

52 Karpati G, Engel WK. (1968) Histochemical investigation of fiber type ratios with the myofibrillar ATPase reaction in normal and denervated skeletal muscles in guinea pig. *Am J Anat* **122**, 145–155.

53 Resnick JS, Engel WK, Griggs RC et al. (1968) Acetazolamide prophylaxis in hypokalemic periodic paralysis. *N Engl J Med* **278**, 582–586.

54 Griggs RC, Engel WK, Resnick JS. (1970) Acetazolamide treatment of hypokalemic periodic paralysis. *Ann Intern Med* **73**, 39–48.

55 Dalakas MC, Engel WK. (1983) Treatment of "permanent" muscle weakness in familial hypokalemic periodic paralysis. *Muscle Nerve* **6**, 182–186.

56 Askanas V, Engel WK. (2003) Toxicity of long-chain fatty acids (LCFAs) in muscle carnitine deficiency and other LCFA endodissolutions? Dietary LCFA restriction associated with dramatic long-term improvement. *Neurology* **36**, 94.

57 Engel, WK. (1986) Toxic role of long-chain fatty-acids in muscle carnitine deficiency and other LCFA endodissolutions: dietary LCFA retriction associated with dramatic long-term improvement. *Neurology* **36** (Suppl 1), 94.

58 Askanas V, Engel WK, Kwan HH et al. (1985) Autosomal dominant syndrome of lipid neuromyopathy with normal carnitine: successful treatment with long-chain fatty-acid-free diet. *Neurology* **35**, 66–72.

59 Prockop LD, Engel WK, Shug AL. (1983) Nearly fatal muscle carnitine deficiency with full recovery after replacement therapy. *Neurology* **33**, 1629–1631.

60 Engel WK, Hanna CJ, Misra AK. (1990) HTLV-I-associated myelopathy. *New Engl J Med* **323**, 552.

61 Engel WK, Misra AK, Alexander SJ et al. (1990) Syndrome of continuous motor unit activity responsible to immunosuppression suggests dysimmune pathogenesis. *Neurology* **40**, 118.

62 DeVivo DC, Engel WK. (1970) Remarkable recovery of a steroid-responsive recurrent polyneuropathy. *J Neurol Neurosurg Psychiatry* **33**, 62–69.

63 Engel WK, Borenstein A, DeVivo DC et al. (1972) High-single-dose alternate-day prednisone (HSDAD-PRED) in the treatment of dermatomyositis/polymyositis complex. *Trans Am Neurol Assn* **97**, 272–275.

64 Engel WK, Resnick JS. (1966) Late-onset rod myopathy - a newly recognized, aquired and progressive disease. *Neurology* **16**, 308–309.

65 Engel WK. (2007) Late-onset rod myopathy with monoclonal immunoglobulin can be treatable with IVIG. *Neuromuscul Disord* **17**, 885.

66 Engel WK. (1977) Rod (nemaline) disease. In: Goldensohn ES, Appel SH (eds), *Scientific Approaches to Clinical Neurology*, Lea Febiger, Philadelphia, pp. 1667–1691.

67 Mahajan S, Engel WK, Luthra I, Gupta V. (2011) Adult-onset rod myopathy syndrome (AORMS): sustained benefit from IVIG plus rituximab. *Ann Neurol*, in press.

68 Engel WK, Lichter AS, Galdi AP. (1982) Polymyositis: remarkable response to total body irradiation. *Lancet* **1**, 658.

69 Engel WK, Cuneo RA, Levy HB. (1978) Polyinosinic-polycytidylic acid treatment of neuropathy. *Lancet* **1**, 503–504.

70 Engel WK, Adornato B. (1993) Fever-responsive neuropathy (FRN) benefited by long-term interferon alpha-2A (Ib) treatment. *Can J Neurol Sci* **4**, S44.

71 Engel WK. (2007) Fever-responsive dysschwannian neuropathy (FRDN): Interferon-alpha 2a (Iα) treatment has produced remarkable recovery from total quadriplegia, the benefit now persisting 4 years beyond the 14 years of therapy. *Neuromuscul Disord* **17**, 885.

72 Engel WK. (2011) Remarkable benefit persisting undiminished for 8 years after stopping 14 years of In-

terferon-α 2A (Inf-α) treatment for fever-responsive dysimmune neuropathy (FRDN): possibly a combined antidysimmune plus antiviral effect, and thus a putative model for future "combined antidysimmune" therapies. *Neurology* **76**, A520.

73 Engel WK, Askanas V. (1976) Letter: overlooked avian oncornavirus in cultured muscle–functionally significant? *Science* **192**, 1252–1253.

74 Engel, WK (1969) Motor neuron histochemistry in ALS and infantile spind muscular a trophy. In Norr is FH Jr., Kurland LT (Eds) *Motor Neuron Diseases*, pp 218–234. Grune & Stratton, New York.

75 Renton AE, Majounie E, Waite A, et. al. (2011) A hexanucleotide repeat expansion in C90RF72 is the cause of chromosome 9p 21–linke ALS-FTD. *Neuron* DOI: 10.10.16, neuron. 2011.09.010.

CHAPTER 3

Aging of the human neuromuscular system: patient vignettes

W. King Engel[1,2], Shalini Mahajan[2], and Valerie Askanas[1,2]

[1]Departments of Neurology and Pathology, University of Southern California Neuromuscular Center, University of Southern California Keck School of Medicine, Los Angeles, CA, USA
[2]Good Samaritan Hospital, Los Angeles, CA, USA

Complex, probably-neurogenic coexisting disorders

Vignette 1. Type-2 muscle-fiber atrophy, neoplasm-related cachectic atrophy, plus sensory-motor neuropathy

Proximal muscle weakness in an elderly patient associated with a normal electromyogram (EMG) can be caused by type-2 muscle fiber atrophy, which is diagnosable only on muscle biopsy. One should seek an identifiable cause, such as cachexia, disuse, glucocorticoid toxicity, a "remote" neoplasm, hyperparathyroidism, subtle denervation, or suprasegmental central nervous system (CNS) abnormality. This mainly-sensory nerve neuropathy can cause slowed sensory nerve conductions, if involving large diameter fiber, ± small diameter ones.

Nine months ago, a 62-year-old man began having difficulty climbing stairs and getting up from a low chair or a squatting position. He fatigued easily and needed frequent periods of rest during his daily activities. His arms tired easily carrying bags of groceries or holding his 18 kg grandchild. He had no symptomatic weakness in his distal limbs. He had slight distal sensory symptoms, no muscle pain. He had been a chronic smoker, but had stopped 10 years ago.

Examination: He had moderate bilateral proximal lower-limb weakness, especially in the ileopsoas, quadriceps, and glutei, and slight–moderate weakness in his proximal upper limbs. He had slightly reduced vibration and pain sensations in his feet. Cranial-nerve functions were normal. Tendon reflexes were reduced throughout, ankle jerks were absent, and plantars were unresponsive.

Studies: Creatine kinase (CK) was slightly elevated (380 IU/L; upper normal for men is 370 IU/L). Liver-function tests and other blood chemistries were normal. The serum *anti-neuronal/anti-Hu antibody* test was positive. Immunofixation showed a *monoclonal IgG-kappa band*. Sensory and motor nerve conduction velocities were slightly slowed (dysschwannian) in the lower limbs, and EMG was normal. Cerebrospinal fluid (CSF) protein was slightly elevated (48 mg/dL; upper normal is 45 mg/dL), without detectable lymphocytes or tumor cells. Repetitive neuromuscular junction stimulation at low and high frequency was normal.

Quadriceps muscle biopsy showed prominent *type-2 muscle-fiber atrophy* (especially of the type 2B fibers) prominent in degree and extent, and slight recent denervation (see Chapter 1 in this volume). Imaging of his chest disclosed a small lesion, which upon biopsy was a solitary bronchogenic small-cell carcinoma. Other studies did not disclose any metastases. Surgical resection of the chest lesion was considered complete.

Diagnosis: This patient had type-2 fiber atrophy, probably as a remote "paraneoplastic" effect of the

---

Muscle Aging, Inclusion-Body Myositis and Myopathies, First Edition. Edited by Valerie Askanas and W. King Engel.

lung carcinoma. Possible links between the neo-plasm and the type-2 atrophy are detailed in Chapter 1. They include: a *paraneoplastic dysimmune* or another type of *autogenic toxic neuropathy*, and hyponutrition/cachexia. Although his more prominent fatigue than weakness was characteristic of type-2 atrophy, the diagnosis was based on the muscle biopsy histochemistry. His hyporeflexia and slightly elevated CSF protein probably were caused by subtle sensory dysimmune peripheral neuropathy, with a motor component. On the first clinical examination, the differential diagnosis included polymyositis; motor neuropathy; facilitating myasthenic syndrome of Lambert–Eaton; and a possible component of brain or high-spinal-cord or meningeal metastases.

Treatment: Treatment was to identify and correct the cause, in this case by tumor-excision surgery. This patient's bronchogenic carcinoma might or might not have been completely removed. Resection of a tumor often does not stop a remote effect of that tumor. If the type-2 fiber atrophy continues after "complete resection," as occurred in this patient, possibilities include the following: (a) tumor cells are persisting at the original site or in undetected metastases that are, speculatively, still secreting *cachexins* or other adverse proteins. These may include *parathyroid-hormone-related-peptide* (PTHrP), which can induce cachexia by a mechanism independent of pro-inflammatory cytokine action. For example, it might (i) provoke production of cachexins by other cells, and/or (ii) still be programming lymphocytic production of toxic antibodies. (b) Alternatively, there might be lymphocytes and/or macrophages, previously "programmed" by the tumor cells, that are still secreting circulating toxic antibodies and/or "*cachexins*" (such as tumor necrosis factor α and interleukin-6, or PTHrP).

Comment: A common association of type-2 fiber atrophy (discussed in Chapter 1) is an aspect of a lower-motor-neuron abnormality resulting in functional "dysinnervation," as may be part of the pathogenic mechanism in this patient. Note that routine diagnostic EMG cannot quantify the size of the type-2 muscle-fiber fast-twitch units because they are activated only by vigorous contraction, whereas slow-twitch type-1 motor-units are activated by early slight contraction and usually are the only ones quantified.

Myopathic disorders

Vignette 2. Sporadic inclusion-body myositis

In a patient who has had gradual onset of proximal and distal muscle weakness at age 50 or older, especially involving the quadriceps, ankle extensors, and flexors and/or extensors of the distal phalanges of the fingers and toes, slightly to moderately elevated CK and no family history, one should consider *sporadic inclusion-body myositis (s-IBM)*. Muscle-biopsy histochemistry, utilizing our special staining techniques (see Chapters 7 and 10 in this volume), is virtually always diagnostic.

A 60-year-old man has had very gradual onset for at least 5 years, and probably 8 years, of progressive neuromuscular fatigue, difficulty ascending stairs and arising from sitting. Now, one or both legs can suddenly give way while walking, or even while standing. He also has a slight foot-drop bilaterally. In the upper limbs he has moderate weakness of the fingers in gripping keys and picking up small things, and in using his proximal upper-limb muscles. He has developed general exercise intolerance. He recently has had occasional *difficulty swallowing*, needing liquid to wash the food down. He has not had muscle cramps, pain, or sensory symptoms. Family history is negative for neuromuscular disease.

Examination: There was prominent weakness and atrophy in the quadriceps muscle, and moderate weakness of the glutei, and of the toe and ankle extensors. He also had prominent weakness of the flexors of the distal finger phalanges (namely, flexor digitorum profundus, especially of fingers 4 and 5) and contrastingly good strength of the flexors of the metacarpal-phalangeal joints (flexor digitorum sublimus). Finger extensors were moderately weak, as were biceps, triceps, and deltoid muscles. There were no fasciculations. Cranial-nerve functions, except for the dysphagia, were normal. Speech, sensory, and cerebellar functions were normal. Tendon reflexes were moderately–prominently reduced throughout. Plantar responses are not interpretable because extension of all the toes was weak.

Studies: Serum CK was slightly elevated at 512 IU/L (upper normal is 397 IU/L). Nerve conductions were normal. EMG showed small motor units (*BSAPs, "brief-duration, small-amplitude, overly abundant motor-unit potentials"* [1]), plus recent denervation (fibrillations and positive waves).

Muscle biopsy showed five types of abnormality, as follows (see Chapters 7 and 10): (a) a few to a moderate number of muscle fibers, each containing one or a few small *vacuoles* (which were sometimes red-rimmed with the Engel trichrome stain); (b) mononuclear lymphocytic inflammatory cells (notably CD8 lymphocytes) around muscle fibers, and sometimes invading muscle fibers that were otherwise only minimally abnormal; (c) small inclusions, one or a few per fiber on cross-section, (i) that were congophilic (indicating abnormal protein aggregated in the β-pleated sheet conformation of amyloid); and (ii) by immunolocalization contained either amyloid-β protein and or hyperphosphorylated tau protein (p-tau) (each colocalizing with any of about 20 other proteins, including α-synuclein), that are also typical of Alzheimer and/or Parkinson brain). (Amyloid-β and p-tau accumulations are typical of Alzheimer brain, and α-synuclein accumulations typical of Parkinson brain.) (d) A few small angular muscle fibers that suggest a recent-denervation component (which could be neurogenous or myogenous deinnervation or dysinnervation). (e) Stained squiggles that contain p-tau protein, which are much better displayed by the P62 antibody than TDP-43, and by electron-microscopy are seen as paired helical filaments.

Treatment: There is no enduring treatment for stopping the gradual progression of s-IBM. How-ever, some patients can have useful transient benefit in response to small or medium doses of oral glucocorticoid treatment, in the range of 15–45 mg single dose on alternate days (see Chapter 7). But note, if the patient or a close family member has diabetes-2 (type-2 diabetes), a glucocorticoid can bring out diabetes-2. Dysphagia sometimes is benefited by IVIG.

Comment: Identifying s-IBM is clinically important, for example to distinguish it from amyotrophic lateral sclerosis (ALS), a fatal diagnosis that had been given erroneously to several of our s-IBM patients.

Vignette 3. Dermatomyositis

Dermatomyositis causes a moderately or rapidly progressive muscle weakness, with or without skin manifestations. Muscle biopsy is nearly always diagnostic. Treatment is typically begun with a *glucocorticoid*, usually *prednisone*, and it is often effective in restoring good to excellent strength.

In patients who have diabetes-2 in themselves or in a close family member, a glucocorticoid should be avoided or used with great caution, and, if used, blood glucose and hemoglobin A1c should be constantly monitored to try to avoid worsening or precipitating diabetes. Alternative immunosuppressant treatments include intravenous immunoglobulin (IVIG), Imuran/ azathioprine, possibly rituximab, and others (see Chapter 2). If the patient is an adult, one should search for an occult neoplasm that could be causing the dermatomyositis as a remote effect: if found, a neoplasm should be treated aggressively.

For 6 months a 52-year-old woman has had *progressive difficulty climbing stairs* and getting up from a chair. She has been much weaker over the last 3 months, and now unaided cannot arise from a chair or walk, and is also very weak proximally in the upper limbs. She has some tenderness of muscles and occasional deep aching pain in her thighs. She has no sensory symptoms or imbalance. She has a moderate violacious rash on her face, especially around her eyes, and upper chest. Family history is negative.

Examination: This revealed prominent bilateral weakness of hip flexion and extension, and moderate–prominent weakness of knee extension and hip adduction. There is also prominent weakness of proximal upper limbs. Distal limb strength was only slightly decreased. Tendon reflexes were decreased throughout. Plantar responses were normal. Sensory and cerebellar functions were normal.

Studies: Serum CK was high 3200 IU/L (upper normal for women was 240 IU/L). Serum aspartate aminotransferase (AST), alanine aminotransferase (ALT), and lactate dehydrogenase (LDH) were also rather highly elevated. But, the serum liver-enzyme γ-glutamyl transpeptidase (GGTP; which can leak from liver but not from muscle) was very normal: this indicates normal liver function and demonstrates that the elevated AST, ALT, and LDH were due to leakiness of abnormal muscle fibers (which was also indicated by the high serum CK-MM, a skeletal-muscle enzyme). Sedimentation rate was 42 mm/hour (upper normal is 20 mm/hour for women). Complete blood count and thyroid tests were normal.

EMG of the quadriceps and biceps showed increased recruitment of abnormally small, sometimes polyphasic, motor-unit potentials, Those "BSAPs" and "BSAPPs" [1], evident during slight voluntary contraction, indicated "fractionated" motor units, which can be caused by either a myopathic or a distal-axonal-twig neuropathic disturbance (see Chapters 1 and 2). It also showed spontaneous fibrillations and positive waves at rest, indicating separation of viable muscle fibers from their motor-neuron control (on a neuropathic or myopathic basis), which would normally prevent such spontaneous activity. Nerve conductions were normal.

Muscle biopsy of the quadriceps showed changes characteristic of dermatomyositis: (a) necrotic fibers and fibers being phagocytosed; (b) "regen-degen" muscle fibers, many of which are multivacuolated and many are positively stained with the alkaline phosphatase reaction; (c) a perifascicular accentuation of these two types of abnormalities at borders of the fascicles (bundles) of muscle fibers; (d) alkaline phosphatase-positive proliferating perimysial connective-tissue (in muscle biopsies, this is unique to dermatomyositis, lupus erythematosus, and sometimes polymyositis, and perhaps some other collagen-vascular diseases); (e) mononuclear inflammatory cells, mainly lymphocytes and some macrophages, which are around muscle fibers, and sometimes are invading fibers that otherwise are only minimally abnormal (but never completely normal morphologically); (f) perimysial lymphocytic inflammation and fibrosis; (g) immunoglobulin deposition in intramuscular blood-vessels (see Chapter 2) [2]. The moderate to prominent alkaline phosphatase positivity of perimysial connective tissue is virtually diagnostic (see above). In this patient, search for a remote neoplasm was negative, although in older patients with dermatomyositis there is sometimes an associated remote neoplasm, which might be discovered initially, or only months after the first clinical presentation of weakness.

Treatment: The patient, who had no diabetes-2 herself or in a close relative, was started on 60 mg of single-dose alternate-day oral prednisone, with potassium supplement. Our "prednisone-accompanying" dietary instructions were to omit caffeine and sodium, and to limit calorie intake (prednisone, being a glucocorticoid, causes adrenergic stimulation/insomnia, sodium retention, and increased appetite). For this patient, since she was currently progressing rather rapidly, was very weak, and was not a fertile female, we added Imuran/azathioprine, which we then personally monitored by obligatory absolute neutrophil counts, initially done weekly, that were obtained locally by the patient and the results faxed immediately to us. (See Chapter 2 for an explanation of the illogicality of a "white blood cell count" and the possibility of incorrect management based on it.) We also initially gave her IVIG, 0.4 g/kg on five consecutive days, and then on two nonconsecutive days weekly for the next 16 weeks. She has had a cumulatively excellent response, with improvement of strength and elimination of pain in her legs. Concurrently, her CK returned to nearly normal. In treating this type of patient, we follow the *clinical response*, primarily *strength* and *endurance, not* the CK level itself. (A rising CK indicates worsening; a falling CK reflects improvement *if the patient is also becoming stronger*; however, if the patient is weakening, a falling CK suggests there is ongoing progressive disease producing so much muscle damage that there is less muscle from which CK can leak.) Note: dermatomyositis patients often have a good response to IVIG, which can be more effective and safer to give, but it is more complicated and costly. IVIG can be used in two general ways: (a) initially along with *prednisone*, with or without *Imuran*, for a probably-faster onset of benefit, or (b) added later if the response to prednisone with or without Imuran is less than satisfactory.

Comment: *Alkaline phosphatase-positive proliferating endomysial connective tissue* in muscle biopsies is unique to dermatomyositis, lupus, and some other collagen-vascular diseases. We think it is probably produced by proliferating disease-characteristic connective-tissue fibroblasts. Azathioprine has had proven benefit for dermatomyositis in a few patients. Occasional patients have side-effects with generic azathioprine, but good tolerance and benefit with brand Imuran (some are intolerant to both). If the patient had been unresponsive, we would have considered *rituximab*. If the patient had remained unresponsive and seriously weakened, we would have considered *total-body irradiation* [3], if available (see Chapter 2). In some patients we have found total-body irradiation to be cumulatively, dramatically beneficial.

Vignette 4. Polymyositis with disease-associated high IgG

In a dysimmune disease, if the patient's serum IgG is already too high, repeated plasmaphereses can be beneficial, and presumably safer then IVIG.

A 51-year-old woman had had slowly progressive, painless proximal muscle weakness for 8 years. She could not lift her arms to shoulder level; and walking more than 20 m was very difficult, as was arising from a chair or entering a car. Her serum CK was very high, 7700 IU/L (upper normal was 240 IU/L). Muscle biopsy showed a lymphocytic inflammatory myopathy, typical of polymyositis. Prior to our involvement, she had failed therapeutic attempts with prednisone, mycophenolate, and etanercept.

Treatment: We considered IVIG treatment, but her own disease-produced serum IgG was already very high, 2900 mg/dL (normal is 650–1650 mg/dL). From our experience with numerous patients given IVIG, we have observed that the serum IgG can, for more than 24 h, be as high as 3000–4500 mg/dL, and – undesirably – sometimes higher. Therefore, rather than adding to her already-high serum IgG, which might have produced blood thickening and possibly vascular occlusion, we did the opposite, using *repeated daily plasmaphereses* (see Chapter 2) to remove her high IgG, per the following schedule: week 1, plasmaphereses on Monday, Tuesday, Thursday, Friday; week 2, Monday, Tuesday, Friday; week 3 and thereafter, two nonconsecutive days per week, and later reducing to once per week as needed. The patient had cumulatively dramatic benefit. She could jog 5 km, and perform strenuous

yoga poses. Because her own pathologically elevated IgG, produced by abnormal B-lymphocytes, was apparently toxic to her muscle, this woman (who is post-menopausal) seems to be a candidate for *more definitive treatment* with the anti-B-lymphocyte drug *rituximab* (pregnancy class C).

Comment: As good as *plasmaphereses* can be, their use does not produce an enduring benefit: it is more like *repeatedly bailing out a leaky boat*. For a patient having plasmaphereses, medicines should be given after, not before, the phereses.

Vignette 5. Oculo-pharyngeal muscular dystrophy

This is an autosomal dominant hereditary muscle disorder characterized by ptosis, dysphagia and proximal-limb weakness. The mutation is a GCG polyalanine trinucleotide expansion in the poly (A)-binding protein nuclear 1 (*PABPN1*) gene. Genetic testing for this can confirm the diagnosis. There is no effective treatment for the genetic muscle weakening. If pharyngeal constriction is demonstrable by a cine-swallowing test, progressively severe swallowing difficulty can often be satisfactorily improved by gradual dilation of the pharyngeal constriction using a bougie, performed by a gastroenterologist or otolaryngologist. Prominent drooping of the eyelids can be repaired by ophthalmologic surgery (but inadvertent overcorrection can result in dangerous corneal exposure). (See Chapter 2 for an example of a patient with oculo-pharyngeal muscular dystrophy who developed a late-onset, initially unidentified, treatable polymyositis.)

For 20 years a 54-year old woman has had slowly progressive ptosis of both upper eyelids, difficulty swallowing food, and slightly nasal speech. Her gradually drooping upper eyelids are now interfering with her vision, and it is a constant effort for her to keep the eyelids open; in fact, she has already had two eyelid surgeries to correct the ptosis, each producing useful temporary benefit. She has not had double vision. She now frequently gets small pieces of food stuck in her throat; especially troublesome are pieces of meat, bread, and lettuce. Small dry particles such as nuts can produce aspiration and coughing. For the last few months, she has developed moderate difficulty arising from the floor or a chair, due to gluteal and quadriceps weakness. She has no difficulty breathing and no sensory symptoms.

Her mother, mother's sister, and mother's father had similar eyelid and swallowing abnormalities. Her mother became wheelchair-dependent in her 60s. There is no significant diurnal variation of the patient's weakness, but her limbs have been fatiguing more often in the past 3 years.

Examination: There was bilateral ptosis, which did not worsen during 2 min of sustained up-gaze. There was moderate weakness of the neck flexors, fingers, glutei, quadriceps, and hip adductors. Extraocular movements of the globes were normal. Speech was slightly nasal. Swallowing water in the presence of the physician required extra attempts. Tendon reflexes were reduced throughout. Plantar reflexes, and sensory and cerebellar examinations, were normal.

Laboratory: Blood counts and chemistries, including thyroid tests, were normal. Antibodies to the nicotinic acetylcholine receptor and to striated muscle were negative (the former are typically positive in myasthenia gravis (MG), and the latter would suggest the presence of a thymoma).

Nerve conductions were normal. Also normal was low-frequency repetitive neuromuscular-junction stimulation (distinct from MG, which typically shows a decremental response). EMG showed BSAPs [1] on voluntary contraction in the upper and lower limbs, and also slight signs of recent denervation.

Biceps muscle biopsy showed a very few small angular atrophying muscle fibers; rare fibers were necrotic and being phagocytosed, and there was slight established reinnervation. There were no "ragged-red fibers." There was no inflammation. Genetic testing revealed the typical GCG trinucleotide expansion in both the patient and her mother.

Treatment: There is no effective treatment for this genetic muscle weakening. Severe swallowing difficulty can often be satisfactorily improved by *esophageal dilation using a bougie*. If it is too severe, a *feeding gastrostomy* can be installed for safe intake (with it sometimes the patient can still cautiously take small amounts of favorite food and drink). Prominent eyelid drooping can be surgically repaired, with caution to not overcorrect.

Comment: Anatomically, a more precise name for this disease would be *palpebro-pharyngeal muscular dystrophy* because, although there is prominent weakness of eyelids, there is no weakness of eye-globe movements.

Vignette 6. Myofibrillar myopathy, plus a treatable dysimmune neuropathy (CIDP)

Myofibrillar myopathies are a heterogeneous group of muscle diseases with various ages of onset and clinical presentations. All are characterized by a distinct, and diagnostic, muscle-biopsy morphologic phenotype. The majority of patients are sporadic. However, there are hereditary patients having an autosomal dominant or autosomal recessive pattern, that include a number of different mutations of several different genes encoding various myofibrillar proteins, as well as genes encoding intermediate-filament desmin, αB-crystallin, and plectin. These have been identified mainly by the Mayo Rochester group. Myofibrillar myopathy patients generally have a slowly progressive course leading to severe muscle weakness and disability. Sometimes there is an associated motor or sensory peripheral neuropathy, which in two sporadic patients we have found clearly responsive to IVIG and therefore representing a treatable dysimmune phenomenon. There is no widely effective treatment for the myofibrillar myopathy itself, but certainly a treatable dysimmune aspect should be sought.

This patient is a 74-year-old woman who has had, for the past 7 years, slowly progressive proximal, and slightly distal, muscle weakness. She had difficulty walking, ascending steps, and performing even slight household activities. She was easily fatigued, needing frequent rests during the day. Her symptoms began gradually, but have become prominent in the last 2 years. Family history was negative for any neuromuscular disorder. The patient was not diabetic, but both of her parents had diabetes-2.

Examination: There was moderate to prominent proximal>distal muscle weakness in all limbs. The tendon reflexes were diminished throughout and absent at the ankles. The vibration sense was absent at the toes and decreased at the ankles; there was a stocking distal distribution of diminished pinprick sensation in both feet and lower legs.

Studies: Serum CK was slightly elevated (475 IU/L) and an IgG-kappa monoclonal antibody was present. Other blood chemistries and hemogram were normal. CSF protein was elevated, 94 mg/dL (normal <46 mg/dL), strongly suggesting a dysimmune neuropathy. Nerve conductions velocities were slow, and indicative of a dysschwannian neuropathy. Her EMG showed (a) a BSAP pattern indicating fractionated motor units, which can be myopathic or neuropathic, and (b) fibrillations and positive waves indicating recent denervation (neurogenous or myogenous).

Muscle biopsy showed abnormalities diagnostic of myofibrillar myopathy, including presence on Engel trichrome staining (see Chapter 1) of regions of degenerative myofibrillar material and absent cross-striations, appearing amorphous and hyaline, reddish or dark-purplish in color. In these same regions there was absence of the usual intermyofibrillar oxidative enzyme activity of mitochondria and reticulum. A few muscle fibers had vacuoles possessing some autophagic features. No lymphocytic or macrophagic inflammation was detectable. There were a few small angular, atrophic muscle fibers and some muscle-fiber type-grouping indicating, respectively, recent denervation and established reinnervation.

Treatment: Because of the sensory abnormalities, dysschwannian nerve conductions, elevated CSF protein, aspects of denervation-reinnervation in the muscle biopsy, and the diabetes-2 in both parents, we considered that our patient probably had coexisting "*genetico-diabetoid-2 dysimmune neuropathy,*" a type of chronic immune dysschwannian polyneuropathy (CIDP) (sometimes less precisely called chronic inflammatory demyelinating polyneuropathy, Chapter 2). We therefore treated her using *IVIG*, and she was remarkably benefited: her walking ability and endurance *greatly improved*, she did not require frequent rests, and was able to ascend steps much more easily.

Comment: Even though there is no specific treatment for myofibrillar myopathy, this patient greatly benefited from treatment of her coexisting dysimmune motor-sensory neuropathy. This exemplifies the need for carefully seeking treatable aspects in each patient (see Chapter 2).

Neuromuscular junction disorder

Vignette 7. Myasthenia Gravis (MG)

MG, originally deserved the name "gravis" for its often fatal respiratory outcome, but now it is usually (but not always) well treatable. Once diagnosed, MG should be aggressively treated with a *glucocorticoid* or *other immunosuppressant*, and not just symptomatically with an anti-cholinesterase such as pyridostigmine/Mestinon (unless the patient is only mildly affected and easily responsive). We also feel that moderate or severe MG should not be treated with primary or adjunctive pyridostigmine because that can actually weaken the patient when in excessive dosage for that specific patient. That weakening is more likely to happen if given concurrently with prednisone) [4]. Acute and/or severe myasthenic weakness ("crisis") is treatable by emergency admission to intensive-care (intubation, ventilation, and nasogastric feeding as needed), stopping any pyridostigmine, starting a) plasmaphereses (which remove both toxic MG antibodies and any weakening effects of "excessive" pyridostigmine), or b) IVIG infusions. Usually high-dose prednisone is started (see Chapter 2), with or without Imuran, or Imuran alone if the patient or a close relative has diabetes. Rituximab is now being used for some difficult patients. In every MG patient, even in aging patients, thymoma should be sought and, if found, surgically removed to treat the MG and remove the tumor. Surgery has been most complete by trans-sternotomy to allow visualization and removal of the entire anterior mediastinal contents. Now, some thymectomies, especially for fragile surgical candidates, are being done by minimally invasive multiple-probe surgery, but the completeness of this technique and long-term benefit are still being evaluated.

A 58-year-old man has had, for the last 8 months, diffuse muscle weakness, easy fatigability, drooping of the eyelids, and sometimes double vision in the early evening. In the mornings he feels better. For the past month he has had at least three episodes of choking and coughing while eating dinner. (Note: patients often minimize such chokings and aspirations, whereas the spouse often gives a more accurate account of their frequency and severity.)

The patient does not have sensory symptoms. As usual with adult-onset MG, there was no family history of neuromuscular disease.

Examination: There was bilateral ptosis, mild bifacial weakness (can't whistle; a snarl-type of horizontal smile), diplopia, especially on lateral gaze to each side (attributable to bilateral sixth-nerve weakness) and, as part of the clinical exam, definite difficulty swallowing water. He was short of breath and vital capacity was very low at 1.2 L. There was also moderate proximal weakness in the upper limbs, and hip flexors: these worsened with briefly repetitive maximal effort. Sensory examination was normal. Tendon reflexes were slightly brisk throughout (as is usual in MG), and both plantar responses were flexor.

Studies: Acetylcholine receptor binding and blocking antibodies were positive, as was the *anti-striated-muscle antibody*. Other immunological parameters were normal, as were thyroid function tests. *Repetitive nerve stimulation* at low-frequency (3 Hz) showed an 18% decremental response of the compound-motor-unit potential indicating MG (normal is <11% decrement). Nerve conduction studies were normal. Computed tomography (with contrast) of the mediastinum revealed a mass, presumably thymoma.

Treatment: Following three daily plasmaphereses, the patient was concurrently started on (a) prednisone at 60 mg single dose daily (which subsequently was gradually converted to single dose on alternate days) and (b) 2.5 mg/kg Imuran divided-dose daily (evolving to 3 mg/kg daily as needed and tolerated; see Chapter 2). A thoracic surgeon performed a presumably complete excision of the histologically confirmed thymoma. Improvement was evident beginning 12 h after the first plasmapheresis, and gradually incremented. The patient was nearly back to normal within 6 weeks.

Comments: MG usually can be very well treated, but it requires a coordinated effort and very careful monitoring. Slightly increased tendon reflexes are typical of MG. Removal of the thymoma eliminates the thymic epithelial cells that possess nicotinic receptors [5], which we have proposed to be the provoking origin of the MG dysimmune mechanism [4], possibly from viral infection of them.

Neurogenic disorders

Vignette 8. "Multi-microcramps" (not "fibromyalgia") and a cramps-fasciculations syndrome

"Multi-microcramps" can be the clinical presentation of a neuropathy, manifesting as diffuse muscle pains, stiffness, and/or fatigue, occurring especially during and after a day of vigorous exertion, often worse in the evening, resulting in *"painful insomnia,"* i.e. difficulty achieving sleep or awakening during sleep [6]. Such symptoms are often dismissed as mysterious "fibromyalgia" (see Chapter 2). Muscle-biopsy histochemistry (see Chapter 1) is the best way to identify the typical neurogenic basis of this multi-microcramps disorder, as evidenced by recent denervation and established reinnervation. EMG studies are less precise, but might reveal nerve irritability in the form of microcramps or macrocramps, and sometimes fasciculations. The motor-nerve distal-twig location of the pathology can cause a neurogenic type of "BSAP" EMG pattern. Motor and/or sensory nerve conductions can be normal or somewhat slow. For treatment, first we stop all caffeine and any other "herbal" or other stimulants, and try to switch out any beta-agonists. Then, according to our experience, treatment with bedtime very-low-dose clonazepam/Klonopin (off-label, 0.5–2 mg) is often extremely beneficial for rapidly reducing the intensity and frequency of the symptoms (and sometimes is mildly soporific), overall resulting in a much better quality of life. Presumably it is suppressing the causative distal-twig nerve instability/irritability, thereby reducing the "microcramps." This can provide reduced discomfort during the day and more restful sleep at night. At a given dose, it either provides relief the first night – e.g., "the first good night's sleep I've had in months" – or it doesn't. Some patients who also have troublesome daytime muscle cramps, or fasciculations, benefit from 0.25–0.5 mg during the morning without engendering sleepiness.

Clonazepam is usually more effective, and it is cheaper than pregabalin, duloxetine, gabapentin, or ropinirole, or hypnotics. Complex trials are not required to demonstrate clonazepam's effectiveness. No drug build-up is needed, but initial incremental dose-finding is appropriate. Although clonazepam is not US Food and Drug Administration (FDA)-approved for multi-microcramps, it can be effective and safe, producing much less-pained, better-slept, grateful patients. Pharmacologically, clonazepam acts especially on integrated pentameric γ-aminobutyric acid (GABA)-gated chloride channels to facilitate GABA-mediated chloride conductance, causing hyperpolarization (inhibition of excitability) [6].

There seems to be a continuum of clinical manifestations encompassing microcramps, macrocramps, and fasciculations, all due to spontaneous firings from anywhere in the lower motor neuron: soma, axon–Schwann-cell complex, or distal axonal twigs. *Multi-microcramps* we consider to be caused by rather diffuse, repetitive firings of many distal axonal twigs, each activating a very few of its muscle fibers [6]. *Macrocramps* can involve somewhat larger regions of a muscle such as to produce i) a focal painful and tender "sausage," or ii) nearly an entire muscle such as the gastrocnemius or tibialis anterior. Cramps are caused by concurrent activation in the same muscle of a variable number of motor neurons, each activating most or all of its family of approximately 200 muscle fibers. *Fasciculations* probably involve spontaneous firing of only one, or a very few, motor neurons at a time, each activating some of its muscle fibers.

For the last 2 years, and especially the last 4 months, this 60-year-old man has had progressively painful tightness and "stiffness" in his calves, thighs, and arms. Upon awakening in the morning, he has increased muscle "tightness" and stiffness, and after 15–20 min and a prolonged hot shower he feels "looser" again. He now is having the painful tightness and stiffness after even slight exercise, and those symptoms are worse with more prolonged exercise. Frequently they are so painful that he has to limit his exercise. He obtains some relief by stretching his painful muscles for a few minutes. The frequent painful muscle symptoms make getting to sleep and staying asleep very difficult, resulting in a general painful sleep deprivation. He has no subjective or objective weakness and no numbness or tingling. In retrospect, from age 17 he often has

had mild muscle cramps after prolonged exercise. He has no thyroid disorder. There is no family history of any neuromuscular disease, or diabetes-2.

Examination: Examination reveals slight hyperreflexia diffusely (probably due to a pathologic *hyperexcitability* of his lower motor neurons). In *resistance testing*, muscle strength is normal.

Studies: *Voltage-gated K^+ channel antibodies* twice were negative (a test that might have identified a toxic antibody detectable in some similar patients). Also, anti-glutamic acid decarboxylase (GAD) antibodies (which are detected in some patients with "stiff-person syndrome") were negative. Thus his presumed pathologic antibody remains unidentified. Thyroid and parathyroid hormones were normal. Serum potassium, sodium, magnesium, and ionized calcium were normal. Lumbosacral and cervical spine magnatic resonance imaging (MRI) scans were unremarkable.

Nerve conductions showed mild–moderate dysschwannian neuropathy in the lower and upper limbs. The EMG showed frequent small-amplitude spontaneous bursts of motor-unit activity.

Treatment: Oral *Klonopin/clonazepam* has produced good to dramatic symptomatic relief from the painful muscle stiffness and cramps, achieving "70% improvement" according to the patient. This was obtained immediately by taking 1 mg at bedtime and 0.5 mg in the morning. These doses did not cause him any daytime sleepiness side effect. For putatively more definitive and rather rapid anti-dysimmune benefit, plasmaphereses (for hemodynamically stable patients) could be added, but the patient declined. Note: in general, the benefits from plasmaphereses are often very good but usually persist less than 1–2 weeks after the last pheresis. These hospital-based out-patient treatments are inconvenient, expensive, and can cumulatively damage veins. IVIG treatments can also benefit, but they also must be given repeatedly, because IVIG benefit begins to wane within 7–14 days after the last dose. Oral anti-dysimmune therapies that we have found beneficial are Imuran/azathioprine plus low-dose alternate-day prednisone, and previously used cautious and closely-monitored oral cyclophosphamide [8].

Comment: *Symptomatic treatments* are: (a) *omit* intake of all stimulants and (b) consider treating with low-dose clonazepam/Klonopin [6, 7]. (Note: *quinine* has been an effective treatment of muscle cramps for at least a century, but recently the FDA has more actively expressed concerns about possible significant side effects. We wonder whether such side effects have actually not been caused by the *low doses of quinine used for muscle cramps*, but rather from the 3–6-fold higher daily doses currently recommended for malaria.)

Multi-microcramps appears to be an autoimmune disorder, sometimes, but not always, caused by an identifiable toxic antibody against voltage-gated potassium channels that are located very distally twigs of the motor axon's pre-synaptic region, causing unstable, aberrant firing of those affected twigs. Antibody negativity, as in this patient, is certainly not an absolute contraindication for anti-dysimmune treatment, given that: (a) antibody positivity is basically a *quantitative testing* (it is conceivable that a *sub-threshold amount* of a toxic antibody could cause clinically evident damage; thus, absence of a *detectable* toxic antibody is not proof of absence of an *undetectable but still toxic amount of an antibody*) or (b) in some patients an abundent but still unknown type of antibody may be causative.

This group of patients can often be improved by repeated plasmaphereses or repeated IVIG infusions. While improvement with either of these treatments is essentially diagnostic of toxic circulating antibodies, with or without toxic cytokines, their benefits are only transient. More sustained improvement, sometimes accumulating dramatically, requires stopping production of those toxins from B-lymphocytes (±macrophages), such as was done very successfully with: (a) oral cyclophosphamide + oral prednisone + plasmaphereses, for a severely crippled similar patient who in 1990 we designated "syndrome of continuous motor-unit activity" [8] (and some have called neuromyotonia), and we demonstrated that her complex was an excellently treatable autoimmune disorder [8]; (b) oral Imuran/azathioprine (plus low-dose alternate-day prednisone to boost the circulating neutrophils); or (c) putatively rituximab. Other causes of general muscle "stiffness" include "*stiff-person syndrome*," which has more axial stiffness and is often associated with detectable toxic antibodies

against *GAD*. *Radiation plexopathy* can cause *focal* muscle stiffness and visible myokymia.

Vignette 9. Primary hyperparathyroidism

Neuromuscular symptoms of weakness, or even general symptoms of fatigue and tiredness, especially in older patients, should always raise the possibility of hyperparathyroidism. If a parathyroid adenoma (or adenomas) is identified by ultrasound or a sestamibi nuclear scan, or CT it can be easily surgically excised, typically resulting in excellent clinical benefit. The therapeutic possibility of surgically removing overly active parathyroid hormone (PTH)-producing cells that are not grouped into an easily detectable adenomatous lump is discussed in Chapter 2.

A 56-year-old woman has had, for 10 months, progressive weakness of her legs causing difficulty ascending stairs, and getting up off a bed, a chair, or the floor. She also has had some difficulty walking and has to make a conscious effort to lift her legs when walking on uneven surfaces. Although she used to be an enthusiastic jogger, she now can walk less than one block before her legs fatigue and she has to stop. She has also been feeling very fatigued generally, with an overall low level of energy. Endurance seems more diminished than brute strength. There are no sensory symptoms, and no cardiac or respiratory abnormalities; nor is there any abnormality of swallowing or speaking. She has passed three renal stones in the past 12 months.

Examination: She had bilateral moderate weakness of proximal leg muscles, e.g. hip flexion, extension and adduction, and knee extension. She also has had mild–moderate weakness of her deltoids, biceps, and triceps. Tendon reflexes were reduced throughout. Sensory exam was normal.

Studies: "Intact" PTH levels were persistently elevated, ranging from 86 to 102 pg/mL (normal is 14–72 pg/mL). Serum *total* and *ionized calcium values* were variably high, both ranging between high-normal and slightly above-normal. *Total calcium* was 10.5–11.2 mg/dL (normal 8.6–10.6 mg/dL), and *ionized calcium* being 1.31 and 1.34 mmol/L (normal is 1.12–1.32 mmol/L). CK was slightly high 441 IU/L (normal <397 IU/L). Thyroid tests were normal.

EMG did not detect recent denervation, and motor-unit action potentials were of normal size (note that routine EMG does not allow quantitation of the size of the later-activated type-2-fiber fast-twitch motor units, but only of the earlier-activated type-1-fiber slow-twitch motor units) [9]. Nerve conductions were normal. Muscle biopsy histochemistry showed moderate–prominent *type-2 fiber atrophy*, slight *recent denervation*, and slight– moderate *established reinnervation*.

Imaging: Although the soft-tissue sestamibi radionuclide scan of the neck seeking a PTH adenoma was negative, ultrasound revealed an *adenoma* in two of the four parathyroid glands (usually there is only one adenoma).

Surgical treatment: A surgeon removed *both* of the parathyroid adenomas during intraoperative real-time monitoring of the PTH levels in the individual outflow veins from the four parathyroid glands. The two adenoma-containing glands had a high output of PTH and were thereby precisely localized and excised. Within hours post-surgery, the patient evidenced the beginning of her cumulatively dramatic recovery, eventuating in complete relief of muscle fatigue and weakness, and dramatically improved walking. She now ascends stairs easily, can walk at least 5 miles a day, and has resumed her teaching job.

Comment: This highly treatable disorder can be easily overlooked, especially when the serum total and ionized calciums are not elevated, and/or the serum PTH is fluctuating between high normal and elevated. The *mechanism by which high PTH damages motor nerves and muscle fibers* is not known; speculatively, it could be by: (a) a hypothetical direct toxicity of PTH on the neuromuscular apparatus; (b) a *hypothetical autoantibody* having both agonist action on the parathyroid cells and detrimental action on neuromuscular function; or (c) increasing toxic circulating proinflammatory and cachectogenic cytokine network components, such as tumor necrosis factor α and interleukins-6, -5, and -8, perhaps impairing energy utilization of a motor-unit component.

Vignette 10. Multifocal motor neuropathy with conduction block - a pseudo-ALS

Multifocal motor neuropathy with conduction block can involve one or more limbs. It may or may not be associated with *IgM anti-GM1 antibody*. One should also look for other dysimmune abnormalities through immunofixation electropheresis, quantitative immunoglobulins, and testing for immune complexes, antinuclear factor, and rheumatoid factor. Response to IVIG treatment is often excellent or good and, more recently, the immunosuppressant rituximab has sometimes been successful.

A 62-year-old man has had, for 1 year, progressive asymmetric weakness of his right shoulder and hand, and of his left leg. He was unable to lift the right arm above shoulder level and had difficulty shaving. He also had difficulty holding objects in his right hand and was not able to pick up small objects, turn keys, or open jars. He had a slight limp in his left leg. For the last 6 months, he has observed occasional twitches (fasciculations) of muscles in his right arm and forearm, and in his left thigh and calf. He often is awakened at night by calf muscle cramps. He has no numbness or tingling, and no difficulty with balance, speech, or swallowing. He is quite anxious because he has been told he has "ALS" and less than 2 years to live. There is no family history of any neuromuscular disorder.

Examination: There are muscle fasciculations in the right arm and forearm, and left thigh and calf. The right arm and forearm muscles were moderate weak and atrophic. He has slight–moderate weakness of his right hand muscles. There is a slight proximal left lower-limb weakness and a left foot drop. All tendon reflexes were absent or prominently reduced. The plantar responses were flexor on the right and not applicable on the left due to toe weakness. Sensory examination and cranial nerves were normal.

Studies: *Serum IgM anti-GM1 antibody titers were elevated*. Serum blood counts, general chemistries, vitamin levels, and thyroid and parathyroid tests were normal. CSF protein was 68 mg/dL (normal up to 45 mg/dL). Nerve conductions showed an asymmetric dysschwannian motor polyneuropathy, with "conduction blocks" involving his upper more than his lower limbs. EMG showed, in the weak muscles, recent denervation and established reinnervation.

Treatment: IVIG infusions on two nonconsecutive days every week have been producing a cumulatively very good response, evidenced as moderate, and still incrementing, return of strength in his previously weakened muscles. After 6 months of IVIG he now considers that he is "nearly normal functionally." Because we estimate that he may still show further improvement we are continuing the IVIG treatments, and we are also considering phasing in rituximab, which initially would overlap with the IVIG program so as to not lose the IVIG benefit. This will require careful monitoring of absolute neutrophil counts and other safety parameters (see Chapter 2).

Comment: This patient's remarkable clinical improvement demonstrates that he is a very gratifying example of *"pseudo-ALS"* (see Chapter 2). Another example of *pseudo-ALS* is given in Vignette 21.

Vignette 11. Sensory-predominant dysimmune polyneuropathy

A nonhereditary "sensory polyneuropathy" affects sensory nerve fibers much more than motor nerve fibers. The sensory component can involve (a) large-diameter nerve fibers conveying position and vibration sense, and/or (b) small-diameter nerve fibers conveying pain and temperature sensations. It may be associated with a postural or action tremor, presumably due to lack of subconscious normal position-sense information caused by impaired large-diameter peripheral sensory nerves. This type of sensory polyneuropathy is often, as in this patient, associated with a presumably pathogenic immune abnormality manifest in a) the serum or urine as a *monoclonal band* (or of a free light-chain or a free heavy-chain), or a *polyclonal increase* of an immunoglobulin; or b) in the CSF as one or more oligoclonal bands.

A 60-year-old man has had, for 14 months, slowly progressive imbalance, especially in the dark and when closing his eyes during showering. He has suffered two severe falls going down stairs in his home. For the last 6 months, he also has been having severe pain, tingling, and numbness, initially, of his toes, which has now ascended to above his ankles. He has developed a moderate *intention tremor* of his fingers (probably a large-fiber sensation-deprivation tremor). He has no weakness when looking at the muscle he is attempting to contract, but with his eyes closed his effort fluctuates irregularly, presumably due to lack of peripheral-nerve positional-sense feedback. Family history is negative, and there is no diabetes in himself or his family.

Examination: Tandem gait is impossible, and the Romberg test is very positive. There is complete absence of vibratory sensation at the toes and ankles, and absent position sense in the toes. In his feet and lower half of the legs there is prominent hypersensitivity to pain stimuli (tested using a round toothpick), and decreased sensitivity to touch. Tendon reflexes are absent at the ankles and knees, and prominently reduced in the upper limbs. Plantar reflexes are unresponsive, presumably due to sensory loss in the soles.

Studies: Serum IgG was high, 2568 mg/dL (normal is 650–1650 mg/dL). By immunofixation electropheresis, the patient had an *IgG-kappa monoclonal band* (not to be dismissed as a "normal" aging phenomenon) and *free kappa light chains* in the urine). Serum complement C3 and C4 levels were low. CSF protein was elevated at 93 mg/dL (normal up to 45 mg/dL). Sensory nerves were totally unresponsive in the lower limbs, and in the upper limbs they manifested a prominent *dysschwannian sensory neuropathy*. Motor nerves had *slight–moderate dysschwannian abnormality* in the lower and upper limbs. EMG showed slight recent denervation and reinnervation in the lower limbs, and was normal in the upper limbs.

Biopsy of the clinically strong quadriceps showed slight–moderate *recent denervation* and moderate–prominent *established reinnervation*.

Treatment: IVIG (which can be a 10 or 5% solution of human IgG) was *not given* because the serum IgG was already too high; infusing more might make the blood too thick, increasing its viscosity, possibly predisposing to small-vessel occlusions. Because the patient was hemodynamically stable, a series of *plasmaphereses* was begun. The initial schedule was: week 1, phereses on Monday, Tuesday, Thursday, and Friday; week 2, phereses on Monday, Tuesday, and Thursday; week 3 and subsequently, two plasmaphereses on nonconsecutive days each week for 6 weeks, or longer as needed. He has had an excellent response, beginning very slightly within 24 h, and followed by a cumulatively very significant benefit. Improvement initially was of the numbness, paresthesias, and pain of his feet and legs, and then of his balance, and slight–moderate improvement of the intention tremor. Note that although benefit from repeated plasmaphereses is able to be summated, it is, nevertheless, evanescent: it begins to wane within about 1–2 weeks after the last pheresis. Accordingly, after the first 3 weeks of plasmaphereses this patient was started concurrently on long-term Imuran/azathioprine plus a low single-dose (10 mg) alternate-day prednisone, with careful monitoring especially of the absolute neutrophils (by weekly complete blood-cell count plus differential), and for 6 months monthly liver functions (including GGTP levels). He continued to show good improvement. After 3 months, the plasmaphereses were gradually less frequent and then stopped, while he was carefully watched for any clinical regression.

Comment: A patient's *IgG-kappa or other monoclonal band* should *not* be dismissed as "normal in aging;" it is an important dysimmune parameter that is *more common* in aging but is *not* normal. The likelihood that the monoclonal immunoglobulin is the *cause* of a patient's neuromuscular disorder is based on clinical judgment. Careful and prolonged treatment is usually needed to achieve summated improvement, and avoid the Sisyphus phenomenon (see Chapter 2).

Vignette 12. Treatable forms of "diabetic neuropathy": diabetes-2 dysimmune sensory-motor polyneuropathy, and genetico-diabetoid-2 dysimmune polyneuropathy

For many years, and even today, any neuropathy occurring in a diabetes-2 patient has, simplistically, incorrectly, and pessimistically often been called "untreatable diabetic neuropathy." However, our 1993 demonstration of the widely occurring and frequently *gratifyingly treatable diabetes-2 dysimmune polyneuropathy*, usually associated with *elevated CSF protein*, has led to our benefiting many patients dismissed by others. IVIG is especially beneficial

(and corticosteroid is generally contraindicated). *"Genetico-diabetoid-2 dysimmune polyneuropathy"* (GD2DP), our term, is defined in Chapter 2 [10–13]. Similarly, this is also often treatable.

For 10 months, a 68-year-old woman has had frequent falls, caused by tripping over her own feet or on small irregularities of the sidewalk, the ground, or rugs. Lately, she has been using a cane, but it provides less than adequate help with balance, leaving her in peril of falling. She has decreased sensation in both feet, especially the soles, combined with burning pain throughout her feet and lower legs. For 4 years she has had *diabetes-2*, treated with oral agents, and more recently with insulin. Her father and a maternal aunt also had diabetes-2.

Examination: The patient was somewhat obese, 82 kg, and 1.67 m tall. She had bilateral foot drop and weak toe extensors. She also had absent vibratory sense and position sense at her toes, and a gradient sensory loss distally to pinprick and touch in her feet and legs up to the mid-thighs. Tendon reflexes were absent in the lower limbs and only trace in the upper limbs. Plantar reflexes were unresponsive, probably due to the numbness of the soles and the extensor and flexor weakness of all her toes. Her hypertension was well-controlled with telmisartan, ramipril, and sotalol by her cardiologist.

Laboratory studies: CSF: *protein was high*, 116 mg/dL (upper normal is 45 mg/dL); glucose was high 95 mg/dL (upper-normal is 70 mg/dL); and there were two abnormal oligoclonal immunoglobulin bands. She had normal serum quantitative immunoglobulins and did not have a detectable monoclonal band. Nerve conductions showed severe dyschwannian sensory-motor neuropathy in the lower more than the upper limbs. EMG showed recent denervation and established reinnervation, especially in distal lower-limb muscles. Quadriceps biopsy showed both moderate recent denervation and established reinnervation.

Treatment: The patient was given IVIG, according to our most often used protocol, as the most likely, most rapidly beneficial, and safest treatment (see Chapter 2). Throughout, weight reduction was advised. The IVIG involved 0.4 g/kg/day on two nonconsecutive days every week, infusion rate not over

100 mL/h (and slower if her carefully monitored blood pressure rose during an infusion).

Within 1 week she began to show improvement, and at 1 month she had increased ability to move her feet, decreased pain in the feet, beginning return of sensation in her legs and soles, and descent of the level of sensory impairment of her lower limbs. (Glucocorticoid was contraindicated as it typically worsens diabetes.) Her improvement continued to increment over the next 8 months. She was responsive to, and dependent upon, her IVIG therapy as evidenced by her symptoms beginning to return if she omitted one or two IVIG doses. At some future point, we might attempt a very cautious reduction of the IVIG frequency, to a schedule of two and one infusions on alternate weeks, as needed to maintain her improvement; if she would begin to lose the IVIG benefits as a presumed Sisyphus phenomenon (Chapter 2), the twice-weekly IVIG schedule would have to be resumed in an attempt to restore the previously attained benefits. Adding another anti-dysimmune treatment is planned, using brand-name-Imuran/azathioprine (without prednisone) or rituximab, to try to diminish her dependence on IVIG.

Comment: In suspected *diabetic-2 dysimmune polyneuropathy* and in *genetico-diabetoid-2 dysimmune polyneuropathy* patients, CSF exam is important; in general, the *more elevated the CSF protein, the more likely the neuropathic process is dysimmune* (if CNS infection is not a consideration), and the more likely the neuropathic process will respond to IVIG treatment. In both conditions, careful and prolonged treatment is typically needed to achieve summated and sustained improvement, and to avoid the Sisyphus phenomenon. However, *IVIG*, as excellent as it is, being *the best and safest anti-dysimmune treatment*, it does have some logistic encumbrances and certainly needs molecular improvement as a therapeutic agent (see Chapter 2). Note: a *basically Schwann cell disorder* causes motor or sensory symptoms only by *secondarily impairing* the function and, more severely, the cellular architecture of *the encased and nurtured motor or sensory axons*. Thus a *Schwann cell disorder can evolve* to have *concurrent nerve-conduction aspects of a dysneuronal neuropathy* (see Chapter 2).

Vignette 13. Subacute sensorimotor neuropathy, paraneoplastic

For the cause of a subacute sensorimotor neuropathy in an elderly patient, one should consider a possible dysimmune effect of a "*remote paraneoplastic syndrome*." This is commonly associated with small-cell lung carcinoma and anti-Hu antibody positivity in the serum. Other cancers frequently associated with this mechanism are of breast and ovary. As in Vignette 1, treatment of a remote paraneoplastic neuropathy is 2-fold: (a) attacking by radiation, chemotherapy, or surgical excision the presumably provoking neoplasm; and (b) anti-dysimmune treatment, such as IVIG or another treatment, which can be given concurrently with (a). If the (a) approach is technically but not therapeutically successful, that suggests the putative toxic mechanism had become autonomous. If (b) is not beneficial, that suggests the tumor may have directly or indirectly instigated production of circulating nonimmunologic toxic molecules, such as detrimental cytokines.

A 76-year-old former heavy smoker has had 5 months of insidiously increasing burning pains in his feet and lower legs. These are worse at night and severely interfere with sleep, especially on days when he has been standing or walking longer than usual. He also has occasional shooting pains in the feet. He has imbalance when walking, and has had several falls. In one of them he broke his wrist, and in another he had a scalp injury and mild concussion. He also has had, for 3 months, mild weakness of his legs and difficulty keeping his sandals on while walking. He has no difficulty swallowing or speaking. He has had a chronic dry cough for the last 6 years, which has not been investigated. There is no diabetes in himself or his family.

Examination: The patient has absent vibration and position sense at the toes and fingers. In his feet and lower legs there is prominent *hypersensitivity* to light pinprick, which is excessively *painful*. There is moderate weakness of extension and flexion of all toes. All *tendon reflexes* were *absent*. Plantar reflexes were not interpretable, probably because of weakness of the toes and sensory loss in the soles. There is a moderate *intention tremor* of the fingers, probably due to the severely impaired position sense. Tandem gait and the Romberg test were impossible due to his *severe imbalance*.

Studies: Serum *anti-neuronal (anti-Hu) antibody was highly positive*. General blood count, chemistry, and other autoimmune parameters were normal. Serum vitamin levels were normal.

Sensory-nerve conduction responses were unelicitable in the lower limbs, while in the upper limbs they showed moderate dysschwannian plus dysneuronal neuropathy (see Vignette 12). EMG showed slight recent denervation and slight reinnervation. Quadriceps muscle biopsy showed slight–moderate recent denervation and moderate reinnervation. CSF protein was elevated at 61 mg/dL (normal up to 45 mg/dL). Chest X-ray showed hilar lymphadenopathy, and a small lesion in the left lower lung field, biopsy of which disclosed a *small-cell carcinoma*.

Treatment: The carcinoma was excised, and radiation and chemotherapy started. (Note: *certain forms of anticancer chemotherapy can themselves produce a toxic neuropathy*, which complicates interpretation of any worsening of the patient's neuropathy.) For the probable dysimmune component of this neuropathy, the patient was also started on *IVIG* 0.4 g/kg/day, on two nonconsecutive days every week. He showed some improvement, but we do not know which treatment, or treatments, should receive the credit, because *some anticancer treatments* are also *anti-dysimmune*.

Comment: The *paraneoplastic pathogenic mechanism* is probably at least partially dysimmune, although toxic cyokines and other molecules produced by, or provoked by, the tumor cells might also be playing a role. The lack of an excellent benefit from IVIG for this patient suggests that possibly: (a) the nerves had suffered a certain amount of totally irreversible damage, (b) his dysimmune pathogenesis is unusually unresponsive, or (c) the dysimmune component was not the only operative neurotoxic mechanism.

Vignette 14. Remarkable "triple benefits" of IVIG: anti-dysimmune, antiviral, and antibacterial

IVIG has a well-recognized *anti-dysimmune action*, and much less known anti-infection properties, namely *antiviral and antibacterial benefits*. Virtually all of our >300 patients who have received repeating dosings of IVIG for a dysimmune disorder state that they "never" contract the local community viruses that infect family, friends, and coworkers. Accordingly, *IVIG's triple benefit* might be an excellent treatment, perhaps life-saving: a) for *moderate or severe cases of an epidemic or pre-pandemic flu*, especially patients who are unresponsive to "specific" antivirals; and b) for *other bacterially or virally infected patients* not responding to standard therapy.

Ten years ago, a 63-year-old physician colleague had returned from a tourist visit to China with a pulmonary infection. In our hospital, it did not respond to various oral and intravenous antimicrobial treatments, given as an in-patient. Because the diagnostic bacterial cultures were negative, the cause of the infection was suspected to be viral. During those treatment failures, his parenchymal pneumonopathy continued to worsen, progressing to ventilator-dependence in the intensive care unit (at which time he also had developed a complicating bacterial pneumonia and septisemia). By the time we were called to see him, the patient had also developed a prominent progressive peripheral neuropathy causing severe weakness in all four limbs and probably contributed to the respiratory insufficiency. *He seemed near death*.

For a possible dysimmune cause of the neuropathy, one of us (W.K.E.) started IVIG, 0.4 g/kg/day on five consecutive days. Then a series of three infusions per week were repeated for 3 weeks, and subsequently twice weekly. The IVIG greatly benefited the neuropathy as hoped for, and *the previously untreatable lung infection and septisemia were unexpectedly cured*. After 3 months, the patient was off IVIG, and by 6 months was playing singles in tennis (when his colleagues prefered to play doubles).

Comment: This patient demonstrates that we can learn *new, potentially important therapeutic information* from chance occurrences—in this case regarding the combined anti-dysimmune, antiviral, and antibacterial triple benefits of IVIG.

Also in that theme, we should remember that the cumulatively dramatic, and apparently enduring, benefit of *interferon-α2A* in a *fever-responsive dysimmune neuropathy* patient (see Chapter 2) may be due to both the known anti-dysimmune and the known antiviral (e.g., anti-hepatitis C virus) benefits of interferon. That combined information has led to our suggesting that in *all anti-dysimmune treatments perhaps one should consider concurrent antiviral therapy* (see Chapter 2) [14], especially if there is a *serum elevated specific antiviral IgM antibody titer* suggesting an ongoing or recent infection with that virus— however, identification of an elevated IgM anti-viral titer does not need to be an absolute requirement.

Vignette 15. A treatable late-onset dysimmune polyneuropathy superimposed on mild hereditary motor-sensory polyneuropathy (pseudo late-progressive CMT")

An hereditary sensory-motor polyneuropathy, sometimes loosely called Charcot-Marie-Tooth (CMT) syndrome, only rarely first presents in the older population. An exception is some forms of hereditary amyloid neuropathy (see above, and Vignette 17). In developed nations, neuropathies beginning in the elderly are usually: dysimmune (including diabetic-2 and genetico-diabetoid-2 dysimmune neuropathies); other neuropathies associated with diabetes-2; and toxicities from drugs and from the environment. This patient's lifelong high-arched feet and difficulty getting a good fit of shoes (both abnormalities also present in her father, paternal uncle, and paternal grandfather) had provoked, prior to our seeing her, a diagnosis of "untreatable late progressive CMT disease" for her late-onset prominent neuropathic worsening. However, we considered a newer, potentially treatable, dysimmune neuropathy in this patient because her CSF protein was 146 mg/dL, with normal cell count. That possibility was confirmed because our treatment with IVIG has been providing sustained, cumulative benefit. Interruption of the IVIG schedule due to personal obligations caused transient worsening, which reversed 2 weeks after the twice-weekly IVIG schedule was resumed.

A now-86-year-old woman presented to us 7 years ago. She had, beginning at age 66, progressive spontaneous pain in the feet and lower legs, and dysthetic sensations in her soles. Initially she noted a "leathery"-feeling sensation when walking bare-foot, combined with a constant burning sensation, and sometimes feeling like she was walking on broken glass. She would sometimes injure her feet without realizing it, resulting in bruises and cuts. The pains persisted and increased, and were requiring maximal Vicodin medication three times daily to try to diminish them, along with locally supervised nightly quinine to counteract the muscle cramps. At night her feet pain was increased, and painful calf cramps also occurred every night. These caused great difficulty getting to sleep and awakened her from sleep, resulting in *"painful insomnia."* She would *soak her feet in ice water* every evening to temporarily diminish the pain. (Note: we have had at least six other patients, all women, with painful neuropathy who found that ice water or iceing the feet provided some definite but transient relief of their pain.) This patient also had a slight amount of similar pain in her hands. When walking, it was difficult for her to quickly change direction. She has had "weak ankles" and "high arches" from childhood (as did her father, paternal uncle, and paternal grandfather). She was never athletic, would often sprain her ankle, and frequently would have muscle cramps while trying to exercise. There has not been any subjective proximal muscle weakness. She was erroneously told recently she was having "accelerated progression of her CMT" and that there was no treatment. Her father and his brother and sister have diabetes-2, and are being treated with oral agents.

Examination: She has prominent distal sensory loss to touch and pinprick in her feet and lower legs, absent vibratory and position sense in the toes, and some numbness in all the fingers up to the mid-palms. Tendon reflexes were absent throughout. Her feet are floppy at the ankles, and her arches are very high (pes cavus). There is prominent extension and flexion weakness of all the toes and extension weakness at the ankles. Both plantar reflexes are nonresponsive, presumably due to the toe weakness and the sensory loss in the soles. Rapid alternating hand-patting was irregular, probably due to large-diameter sensory nerve fiber impairment.

Studies: Blood glucose, hemoglobin A1c, and dysimmune markers were normal. CSF protein was prominently elevated at 146 mg/dL, with a normal cell count. Sensory and motor nerve conductions were unobtainable in the lower limbs and showed a prominent dysschwannian-plus-dysneuronal sensory neuropathy in both upper limbs. EMG showed slight–moderate recent denervation and moderate–prominent established reinnervation distally in the lower more than upper limbs.

Quadriceps muscle biopsy histochemistry showed moderate recent denervation and prominent established reinnervation. No amyloid was seen by crystal violet staining or with the Askanas Congo red fluorescence (see Chapter 7).

Treatment: Seven years ago we began treatment with IVIG, 0.4 g/kg/day on two nonconsecutive days every week. Initially, improvement became subjectively evident after 2 weeks of IVIG treatment, and the benefits gradually summated. The improvements included elimination of the constant peripheral neuropathic pain, the need to nightly soak her feet in a bucket of ice water, and the nightly muscle cramps (she was able to omit the nightly quinine dosings); and cumulatively much better balance and somewhat better strength, giving her greater security when walking and descending and climbing stairs.

This patient is *very dependent on IVIG treatments*. For example, if due to her personal schedule she has to omit IVIG, the first week is OK; during a second week off IVIG the increased feet pain necessitates one daily Vicodin; and during a third week off she had definitely less energy, and walking and ascending stairs "became very difficult," and descending became "very scary". The resurgent feet pain was "terrible," requiring ice-water soakings nightly, resumption of an evening dose of quinine for cramps, and three doses of daily Vicodin. After resumption of her IVIG treatments, during the first week she was slightly better and by the end of the second IVIG week she was nearly back to her best pre-omission status, which was achieved after the third week of IVIG resumption.

Comment: This patient has a sensory neuropathy (small- and large-fiber), plus a motor neuropathy. In general, if there is significant worsening over age 40 of a chronic, presumably genetic neuropathic process that had been present from childhood, one should look for a recent additional pathogenesis, such as dysimmune, that might be treatable, as exemplified in this patient. She also exemplifies an *excellent*

response to IVIG and a dependence upon it. Note: *all basically dysschwannian neuropathies cause symptoms only by secondarily impairing function of their encased and nurtured sensory and motor neuron axonal extensions.* If the dysschwannian process is severe and/or chronic, a *secondary dysneuronal aspect* will be induced and be evident by nerve-conduction studies and nerve morphology.

Vignette 16. Chronic sensorimotor neuropathy and myelopathy, caused by vitamin B$_{12}$ insufficiency or deficiency

Chronic sensorimotor neuropathy can result from vitamin B$_{12}$ (cobalamin) deficiency, and can easily be treated by subcutaneous B$_{12}$ injections (using insulin syringes with #31 needles). B$_{12}$ deficiency or insufficiency can also cause myelopathy and cerebral involvement.

A 71 year-old man has had, for 1 year, progressively worsening numbness of his feet and legs, gradually ascending up to the mid-thighs. He also had intermittent, sudden electrical-shock-like sensations in his feet. He feels stiffness when walking, and has greater difficulty lifting his feet to ascend curbs and stairs. He stumbles on irregularities of the sidewalk or the ground. He frequently loses his balance, and has fallen a few times while walking and stepping up or down the curb. He has difficulty with balance in darkness or with his eyes closed. He recently developed some difficulty with recent memory. There is no abnormality of swallowing or speaking.

Examination: He is thin but not definitely undernourished. He has increased muscle tone at the knees and slowness of walking, but he has normal power to resist the examiner's force. Sensory examination shows: absent vibratory sense and position sense at his toes and ankles, and a moderately prominently decreased sensitivity to touch and pinprick in his feet and legs up to mid-thighs. Romberg test is positive. Tendon reflexes were increased at the knees and absent at the ankles. Plantar reflexes are extensor bilaterally.

Studies: There was not a macrocytic anemia, but it is known that the *folic acid supplementation* that he, and many other persons, take in multivitamins and other supplements can *mask* the macrocytosis indicator of a B_{12} deficiency (see Comment below). In this patient, the serum vitamin B_{12} level was low, 150 pg/mL (normal is 225–1000 pg/mL), and the *folic acid level was moderately elevated*. Serum *anti-parietal-cell antibody* and *anti-intrinsic factor antibody* were very high, and methylmalonic acid was elevated.

Nerve conductions showed a combined dysschwannian and dysneuronal sensorimotor polyneuropathy in the lower more than the upper limbs. EMG in the lower limbs distally showed slight–moderate recent denervation and slight established reinnervation. Quadriceps muscle biopsy showed slight–moderate recent denervation and reinnervation.

Treatment: We began high-dose vitamin B_{12} (cyanocobalamin), 1000 µg, self-injected (or spouse-injected) subcutaneously once daily, in alternate anterior thighs, using disposable insulin syringes with #31 needles (methylcobalamin can also be used). (Our impression is that, compared to the old-fashioned method of once-monthly B_{12} injections with a larger needle in a buttock muscle, this subcutaneous method is much simpler, less painful, does not require a visit to a physician's office, and probably is more effective.) This patient was also continued on oral folic acid (1 mg twice daily). In general, after 4–12 weeks of daily B_{12} injections, if the benefit is estimated to be maximal, the frequency might be reduced, for example, to about one to three times weekly, depending on the clinical status, as was done in this patient after 12 weeks. The benefit was as follows. Within 1 week after starting B_{12} injections this patient had less fatigue and more energy. By about 3–6 weeks, he noted gradual return of sensation in his thighs and upper legs, and slightly in his feet. Balance also began to improve, as did his walking, and memory. By about 8 weeks of treatment, the electrical-shock sensations were gone from his feet and his other sensory symptoms were further improved. Note: we have been using high-dose, initially daily subcutaneous B_{12} for 25 years and not noted any related side effects.

Comment: The normal *gastric parietal cells* secrete into the stomach lumen the intrinsic factor necessary for B_{12} absorption farther down in the terminal ileum. The normal liver reportedly stores a 3–6-year supply of B_{12}. The typical cause of B_{12} deficiency is *autoimmune inactivation* of those parietal cells or their intrinsic factor (often associated with positive serum antibodies against parietal cells and/or intrinsic factor). Anti-dysimmune treatment is not useful because by the time a patient has the neurologic abnormalities the parietal-cell function had been completely destroyed 3–6 years before. Importantly, it is known that the *folic acid supplementation* he, and many other persons, are taking in multivitamins and other supplements can mask a B_{12} deficiency – and probably a B_{12} insufficiency – by correcting the hematologic *macrocytosis of pernicious anemia* (typical in ordinary B_{12} deficiency) while not stopping the progressive *neurologic aspects* of B_{12} deficiency. This is a concern because folic acid is found in most multivitamins and is added to a number of foods. Not related to this patient, it is known that B_{12} deficiency can result from Crohn's disease, or other gastrointestinal disorders, and especially if there was surgical removal of some of the upper gastro-intestinal tract. Note: regarding another aspect, one should remember that (a) the blood red cell mean corpuscular volume (MCV) is raised by certain anti-dysimmune and anticancer chemotherapies, such as azathioprine and cyclophosphamide, and (b) that macrocytosis can persist, despite B_{12} and folic acid treatment, for years after chemotherapy is discontinued.

Vignette 17. Amyloid neuropathy, dysimmune, due to B-lymphocyte dyscrasia

Nonhereditary amyloid neuropathy usually presents as a painful sensory neuropathy, often with some autonomic dysfunction. It usually begins in elderly or mid-age patients, but sometimes in younger adults. It is typically due to a B-lymphocyte overproduction of the variable region of an immunoglobulin light-chain. While this can occur with multiple myeloma, none of our nonhereditary amyloid patients has had myeloma detectable by bone marrow, bone X-ray survey, or radionuclide scanning. A radionuclide scan with 99mTc sestamibi scintigraphy (done technically like a bone scan but focused on the soft tissues of the limbs and heart) can demonstrate, in muscle such as in the thighs, amyloid-based uptake that tends to obscure the bone image [15]. Amyloid in the heart can also be imaged in this non-invasive way. Definitive diagnosis of amyloidosis is made by muscle biopsy histochemistry. There is no established treatment for removing the aggregated amyloid, but anti-B-lymphocyte measures can be tried to stop production of the putatively toxic pre-amyloid immunoglobulin fragments. If production of pre-amyloid fragments could be stopped, aggregated tissue amyloid can be slowly catabolized by macrophages and circulating proteinases. Symptomatically, control of pain, hyponutrition, orthostatic hypotension, cardiac insufficiency, and any other aspects deserves attention.

A 65-year-old man for 2 years has been having increasingly severe, nearly constant pains in his feet and lower legs, causing him to frequently remove his socks and rub those areas, which were also moderately numb to the touch. He had similar, but not as severe, pains and numbness in his hands, with accentuation in the median nerve/carpal tunnel distribution. For the last 8 months he has been having difficulty with balance and walking, especially in the dark. He has an intention tremor of his hands (probably due to peripheral nerve sensory deprivation), and impaired fine movements of his fingers. He also reports urinary overflow incontinence, diarrhea, and impotence. He has exercise intolerance associated with weakness, pain, imbalance, and cardiac difficulty. He feels unusually hot during the summer. He has a feeling of generalized muscle weakness. His voice is slightly hoarse. He is somewhat short of breath during exertion. His appetite is decreased and he has involuntarily lost 9 kg. There is no family history of neuromuscular disease.

Examination: His recent weight loss is evident. He is 1.82 m tall and his 2.4 L maximal vital capacity (per our commercial hand-held respirometer) is moderately reduced. He is unable to tandem walk, and the Romberg test is positive. Sensory examination reveals prominent hypersensitivity to pinprick testing, distal to his knees and on the dorsum of his hands. He also has absent vibration and position sense in the toes and absent vibration at the ankles. There is moderate loss of touch sense of the toes, feet, and lower legs; and there are similar but less prominent abnormalities in the hands and forearms. The patient is hoarse, and the other cranial nerves are normal. Strength is slightly reduced generally, but

he can perform somewhat better when looking at the regions being tested, attributable to his position-sense impairment. There is moderate weakness of flexion and extension of the toes and ankles. Tendon reflexes are absent at the ankles and knees, and much reduced in the upper limbs. Plantar reflexes are unresponsive, probably due to the sensory loss of the soles and partly to first-toe weakness.

Laboratory testing: There is a serum IgG-lambda monoclonal band, and free lambda light chains are in the blood and urine. CSF protein is slightly elevated, 67 mg/dL. Search for myeloma was negative. Sensory nerve conductions were unobtainable in the lower limbs and showed a mixed dysschwannian-dysneuronal neuropathy in the upper limbs. Motor nerve conductions were slightly decreased. EMG revealed slight–moderate denervation and established reinnervation in distal limb muscles. Quadriceps biopsy showed slight recent denervation and established reinnervation. *Extracellular amyloid deposits*, identified by crystal violet and the Askanas fluorescent Congo red stainings (see Chapter 10), were found in the connective tissue septae and walls of some blood vessels, but not inside the muscle fibers.

Treatment: There is no treatment for removing established amyloid. In this type of B-cell dyscrasic amyloidosis anti-B-treatment should be considered (*v.s.*).

Comment: See also the section on Amyloidoses in Chapter 2.

Vignette 18. Amyloid neuropathy, hereditary, due to transthyretin mutation

An hereditary amyloid neuropathy should also be considered in an older patient with a sensory greater than motor polyneuropathy, especially if there is also cardiac involvement (e.g., cardiomyopathy) and/or autonomic dysfunction. There could be an autosomal dominant genetic pattern of similarly affected persons—e.g., if the amyloid is caused by the TTR-Met30 mutation of *transthyretin (TTR)*, that is easily tested for. As with other sensory more than motor polyneuropathies, all treatable causes such as dysimmune, anti-MAG, and diabetes-2, should be sought. A soft-tissue radionuclide scan, which we introduced many years ago [15], can be very helpful in detecting familial and sporadic systemic amyloid in the heart, and to some extent in limb muscles (see Vignette 17 on sporadic amyloid neuropathy). For TTR-mutant amyloidosis, liver transplant is sometimes used to remove the organ (liver) where the cytotoxic mutant transthyretin is being synthesized.

A 62-year-old man has had, for the last 3 years, pain, numbness, and tingling in his feet that progressively ascended to his mid-thighs, and is now appearing in his fingers and hands. He also has muscle cramps, predominantly in his legs, but also involving his hands. He has noted muscle atrophy and weakness of his distal and proximal muscles, in the lower limbs more than upper limbs. He has difficulty walking, imbalance, and difficulty raising his arms overhead. For the last 6–7 months he has had some difficulty swallowing. He has been having very troublesome episodes of diarrhea and constipation, and impotence.

His blood pressure fluctuates, causing orthostatic hypotension. A severe syncopal episode 2 years ago necessitated a cardiac pacemaker implant, at which time he was also found to have *infiltrative cardiomyopathy*, a known concomitant of mutant-TTR amyloidosis. Heart transplant has been considered.

His father and two brothers, and two of their daughters, have similar clinical features, and, like the patient, have the same TTR-Met30 mutation. This mutation is commonly associated with an *autosomal dominant amyloid polyneuropathy*.

Examination: This revealed a distal sensory loss to pinprick and touch in his feet and hands, with a very dysthetic, painful quality of the pin stimulus. He also has absent vibration and position sense loss at his toes and ankles. There is moderate distal weakness in his lower and upper limbs, and slight–moderate proximal weakness. Tendon reflexes are absent throughout. Plantar reflexes are unresponsive, probably due to the numbness of his soles.

Laboratory studies: The patient has a slight normocytic anemia. Sestamibi nucleotide imaging disclosed abnormal uptake in muscle tissue of the thighs, and the heart. Nerve-conduction studies show a sensory-motor mixed dysneuronal dysschwannian polyneuropathy. EMG showed in distal

muscles slight–moderate recent denervation and moderate established reinnervation. Quadriceps muscle biopsy showed prominent recent denervation and established reinnervation. Crystal violet and the Askanas fluorescent Congo red stain (see Chapter 10) showed positive extracellular β-pleated-sheet amyloid staining, located exterior to the muscle fibers. It was in connective tissue regions, especially the perimysium, and in the walls of a few medium-sized blood vessels.

Treatment: Because diflunisal/Dolobid was proposed by others as possibly able to prevent and remove deposited transthyretin amyloid, we have given that to him for 6 months, but during this time his symptoms slightly progressed. The patient is considering a liver transplant, like his brother had. Transplantation has significant risks but has been shown to benefit some mutant-TTR patients. Also some patients with cardiac amyloidosis can benefit from a heart transplant.

Comment: The rationale for liver transplantation is as follows. The mutant-TTR, which is presumably toxic to molecular components of peripheral nerve and various other tissues, is, like many other proteins, synthesized in the liver. Removal of the factory producing that mutant toxin should stop accumulation of mutant-TTR pre-amyloid and amyloid. If the amyloid production and deposition can be stopped, there is experimental evidence in animals indicating that macrophages and tissue proteases can gradually remove abnormal amyloid fibrils, and also the presumably toxic pre-amyloid monomers and oligomers; that removal might be is a slow process. (Note that we think that the amyloid-associated molecular cytotoxicity affecting peripheral nerves is due to the "invisible," (even with the electron microscope.) monomers or oligomers of the mutant-TTR; see Chapter 2 [16].)

Vignette 19. Carpal-tunnel median-nerve, and forearm ulnar-nerve, pressure neuropathies: somewhat common in aged persons and often very treatable

Carpal tunnel syndrome is a common focal nerve constriction-pressure problem that is often overlooked and frequently able to be well treated. It is caused by compression of the median nerve within the carpal tunnel at the wrist. Carpal tunnel syndrome can be diagnosed by clinical findings and confirmed by the presence of electrical conduction block or focally decreased median nerve-conduction velocities across the wrist, while being normal elsewhere along the nerve. Patients are predisposed by obesity, diabetes, various general neuropathies, cervical radiculopathies, arthritic change in the carpal bones of the wrist, or if the wrist is extended repeatedly from physical activity. Treatment can be (a) conservative, by using a splint to hold the wrist slightly flexed or (b) surgical, by freeing the nerve in the carpal tunnel. Numbness, tingling and pain occur in the medial third of the palm, and in the ventral aspect of the fifth and medial side of the fourth finger. One should distinguish carpal tunnel abnormality from cervical radiculopathies, including "ponderous purse disease," which also can cause hand symptoms and signs, and early aspects of a general disorder such as a peripheral neuropathy.

Ulnar pressure neuropathy is a much less common disorder. It is often caused by unrecognized pressure on the mid-forearm, such as by the edge of a hard table pressing on the nonwriting forearm during handwriting a manuscript (less often done nowadays), or the arm over the back of a hard chair, or pressure on the ulnar groove at the elbow. The treatment of ulnar pressure neuropathy is to recognize and prevent the provoking pressure. Sometimes in an early general peripheral neuropathy or ALS, simple ulnar-pressure neuropathy is mistakenly diagnosed, resulting in ineffective ulnar-nerve transposition surgery.

A 63-year-old moderately obese secretary has had, for 2 years, bilateral intermittent numbness and tingling in her thumb, index and middle fingers, and lateral 2/3rds of the palms. Her symptoms were worse under several circumstances – at work, activities involving considerable typing; while driving with her hands up on the steering wheel; and upon awakening in the morning. These positions involve the wrists being in the extension position. The symptoms have progressed from being intermittent and relieved in a few minutes by keeping the wrists flexed, to a constant sensation of discomforting paresthesias in her fingers and sharp stabbing pain at her wrists that prevented her from working. She now also has difficulty opening jars and cutting food with a knife, and she has noticed small twitches (fasciculations) in her thenar muscles. She tried wearing splints at night to keep her wrists flexed, but found them too annoying. She has no neck pain and no symptoms in the other parts of her arms, nor in her lower limbs.

Examination: She is moderately obese, 90 kg, and has osteoarthritis affecting the wrists. There is decreased sensitivity to pinprick and touch in the median nerve distribution of both hands, i.e., the lateral half of the palm and the ventral thumb, and index and middle fingers. Tinel's and Phalen's are positive. There is moderate weakness of the opponens and flexor muscles of the both thumbs. There was no weakness proximal to the wrists or in the lower limbs. Tendon reflexes were normal, plantar reflexes were flexor.

Studies: Blood chemistries including thyroid and parathyroid tests are normal. Nerve conductions showed severe bilateral dysschwannian neuropathy of the median nerves, with prominent conduction block across both wrists. Nerve conductions across the elbow and elsewhere were normal. EMG showed, in both hands, slight–moderate recent denervation in the opponens pollicis and abductor pollicis brevis. Nerve conductions and EMG in the lower limbs were normal.

Treatment: The patient had separate bilateral carpal tunnel release surgeries. She rapidly had significant improvement during the following few weeks, and she was able to return to work.

Comment: For therapeutic purposes, it is important to distinguish between a focal mechanical neuropathy and a generalized neuropathy, or the coexistence of both. One should consider various peripheral neuropathies (such as potentially treatable dysimmune diabetes-dysimmune and B_{12} insufficiency neuropathies), because even subtle ones probably can predispose to mechanical neuropathies of the median and ulnar nerves, as well as to cervical and lumbosacral radiculopathies from mechanical "spondylotic" changes.

Vignette 20. Sporadic ALS

The diagnosis of typical sporadic ALS (sALS) is based on several diagnostic criteria, including clinical and electrophysiological evidence of upper and lower motor neuron degeneration, in the bulbar and multiple spinal regions. Unfortunately, ALS still carries a dismal prognosis: the survival rate is $\leq$ 3–5 years after onset, with only rare exceptions. sALS accounts for about 90% of all ALS patients. Of the 10% hereditary cases of ALS (hALS), about 20% are due to a mutation of the autosomal-dominant *SOD1* gene. Other mutated genes associated with hALS are *TDP-43*, *FUS* [17], and most recently the gene C9ORF72 [22] (see Chapter 2). The last gene may be related to some patients with hALS and sALS, and it raises the question of defective RNA metabolism, as previously suspected [23]. Although there is no definitive treatment for sALS or hALS, enthusiastic and aggressive supportive management is crucial and can positively affect quality of life for the patients, families, and caregivers. These measures include percutaneous endoscopic gastrostomy feeding tube placement for nutrition, respiratory support, speech synthesizer, a communication "speakeasy," a saliva-drying agent, and active and passive physical therapy, as tolerated. A possibly treatable aspect of "pseudo-ALS" should be considered in each patient.

A 54-year-old executive has had for 3 months intermittent difficulty swallowing food and saliva, especially meat and large boluses—he has to wash them down with water. His speech has become slower, spastic, and somewhat nasal, and his left upper arm and forearm have become weaker and thinner over the same period. He has also noticed "twitches" in both arms and one thigh at rest, and the twitches are transiently increased after exercise. Walking is more difficult, and his legs feels "stiffer;" sometimes they have an involuntary spasm, and they fatigue more easily than a year ago. He has no sensory symptoms. General medical history is unremarkable.

Examination: The patient has moderate atrophy of the left upper arm and forearm, and slight atrophy on the right. Fasciculations are evident in all four limbs. He has mild–moderate weakness of both biceps, and left triceps, and both wrist flexors and extensors. The lower limbs are strong to manual testing. He has some face and tongue weakness, and there is atrophy and spontaneous small ripplings of the tongue. Jaw-jerk and Chvostek responses are abnormally brisk. Tendon reflexes are very brisk in all limbs, with sustained clonus at the left ankle. The left and right plantar reflexes are flexor. Sensory and cerebellar examinations are normal.

Studies: Blood chemistry, vitamin levels, and immune parameters are normal. CSF protein is slightly elevated, 75 mg/dL, suggesting impaired blood-CSF barrier. Nerve conductions were normal. EMG of muscles in three limbs diffusely showed prominent recent denervation (fibrillations, positive waves) and slight–moderate established reinnervation (enlarged, polyphasic motor units on slight voluntary contraction); and there were fibrillations in thoracic paraspinal muscles. Muscle-biopsy histochemistry of the clinically normal quadriceps showed prominent recent denervation (small angular atrophic muscle fibers) and slight established reinnervation (type-grouping).

Comment: See Chapter 2 for more information about ALS. In general, the more elevated the CSF protein, the more likely there is a dysimmune mechanism, but exceptions do occur. Sometimes in ALS the plantar response is inexplicably flexor (normal) even when there is generalized hyperreflexia.

Vignette 21. A remarkably treatable man-in-a-barrel syndrome: one type of treatable "pseudo-ALS"

We designate as having "pseudo-ALS," which is a general category, the diagnostically difficult patients who have major features of typically fatal ALS, but also have a discoverable different condition, sometimes one that can be treated. Pseudo-ALS patients are a heterogeneous group, and can present clinically with both upper and lower motor neuron signs, or only lower or upper motor neuron signs. Examples are: fasciculating motor>>sensory neuropathy; coexisting peripheral motor neuropathy and spondylotic cervical myelopathy, and coexisting MG and cervical spondylotic myelopathy; motor neuropathy with conduction block; and multimicrocramps (see Chapter 2). One should be aware of such possibilities, and others, and do an intensive work-up to ensure that (a) no treatable aspect is overlooked, and (b) no patient is incorrectly given a fatal prognosis. If we are uncertain, we try a putatively appropriate treatment. When we first met the patient described below, he had "hanging arms," strong legs, and no abnormality above the neck [18]. This clinical phenotype has been called "man in a barrel" by others and often given the grim prognosis typical of the lower motor-neuron form of ALS [19]. But to the contrary, our patient demonstrates that treatment of this clinical manifestation can sometimes have a cumulative and sustained excellent clinical result.

A now 57-year-old man had developed over a 19-year period, from age 24, progressive weakness and muscle atrophy causing inability to raise either arm, especially his right arm, more than 15 degrees away from his side. Early on, he also became unable to grip a glass of water, and his handwriting considerably worsened. He reported occasional twitches (fasciculations) in both arms, especially after attempting moderately vigorous use of them. The twitches also were more frequent after caffeinated or alcoholic beverages. He has no weakness of the legs, no sensory symptoms, and no difficulty with speech or swallowing. There was no significant general medical history, and no family history of neuromuscular disease or diabetes.

Examination: He has prominent weakness and atrophy of the right deltoid, biceps, triceps, and finger-extensor muscles; and moderate–prominent weakness of the same muscles on the left. Occasional fasciculations were evident in muscles of both upper limbs. Tendon reflexes were absent in both upper limbs and moderately reduced in the lower limbs. Plantar responses were flexor. Sensory and cerebellar examination was normal.

Laboratory studies: Routine hemogram, blood chemistries, and vitamin B_{12}, B_1, B_2, B_6, and D levels were normal, as were our detailed and repeated screenings for dysimmune parameters including a paraneoplastic panel. CSF showed high-normal protein of 44 mg/dL (normal is up to 45 mg/dL); and normal glucose, as well as normal cell count and IgG ("MS") panel. Cervical MRI imaging was normal. Nerve conductions showed a combined motor dysneuronal and slightly dyschwannian neuropathy involving his upper limbs, right more than left.

Sensory nerve conductions were normal. EMG revealed recent denervation and established reinnervation prominently in the very weak upper limbs and slightly-moderately in the clinically strong lower limbs.

Biopsy of the clinically strong quadriceps muscle showed slight but definite recent denervation and slight established reinnervation.

Early follow-ups: During the initial investigations and repeated testings, we noticed that this patient's hemoglobin was gradually falling, to 10.0 g/dL. By positive stool exams for occult blood we were led to a silent asymptomatic 4 cm carcinoma of the transverse colon, which was resected. There has not been any recurrence for 14 years, to date, and the anemia was thereby cured.

Treatment: Because the patient was progressively weakening and a dysimmune process seemed a slight possibility, immunosuppression was tried. Initially, he had an allergic reaction to generic azathioprine plus prednisone; therefore, IVIG was initiated at 0.4 g/kg/day for five consecutive days, every third week. Very early benefit became evident on the next day after the first 5 days of IVIG. After three 5-day IVIG courses he could, momentarily, raise both arms nearly overhead. By 1 year of IVIG treatments he could vigorously raise them fully overhead [18] and he was able to do moderately heavy work, such as putting down 3000 bricks in his patio. Now his hand grip is excellent, but he still cannot fully extend his fingers (this function might be unrecoverable). We have been able to maintain the excellent improvement while very gradually reducing the frequency of IVIG treatments, now to 3 days every 6-10 weeks, plus Imuran 100 mg 3 ×/day.

Comment: The cumulatively dramatic benefit being sustained for 14 years is attributable to the IVIG benefiting a presumably dysimmune pathogenesis, because the patient's weakness begins to return if his IVIG treatments are given 1–2 weeks later than usual. Uncertain is whether there is a perpetuating paraneoplastic "remote effect" dysimmune pathogenesis (see Chapter 2) persisting 14 years after removal of the colon carcinoma, or whether the colon cancer had no influence on this treatable man-in-a-barrel neuromuscular disorder.

Vignette 22. Cervical stenosis: proximal weakness and pain in the upper limbs, with neck pain, and/or spasticity in the legs

Cervical stenosis from spondylosis is a common problem, with various degrees of severity. Focal symptoms in the arms and shoulders with neck pain occasionally, sometimes plus upper motor neuron signs in the lower limbs. These suggest involved cervical nerve roots-sometime plus cervical spinal cord (occasionally misinterpreted as fibromyalgia). A *simple clinical test of neck stretching* [20] with the neck flexed about 15 degrees can be used to seek improvement of symptoms, or inadvertently, mild momentary worsening of symptoms; either result would identify a significant *mechanical component*. *Transient improvement* would be an indication for therapeutic neck stretchings at home or in physiotherapy (after a cervical MRI demonstrates no contraindicating lesion), while *transient worsening* would suggest trying again with the neck somewhat less or somewhat more flexed to seek a favorable position for improvement by neck stretching. A thin night-time pillow is better than a fat one. Sometimes non surgical intervention is the better choice. For patients with significant *cervical stenosis* and/or *foraminal narrowings*, unresponsive to conservative measures, *very cautious neurosurgical intervention* may be beneficial. Evidence of corticospinal tract involvement is a strong point tilting toward surgery.

For 6 years a 64-year-old administrator has been having intermittent pain in her neck that radiates to her right upper arm, and pain and tenderness in the upper right trapezius. For the last 4 months, the right arm has been weak, causing difficulty lifting things to the kitchen counter, holding pots, chopping, or doing her hair. Her hands and left arm are not weak, but she has had occasional tingling in both arms and hands. Her arm symptoms are aggravated when she carries a heavy purse on the right side. The lower limbs seem somewhat "stiff," and her walking and stair climbing are slower. Recently, she has been having some urinary urgency.

Examination: She has neck pain and "stiffness" when turning her head, especially when rotating it to her left, or bending it laterally to the right. There was weakness in right shoulder abduction and elbow flexion. The pains interfere with her sleeping ("painful insomnia"). In the upper right trapezius there is a transverse bundle of tender muscle that the patient says when touched feels like a "sausage," and we agree. She had slightly reduced sensitivity to pain in her right arm in the C-5 nerve-root distribution. Cranial nerve testing was normal. Vibratory sensation was normal throughout. Her right biceps reflex were absent and bilateral triceps, and knee and ankle reflexes were excessively brisk. The plantar responses were extensor. Jaw jerk was normal.

Laboratory testing: Blood and urine testings were normal. Cervical spine MRI showed (a) moderate right neural foraminal stenosis causing compression of the C-5 nerve root and (b) C-4–5 disk indenting the ventral aspect of the spinal cord. Neurologic localization in this patient indicated involvement of (a) lower motor-neuron and sensory axons in the C-5 root to explain the weak biceps and absent reflex, and the sensory distribution on the right arm, and (b) involvement of the corticospinal tracts, evident as hyperreflexia below C-5 level (namely, at the triceps, knee, and ankle reflexes flexes and the extensor plantar reflexes, while above the C-5 level the jaw-jerk reflex was normal). Other possible causes of a similar clinical picture include radiculomyelopathy from: a secondary or primary tumor, abscess, arteriovenous malformation, or post-irradiation of a thymus or cervical nodes; ALS could be considered, but pain is not an aspect of ALS per se, although an ALS patient could have a coexisiting, and possibly treatable spondylotic cervical radiculopathy or myelopathy.

Treatment: A neurosurgeon performed spinal-cord and C-5 nerve-root decompressions, with good results.

Comments: (a) We have found that for a cervical radiculopathy due to spondylosis, without MRI-demonstrable spinal-cord involvement, cautious daily *home neck stretchings* [20] for a few weeks, initially demonstrated and supervised by a physician or experienced physical therapist, can sometimes produce pain relief that persists weeks or months, and occasionally for more than 20 years. (b) "Ponderous purse disease" was identified 20 years ago [21] as a common and treatable cause of neck pain and focal muscle *"sausage cramps,"* and is becoming more pervasive as women's purses become more voluminous and serve as shoulder valises. Computers and paraphernalia for "natural beauty" add to this weighty problem. The obvious treatment involving a much smaller, lighter purse is disdained as more of a pain in the neck than the pain in the neck. (c) The *painful and tender "sausage"* in the upper right trapezius area is a focal transverse muscle cramp caused by nerve-root irritation from the spondylosis: *it is not a mysterious "fibromyalgia"* (see Chapter 2). Clonazepam/Klonopin often is beneficial in relieving the painful cramp and consequently alleviating the "painful insomnia."

Brain disorder

Vignette 23. Normal-pressure hydrocephalus

Frequent falls from loss of balance, memory impairment, and urinary incontinence are three common complaints in older patients, and should not be dismissed as "simply a part of aging." MRI of the head and cervical spine could reveal various treatable neurological/neurosurgical conditions. *Normal-pressure hydrocephalus* is important to be recognized, because treatment might dramatically benefit the patient's quality of life, including safety when walking, and perhaps improve the patient's memory.

A 77-year-old accountant, accompanied in the clinic by his wife, has been having frequent loss of balance and falling for 4 months. During this time he has also been progressively forgetful, and now has difficulty doing simple calculations. His social graces are preserved. He also has occasional urinary incontinence at night. There are no sensory complaints. There is no history of major head injury, although he is falling every 1–2 weeks and has recently broken a wrist and suffered a nose injury, but no unconsciousness.

Examination: He has a wide-based gait. The Mini Mental examination confirmed impaired recent memory. No cranial nerve dysfunction or papilledema was evident. The sensory examination was normal. Tendon reflexes were slightly increased and the plantar responses were extensor.

Studies: Blood count, chemistry, and vitamin levels were normal. Syphilis test was negative. Brain MRI revealed a *communicating hydrocephalus*, with dilated frontal and temporal horns of the lateral ventricles, and slight–moderate periventricular white matter enhancement on contrast. No obstruction or focal mass was evident.

Treatment: *Via lumbar puncture, 60 ml of CSF was removed*. Within a day, there was *improvement* of his mental function, balance, and urinary incontinence. This first improvement lasted about 2 weeks, after which his symptoms gradually returned. After another CSF removal, the patient had the same improvement. Therefore a neurosurgeon installed a *ventriculo-peritoneal shunt*, with a programmable valve that can be adjusted for changes in the intracranial pressure. This is providing more enduring benefit.

Comment: Other possibilities for his presenting symptoms include small strokes (including multi-infarct dementia), chronic subdural hematoma, low-grade tumor metastases, B_{12} deficiency, atypical Alzheimer disease, prion disease, and chronic fungal or other infection.

References

1 Engel WK. (1973) "Myopathic EMG" - nonesuch animal. *New Engl J Med* **289**, 485–486.
2 Whitaker JN, Engel WK. (1972) Vascular deposits of immunoglobin and complement in idiopathic inflammatory myopathy. *New Engl J Med* **286**, 333–338.
3 Engel WK, Lichter AS, Galdi AP. (1982) Polymyositis: remarkable response to total body irradiation. *Lancet* **1**, 658.
4 Engel WK, Warmolts JR. (1971) Myasthenia gravis: a new hypothesis of the pathogenesis and a new form of treatment. *Ann NY Acad Sci* **183**, 72–87.
5 Engel WK, Trotter JL, McFarlin DE, McIntosh CXL. (1977) Thymic epithelial cell contains acetylcholine receptor. *Lancet* **i**, 1310–1311.
6 Engel WK. (2010) Multi-microcramps (MMC) syndrome: a new pathogenic concept of subtle lower motor-neuron (LMN) lability causing very disturbing, continuing muscle pains, sometimes gratifying

treatable – but often misinterpreted as mysterious "fibromyalgia" or "psychogenic". *Neurology* **74**, A465.

7 Mahajan S, Engel WK. (2010) Symptomatic treatment for muscle cramps (an evidence-based review). *Letter to the Editor. Neurology* **75**, 1397–1398.

8 Engel WK, Misra AK, Alexander SJ et al. (1990) Syndrome of continuous motor unit activity responsible to immunosuppression suggests dysimmune pathogenesis. *Neurology* **40**, 118.

9 Warmolts JR, Engel WK. (1972) Open biopsy electromyography. I. Correlation of motor unit behavior with histochemical muscle fiber type in human limb muscle. *Arch Neurol* **27**, 512–517.

10 Engel WK, Prentice AF. (1993) Some polyneuropathies (PNs) in insulin-requiring adult-onset diabetes (IRAOD) can benefit remarkably from anti-dysimmune treatments. *Neurology* **43**, 255–256.

11 Engel WK. (2003) Intravenous immunoglobulin G is remarkably beneficial in chronic immune dysschwannian/dysneuronal polyneuropathy, diabetes-2 neuropathy, and potentially in severe acute respiratory syndrome. *Acta Myol* **22**, 97–103.

12 Engel WK. (2001) Polyneuropathy in type 2 diabetes mellitus. *Lancet* **358**, 2086.

13 Engel WK. (2006) Longer-term (>3 months), IVIG treatment to optimize clinical benefit and cellular protection usually requires an individualized adjustable schedule – not fixed regimentation. *Neuromuscul Disord* **16**, 703–704.

14 Engel, WK (2011) Remarkable benefit persisting undiminished for 8 years after stopping 14 years of Interferon-α2A (Inf-α) treatment for fever-responsive dysimmune neuropathy (FRDN): possibly a combined antidysimmune plus antiviral effect, and thus a putative model for future "combined antidysimmune" therapies. *Neurology* **76**, A520.

15 Kula RW, Engel WK, Line BR. (1977) Scanning for soft-tissue amyloid. *Lancet* **1**, 92–93.

16 Engel WK, Trotter JL. (1979) Plasma-cell dyscrasic amyloid neuropathy: A parasparafucile phenomenon? In: Serratrice G, Roux H (eds), *Peroneal Atrophies and Related Disorders*, Masson Publishing Co, New York, pp. 339–347.

17 Yan J, Deng HX, Siddique N et al. (2010) Frameshift and novel mutations in FUS in familial amyotrophic lateral sclerosis and ALS/dementia. *Neurology* **75**, 807–814.

18 Engel WK. (1995) Rapid and continued improvement from intravenous immunoglobulin treatment of asymmetrical chronic progressive muscular atrophy after 19 years of disease progression. *Ann Neurol* **38**, 333–334.

19 Orsini M, Catharino AM, Catharino FM. (2009) Man-in-the-barrel syndrome, a symmetrical proximal brachial amyotrophic displegia related to neuron disease: a survey of nine cases. *Rev Assoc Med Bras* **55**, 712–715.

20 Engel WK. (1987) A simple, low-tech clinical test and treatment for cervical root compression. *Ann Neurol* **22**, 165.

21 Engel WK. (1978) Ponderous-purse disease. Letter to the Editor. *New Engl J Med* **299**, 557.

22 Renton AE, Mejounie E, Waite A, et al. (2011). A hexahucleotide repeat expansion in C90RF72 is the cause of chromosome 9p 21-linked ALS-FTD *Neuron* DOI: 10.10.16/j. neuron. 2011.09.010.

23 Engel WK. (1991) RNA metabolism in relation to amyotrophic lateral sclerosis. *Adv Neurol* **56**, 125–153.

CHAPTER 4

Mitochondrial changes in aging with particular reference to muscle, and possible clinical consequences

Salvatore DiMauro[1], Eric Schon[1,2], and Michio Hirano[1]

[1]Department of Neurology, Columbia University Medical Center, New York, NY, USA
[2]Department of Genetics and Development, Columbia University Medical Center, New York, NY, USA

Sarcopenia and mitochondria

Considering that skeletal muscle accounts for almost half of the human body mass and is rich in mitochondria, and considering that mitochondrial DNA (mtDNA) is universally considered to be an aging clock [1], it follows that muscle ought to be the ideal tissue in which to study the "catastrophic mitochondrial theory of aging" first proposed on biochemical grounds by Denham Harman in 1981 [2] and confirmed on molecular grounds a decade later by Soong et al. [3]. The latter paper led Anita Harding to title her commentary, only half in jest: "Growing old: the most common mitochondrial disease of all?" [4].

Let us turn the title of this chapter on its head and consider first the clinical consequences of aging on muscle (*sarcopenia*, a Greek term that simply means "muscle atrophy"), then the theoretical and experimental evidence of mitochondrial involvement in the aging process, and finally the therapeutic measures that can be adopted, if not to prevent, then at least to delay and contain the inevitable occurrence of sarcopenia.

The loss of muscle mass in humans starts at about age 40 and proceeds at a rate of approximately 1% per year, such that a 80-year-old individual will have about half the muscle mass of a middle-age person [5–7]. Obviously, there are great individual differences, often related to exercise, which can now be explained by mitochondrial mechanisms (see below). The different mitochondrial content and metabolic makeup of type 1 and type 2 muscle fibers can also explain the different muscle-specific susceptibility to sarcopenia in the rat, as type 1 fibers containing abundant mitochondria are relatively resistant to age-related changes [8]. The more uniform fiber type composition of human muscles masks such differential involvement.

As the number of people older than 65 years is expected to double in the USA over the next 15 years [6], sarcopenia is becoming a serious public health issue, with loss of mobility and increased risk of falls and fractures in the elderly population, and hence the importance of better understanding the pathogenesis and reducing the severity of sarcopenia.

Morphological changes of muscle with aging include atrophy, especially of type 2 fibers, some degree of fiber type-grouping due to loss of motor neurons and denervation, and modest lipid infiltration presumably due to mitochondrial dysfunction (see below). However, the most crucial morphological change associated with aging was described in 1992 by Müller-Hocker, who observed cytochrome

Muscle Aging, Inclusion-Body Myositis and Myopathies, First Edition. Edited by Valerie Askanas and W. King Engel.
© 2012 Blackwell Publishing Ltd. Published 2012 by Blackwell Publishing Ltd.

c oxidase (COX)-negative fibers in diaphragm, limb, and extraocular muscles of normal aged subjects [9]. He also noted that some of the COX-negative fibers reacted intensely with the stain for succinate dehydrogenase (SDH), suggesting excessive mitochondrial proliferation, or – put another way – many COX-negative fibers were ragged-red fibers (RRFs), a typical histochemical feature of primary mitochondrial diseases [10].

In fact, the age-related accumulation of COX-negative RRFs in normal human muscle has complicated the diagnosis of mitochondrial myopathies in elderly individuals, raising the question often asked of the pathologist: "How many RRFs do you need to call a specimen pathological?" To this there is not a simple answer because there is a fine line between normal aging and pathology. This situation is exemplified by nine patients with late-onset proximal or axial weakness, premature fatigue, and high numbers of COX-negative fibers in their muscle biopsies, a myopathy attributed – as it were – to exaggerated aging [11]. However, in clinical practice the diagnosis of mitochondrial myopathy in older individuals is not common.

Mitochondrial abnormalities, in the form of SDH-hyperactive, COX-negative fibers, also increase with age in rat muscles, but the alterations in this species correlate with the type of muscle and probably depend in large measure on fiber type composition: in the vastus lateralis, composed predominantly of type 2 fibers, SDH-hyperintensive, COX-negative fibers were detected at 18 months of age whereas in the soleus muscle, which is richer in type 1 fibers, the same alterations were noted at 36 months of age [8]. As mentioned above, in humans the greater vulnerability of type 2 fibers to sarcopenia is also present but masked by the more admixed fiber type composition, such that we do not have obviously "red" or "white" muscles.

mtDNA as the aging clock

It is remarkable that the "catastrophic mitochondrial theory of aging" was proposed before the first pathogenic mutations in mtDNA had ever been described and it has been strengthened ever since.

This theory was based on several premises pointing to mtDNA as an attractive suspect for the aging process: (a) unlike nuclear DNA, whose genes are diploid in somatic cells, mtDNA is present in thousands of copies in each cell; (b) because it is located in close proximity to the mitochondrial respiratory chain, mtDNA is exposed to the respiratory chain's toxic by-products, reactive oxygen species (ROS); (c) mtDNA fixes new mutations at a higher rate than nuclear DNA; (d) any damage to mtDNA is likely to be functionally deleterious because its structural genes have no 5' or 3' noncoding sequences, no introns, and few intervening spacers; (e) and the repair capacity of mtDNA is significant but probably less robust than that of nuclear DNA.

The mitochondrial theory of aging postulates a pernicious sequence of events. First, in post-mitotic tissues, including muscle, somatic mtDNA mutations, and especially large-scale deletions, gradually accumulate, with a steep increase at about 40 years of age [12, 13], which is – notably – when muscle mass starts declining [5]. Second, as the percentage of somatic mutations increases, due in part to a preferential clonal expansion of mtDNA within individual fiber regions, the efficiency of the respiratory chain decreases, leading to excessive production of ROS and oxidative stress. Third, oxidative stress induces mitochondrial-mediated apoptosis, with gradual loss of muscle fibers, i.e., sarcopenia. A voluminous literature supports the validity of each step, and not just in skeletal muscle but also in other post-mitotic tissues [3, 14]: what follows is a brief review of the main data pertaining to muscle.

Age-related mutations in mtDNA

Initial studies used a specific deletion of 4977 bp (the "common deletion" [15]) as a marker of mtDNA damage, which increased as much as 10,000-fold in the course of the normal lifespan [12] and reached an overall abundance of 0.1% of total muscle mtDNA [12, 13, 16]. A major criticism leveled at the pathogenic role of mtDNA deletions in aging is that these cumulative levels of rearrangements are a world apart from those found in muscle from patients with primary mitochondrial diseases due to mtDNA deletions, such as Kearns–Sayre syndrome (KSS), in whom mutation loads hover around 80% [17].

This objection, however is countered by three arguments. First, the "common deletion" is but one form of mtDNA rearrangement, and numerous other species also accumulate in muscle during aging [13, 18–20]. Second, skeletal muscle is a syncytium and, just as COX-negative and ragged-red areas do not affect the entire length of any fiber but are segmental changes, so too is the distribution and abundance of mtDNA deletions in aging. This has been clearly shown in both rat and human muscle by laser-capture microdissection of COX-negative segments of single fibers, where single clonally expanded rearranged mtDNA species accumulated to concentrations as high as 90% of total mtDNA, well above the pathogenic threshold [5, 21, 22]. The pathogenic significance of these localized molecular and biochemical lesions was supported in rat muscle by the colocalization of fiber atrophy, fiber splitting, and oxidative nucleic acid damage [22]. Third, referring to patients with overt syndromes due to mtDNA deletions may be misleading because the pathogenic threshold for different mutations has been traditionally based on studies of cybrid cells *in vitro* and does not accurately reflect clinical experience. It is conventional wisdom that the pathogenic thresholds for mtDNA deletions and point mutations alike are both high and steep, such that mitochondrial dysfunction does not occur until 80–90% of mtDNAs are mutated and that even small deviations below the threshold are compatible with normal function. However, the high threshold shown by cybrid cells harboring the m.3243A → G MELAS mutation – approximately 90% mutated mtDNA [23] – appears to be much lower *in vivo*, as shown by ^{31}P-magnetic resonance spectroscopy studies of the calf muscle in an oligosymptomatic carrier of the MELAS mutation [24].

Data on the age-related accumulation of mtDNA point mutations in muscle are less abundant, but two common pathogenic mutations, the m.8344A → G mutation (typically associated with MERRF) and the m.3243A → G MELAS mutation, were more abundant in skeletal muscle from aged individuals [25–28] and two muscle-specific mutations in the control region of mtDNA accumulated in normal elderly individuals [29]. It should be mentioned, however, that in another study [13] quantitative PCR of two small regions, one containing the MELAS mutation, the other containing the NARP (m.8993T → G or m.8993T → C) mutation, revealed a much more modest and age-unrelated accumulation of mutations.

Massive accumulation of mtDNA mutations were associated with dramatic premature aging in transgenic mice ("mutator mice") expressing an error-prone version of the catalytic subunit of polymerase γ (polg) [30, 31], but the severe decline in respiratory chain function and ATP production was not accompanied by oxidative stress, leading the authors to conclude that the respiratory chain dysfunction in and of itself induced premature aging [32], possibly through induction of apoptotic markers [31]. Whether the increase in the load of mtDNA point mutations in mutator mice was the cause of premature aging or merely a correlate has generated intense debate [33, 34]. It was noted that the level of somatic mutations in these mice was an order of magnitude greater than in human aging and that the aging features were not specific but shared with other premature aging mouse models not associated with mtDNA mutations [33]. It was also noted that mutator mice could tolerate a 500-fold greater mutation load than normal mice without showing features of premature aging [34]. Thus, the role of somatic point mutations in aging is probably less dramatic than the outward features of the first mutator mouse had led us to believe.

Age-related oxidative stress

As aptly put by Wallace in a comprehensive review of mitochondria in aging, degenerative diseases, and cancer [1], "ROS damage to the mitochondria, mtDNA, and host cells must be one of the most important entropic factors in determining age-related cellular decline."

Having established that mtDNA somatic mutations, especially large-scale deletions, accumulate in aging human muscle, at least segmentally, and almost certainly beyond the pathogenic threshold within individual fibers, it follows that the respiratory chain function must also decline with time. Numerous papers, mostly published in the 1990s, have provided biochemical evidence of such a decline affecting one or more respiratory chain complexes [35–41] and these data have been confirmed by transcriptional profiling [42]. Defects of the respiratory chain hyperpolarize the electrochemical gradient of the electron-transport chain (ETC) and result in excessive production of ROS. Endogenous ROS production is as normal as the release of exhaust fumes from a car motor and it is largely "muffled" by the intrinsic antioxidant defenses of the cell, including the mitochondrial Mn superoxide dismutase (MnSOD) and Cu/Zn SOD, the cytosolic glutathione peroxidase (GPx1), and the peroxisomal catalase. However, when the initial steps of the ETC remain reduced, either because of excessive caloric intake or because of a partial block in the flow of electrons, ROS are produced in excess and exceed the quenching power of the endogenous antioxidants, feeding the vicious cycle of progressive mtDNA mutations but also damaging directly mitochondrial proteins and lipids, including cardiolipin [43].

The correlation between oxidative stress and sarcopenia is documented both directly [22] and indirectly through the rich literature showing the positive effect of caloric restriction (CR) on longevity in multiple species (for review, see [1, 44]) and the life-prolonging effect of upregulating the antioxidant defenses of the organism [45]. More relevant to our review, oxidative stress in muscle of transgenic mice lacking Cu/Zn SOD accelerates the features of sarcopenia [46].

Age-related muscle apoptosis

Apoptosis is a highly conserved cascade of events resulting in cell destruction without associated inflammation or damage to surrounding tissues. The executioner enzymes are cysteine-aspartic proteases (caspases) that are normally present as inactive proenzymes (procaspases). Apoptotic stimuli activate initiator caspases (caspase-8, caspase-9, caspase-12) which, in turn, activate effector caspases (caspase-3, caspase-6, caspase-7) that actually dismantle the cell [43]. The apoptotic cascade can be triggered by extrinsic or intrinsic pathways. In the extrinsic pathway, activation of the Fas receptor and tumor necrosis factor receptor (TNF-R) on the cell surface leads to recruitment of adaptor proteins, such as the Fas-associated death domain (FADD), whose death

effector domain (DED) engages procaspase-8. Active caspase-8 activates the effector caspase-3.

The intrinsic pathways of caspase activation involve the endoplasmic reticulum or the mitochondria. We will only consider here the mitochondrial pathway. The pivotal mitochondrial mediator of apoptosis is cytochrome c, a small electron carrier that can be released into the cytoplasm, where it binds to apoptotic protease-activating factor 1 (Apaf-1), dATP, and procaspase-9 to form the apoptosome, within which procaspase-9 is activated and engages the effector caspase-3 [43]. The release of cytochrome c occurs via the mitochondrial permeability transition pore (mtPTP), which is composed of the inner membrane adenine nucleotide translocator (ANT), the outer membrane voltage-dependent anion channel (VDAC; also known as porin), Bax, Bcl2, and cyclophilin D [1]. Opening of the mtPTP releases into the cytoplasm not only cytochome c but also other cell death-promoting factors, including apoptosis-inducing factor (AIF), SMAC/Diablo, endonuclease G, and the Omi/HtrA2 serine protease. Endonuclease G and AIF enter the nucleus, where they degrade chromatin.

The crucial notion here is that, as ROS accumulate, the propensity to apoptosis increases, thus connecting mtDNA damage, ETC dysfunction, ROS accumulation, and cell death, or sarcopenia [47].

Mitochondrial biogenesis: closing the circle

In recent years, all the different age-related mitochondrial changes have converged on mitochondrial biogenesis and, more specifically, to the peroxisome proliferator-activated receptor γ coactivator 1α protein (PGC-1α for short), a transcriptional coactivator that binds to several transcription factors and induces gene expression [48]. Importantly, PGC-1α is a strong promoter of mitochondrial biogenesis and function [49], and its role in the pathogenesis (and alleviation) of sarcopenia has become increasingly clear. In aged tissues, including muscle, PGC-1α expression declines [50, 51] and, in fact, this phenomenon may precede all the more obvious mitochondrial changes described above and may itself be due to a loss of sensitivity to activators on the part of PGC-1α [52].

In a series of elegant papers, Wenz and collaborators illustrated both the pathogenic role of PGC-1α and its potential therapeutic usefulness [53–56]. First, they used a knock-in mouse model of mitochondrial myopathy, a partial COX deficiency due to a mutation in the assembly gene *COX10*. Promoting mitochondrial biogenesis either by transgenic expression of PG1-α or by administration of bezafibrate (a PGC-1α activator) resulted in improved respiratory chain function and ATP production, delayed appearance of the myopathy, and prolonged lifespan [53]. Next, they explored the effects of upregulating the expression of PGC-1α transgenically in aged mice and they found that all features of sarcopenia, including muscle atrophy, respiratory chain function decline, oxidative stress, apoptosis, autophagy, proteasome activation, and neuromuscular junction damage, were attenuated or retarded. The importance of skeletal muscle in overall energy balance and metabolism was documented by the general health benefits of upregulating PGC-1α expression in muscle only: the mice showed improved exercise performance, bone mineral density, and longer lifespan [54]. Finally, Wenz et al. returned to their transgenic animal models of COX-deficient myopathy to show that enhancing mitochondrial biogenesis indirectly through endurance exercise (which upregulates PGC-1α [57, 58]) also improved muscle performance, respiratory chain function, and increased lifespan [55]. This is a nice experimental confirmation of the beneficial effects of aerobic exercise in patients with mitochondrial myopathy [59].

Although not directly relevant to sarcopenia, a similar protective effect from denervation atrophy was observed in transgenic mice overexpressing PGC-1α: in this case, PGC-1α reduced the activation of FOXO3 and the expression of the atrophy-related ubiquitin ligases atrogin-1 and MURF-1 [60].

Is sarcopenia preventable?

Life elixir is still the stuff of fairy tales, but – having succeeded to prolong life beyond anybody's expectations – it would be ideal to keep our muscles in good health for two excellent reasons: (a) because the frailty that accompanies old age limits mobility and is a major cause of falls and fractures; and (b) because skeletal muscle has an important role in general metabolism, for example insulin-stimulated glucose disposal.

There is little question from the ample literature reviewed above that age-related muscle atrophy and weakness is a mitochondrial "disease," just as predicted by Anita Harding in 1992. There isn't much we can do for mitochondrial myopathies and there isn't much we can do for sarcopenia. However, two sensible approaches to maintain our muscle fitness include diet and exercise.

The beneficial effects of aerobic exercise cannot be overemphasized and regular exercise should be initiated before age 40, when mtDNA mutations start accumulating and muscle mass starts declining.

As mentioned above, there is ample evidence that caloric restriction prolongs life and it is more than likely that overfeeding in rich countries contributes to disease, including sarcopenia. An interesting study examined muscle bioenergetics in 36 young overweight but not obese subjects randomized into three groups and followed for 6 months: controls, 100% of energy requirements; CR, 25% caloric restriction; and CREX, caloric restriction (12.5%) plus exercise (12.5% increased energy expenditure). Needle muscle biopsies showed that members of the CR and CREX groups had increased expression of PGC-1α and other proteins involved in mitochondrial biogenesis (e.g., TFAM, Sirtuin1), increased mtDNA content, and decreased mtDNA damage [61].

This study should be confirmed and extended, but it bodes well as a preventive measure for sarcopenia, even if it requires two of the most unpopular behavioral adaptations in our spoiled society: fasting and exercising.

Acknowledgments

This work was supported by NIH grant HD 32062 and by the Marriott Mitochondrial Disorders Clinical Research Fund (MMDCRF).

References

1 Wallace DC. (2005) A mitochondrial paradigm of metabolic and degenerative diseases, aging, and cancer. A dawn for evolutionary medicine. *Annu Rev Genet* **39**, 359–407.

2 Harman, D. (1981) The aging process. *Proc Natl Acad Sci USA* **78**, 7124–7128.

3 Soong NW, Hinton DR, Cortopassi G, Arnheim, N. (1992) Mosaicism for a specific mitochondrial DNA mutation in adult human brain. *Nat Genet* **2**, 318–323.

4 Harding AE. (1992) Growing old: the most common mitochondrial disease of all? *Nat Genet* **2**, 251–252.

5 Bua E, Johnson J, Herbst A et al. (2006) Mitochondrial DNA-deletion mutation accumulate intracellularly to detrimental levels in aged human skeletal muscle fibers. *Am J Hum Genet* **79**, 469–480.

6 Lang T, Streeper T, Cawton P et al. (2010) Sarcopenia: etiology, clinical consequences, intervention, and assessment. *Osteoporos Int* **21**, 543–559.

7 Arnold A-S, Egger A, Hansdschin C. (2011) PGC-1 alpha and myokines in the aging muscle - A mini-review. *Gerontology* **57**, 37–43.

8 Bua E, McKiernan SH, Waganat J et al. (2002) Mitochondrial abnormalities are more frequent in muscle undergoing sarcopenia. *J Appl Physiol* **92**, 2617–2624.

9 Müller-Hocker, J. (1992) Mitochondria and ageing. *Brain Pathol* **2**, 149–158.

10 DiMauro S, Schon EA. (2003) Mitochondrial respiratory-chain diseases. *New Engl J Med* **348**, 2656–2668.

11 Johnston W, Karpati G, Carpenter S et al. (1995) Late-onset mitochondrial myopathy. *Ann Neurol* **37**, 16–23.

12 Simonetti S, Chen X, DiMauro S, Schon EA. (1992) Accumulation of deletions in human mitochondrial DNA during normal aging: analysis by quantitative PCR. *Biochim Biophys Acta* **1180**, 113–122.

13 Pallotti F, Chen X, Bonilla E, Schon EA. (1996) Evidence that specific mtDNA point mutations may not accumulate in skeletal muscle during normal human aging. *Am J Hum Genet* **59**, 591–602.

14 Cortopassi GA, Arnheim, N. (1990) Detection of a specific mitochondrial DNA deletion in tissues of older humans. *Nucleic Acids Res* **18**, 6927–6933.

15 Schon EA, Rizzuto R, Moraes CT et al. (1989) A direct repeat is a hotspot for large-scale deletions of human mitochondrial DNA. *Science* **244**, 346–349.

16 Cortopassi GA, Shibata D, Soong NW, Arnheim, N. (1992) A pattern of accumulation of a somatic deletion of mitochondrial DNA in aging human tissues. *Proc Natl Acad Sci USA* **89**, 7370–7374.

17 Moraes CT, DiMauro S, Zeviani M et al. (1989) Mitochondrial DNA deletions in progressive external ophthalmoplegia and Kearns-Sayre syndrome. *N Engl J Med* **320**, 1293–1299.

18 Chen X, Simonetti S, DiMauro S, Schon EA. (1993) Accumulations of mitochondrial DNA deletions in organisms with various lifespans. *Bull Mol Biol Med* **18**, 57–66.

19 Melov S, Shoffner JM, Kaufman A, Wallace DC. (1995) Marked increase in the number and variety of mitochondrial DNA rearrangements in aging human skeletal muscle. *Nucleic Acid Res* **23**, 4122–4126.

20 Melov S, Hinerfeld D, Esposito L, Wallace DC. (1997) Multi-organ characterization of mitochondrial genomic rearrangements in ad libitum and caloric restricted mice show striking somatic mitochondrial DNA rearrangements with age. *Nucleic Acid Res* **25**, 974–982.

21 Cao Z, Waganat J, McKiernan SH, Aiken JM. (2001) Mitochondrial DNA deletion mutations are concomitant with ragged red regions of individual, aged muscle fibers: analysis by laser-capture microdissection. *Nucleic Acids Res* **29**, 4502–4508.

22 Waganat J, Cao Z, Pathare P, Aiken JM. (2001) Mitochondrial DNA deletion mutations colocalize with segmental electron transport system abnormalities, muscle fiber atrophy, fiber splitting, and oxidative damage in sarcopenia. *FASEB J* **15**, 322–332.

23 Chomyn A, Martinuzzi A, Yoneda M et al. (1992) MELAS mutation in mtDNA binding site for transcription termination factor causes defects in protein synthesis and in respiration but no change in levels of upstream and downstream mature transcripts. *Proc Natl Acad Sci USA* **89**, 4221–4225.

24 Chinnery PF, Taylor DJ, Brown DT et al. (2000) Very low levels of the mtDNA A3243G mutation associated with mitochondrial dysfunction in vivo. *Ann Neurol* **47**, 381–384.

25 Munscher C, Rieger T, Muller-Hocker J, Kadenbach, B. (1993) The point mutation of mitochondrial DNA characteristic for MERRF disease is found also in healthy people of different ages. *FEBS Lett* **317**, 27–30.

26 Munscher C, Muller-Hocker J, Kadenbach, B. (1993) Human aging is associated with various point mutations in tRNA genes of mitochondrial DNA. *Biol Chem Hoppe Seyler* **374**, 1099–1104.

27 Zhang C, Linnane AW, Nagley, P. (1993) Occurrence of a particular base substitution (3243 A to G) in mitochondrial DNA of tissues of aging humans. *Biochem Biophys Res Commun* **195**, 1104–1110.

28 Fayet G, Jansson M, Sternberg D et al. (2000) Mitochondrial DNA mutations in cytochrome c oxidase

deficient muscle fibers associated with aging. *Neuromusc Disord* **10**, 346.

29 Wang Y, Michikawa Y, Mallidis C et al. (2001) Muscle-specific mutations accumulate with aging in critical human mtDNA control sites for replication. *Proc Natl Acad Sci USA* **98**, 4022–4027.

30 Trifunovic A, Wredenberg A, Falkenberg M et al. (2004) Premature ageing in mice expressing defective mitochondrial DNA polymerase. *Nature* **429**, 417–423.

31 Kujoth GC, Hiona A, Pugh TD et al. (2005) Mitochondrial DNA mutations, oxidative stress, and apoptosis in mammalian aging. *Science* **309**, 481–484.

32 Trifunovic A, Hansson A, Wredenberg A et al. (2005) Somatic mtDNA mutations cause aging phenotypes without affecting reactive oxygen species production. *Proc Natl Acad Sci USA* **102**, 17993–17998.

33 Khrapko K, Kraytsberg Y, de Grey AD et al. (2006) Does premature aging of the mtDNA mutator mouse prove that mtDNA mutations are involved in natural aging? *Aging Cell* **5**, 279–282.

34 Vermulst M, Bielas JH, Kujoth GC et al. (2007) Mitochondrial point mutations do not limit the natural lifespan of mice. *Nat Genet* **39**, 540–543.

35 Boffoli D, Scacco SC, Vergari R et al. (1994) Decline with age of the respiratory chain activity in human skeletal muscle. *Biochim Biophys Acta* **1236**, 73–82.

36 Byrne E, Dennett X, Trounce, I. (1991) Oxidative energy failure in post-mitotic cells: A major factor in senescence. *Rev Neurol* **147**, 532–535.

37 Cardellach F, Galofre J, Cusso, R. (1989) Decline in skeletal muscle mitochondrial respiratory chain function with ageing. *Lancet* **2**, 637–639.

38 Cooper JM, Mann VM, Schapira AH. (1992) Analysis of mitochondrial respiratory chain function and mitochondrial DNA deletion in human skeletal muscle: effect of ageing. *J Neurol Sci* **113**, 91–98.

39 Hseih RH, Hou JH, Hsu HS, Wei YH. (1994) Age-dependent respiratory function decline and DNA deletions in human muscle mitochondria. *Biochem Mol Biol Intern* **32**, 1009–1022.

40 Papa, S. (1996) Mitochondrial oxidative phosphorylation changes in the life span. Molecular aspects and physiopathological implications. *Biochim Biophys Acta* **1276**, 87–105.

41 Trounce I, Byrne E, Marzuki, S. (1989) Decline in skeletal muscle mitochondrial respiratory chain function: possible factor in ageing. *Lancet* **1**, 637–639.

42 Zahn JM, Sonu R, Vogel H et al. (2006) Transcriptional profiling of aging in human muscle reveals a common aging signature. *PLoS Genet* **2**, e115.

43 Marzetti E, Hwang JCY, Lees HA et al. (2010) Mitochondrial death effectors: Relevance to sarcopenia and disuse muscle atrophy. *Biochim Biophys Acta* **1800**, 235–244.

44 Guarente, L. (2008) Mitochondria - a nexus for aging, calorie restriction, and sirtuins? *Cell* **132**, 171–176.

45 Melov S, Ravenscroft J, Malik S et al. (2000) Extension of life-span with superoxide dismutase/catalase mimetics. *Science* **289**, 1567–1569.

46 Jang YC, Lustgarten MS, Liu Y et al. (2010) Increased superoxide in vivo accelerates age-associated muscle atrophy through mitochondrial dysfunction and neuromuscular junction degeneration. *FASEB J* **24**, 1376–1390.

47 Marzetti E, Leeuwenburgh, C. (2006) Skeletal muscle apoptosis, sarcopenia and frailty at old age. *Exp Geront* **41**, 1234–1238.

48 Lin J, Wu, H., Tarr PT et al. (2002) Transcriptional co-activator PGC-1alpha drives the formation of slow-twitch muscle fibers. *Nature* **418**, 797801.

49 Rohas LM, St-Pierre J, Uldry M et al. (2007) A fundamental system of cellular energy homeostasis regulated by PGC-1alpha. *Proc Natl Acad Sci USA* **104**, 7933–7938.

50 Ling C, Poulsen P, Carlsson E et al. (2004) Multiple environmental and genetic factors influence skeletal muscle *PGC1-alpha* and *PGC-1beta* gene expression in twins. *J Clin Invest* **114**, 1518–1526.

51 Handschin C, Spiegelman BM. (2006) Peroxisome proliferator-activated receptor gamma coactivator 1 coactivators, energy homeostasis, and metabolism. *Endocr Rev* **27**, 728–735.

52 Reznick RM, Zong H, Morino K et al. (2007) Aging-associated reductions in AMP-activated protein kinase activity and mitochondrial biogenesis. *Cell Metab* **5**, 151–156.

53 Wenz T, Diaz F, Spiegelman BM, Moraes CT. (2008) Activation of the PPAR/PGC-1alpha pathway prevents a bioenergetic deficit and effectively improves a mitochondrial myopathy phenotype. *Cell Metab* **8**, 249–255.

54 Wenz T, Rossi S, Rotundo RL et al. (2009) Increased muscle PGC-1alpha expression protects from sarcopenia and metabolic disease during aging. *Proc Natl Acad Sci USA* **106**, 20405–20410.

55 Wenz T, Diaz F, Hernandez D, Moraes CT. (2009) Endurance exercise is protective for mice with mitochondrial myopathy. *J Appl Physiol* **106**, 1712–1719.

56 Wenz, T. (2009) PGC-1alpha activation as a therapeutic approach in mitochondrial disease. *IUBMB Life* **61**, 1051–1062.

57 Pilegaard H, Saltin B, Neufer PD. (2003) Exercise induces transient transcriptional activation of the PGC-1alpha gene in human skeletal muscle. *J Physiol* **546**, 851–858.

58 Mathai AS, Bonen A, Benton CR et al. (2008) Rapid exercise-induced changes in PGC-1alpha mRNA and protein in human skeletal muscle. *J Appl Physiol* **105**, 1098–1105.

59 Taivassalo T, Shoubridge EA, Chen J et al. (2001) Aerobic conditioning in patients with mitochondrial myopathies: physiological, biochemical, and genetic effects. *Ann Neurol* **50**, 133–141.

60 Sandri M, Lin J, Handschin C et al. (2006) PGC-1alpha protects skeletal muscle from atrophy by suppressing FoxO3 action and arophy-specific gene transcription. *Proc Natl Acad Sci USA* **103**, 16260–16265.

61 Civitarese AE, Carling S, Heilbronn LK et al. (2007) Calorie restriction increases muscle mitochondrial biogenesis in healthy humans. *PLoS Med* **4**, e76.

CHAPTER 5

Protein degradation in aging cells and mitochondria: relevance to the neuromuscular system

Jenny K. Ngo and Kelvin J. A. Davies

Davis School of Gerontology Ethel Percy Andrus, Gerontology Center, University of Southern California, 3715 McClintock Avenue, Los Angeles, CA, USA

Degradation of oxidized proteins in mammalian cells

The oxidation of proteins is a natural part of aerobic life. Various free radicals, and reactive oxygen species generated as by-products of cellular metabolism, or from environmental sources, can modify the amino acids of proteins, leading to their inactivation. The majority of these modified proteins are either repaired directly, or removed by selective proteolysis. Mammalian cells contain only limited direct repair mechanisms for oxidized proteins. The two most widely studied proteolytic systems to remove oxidatively damaged proteins are the proteasome and the Lon protease.

The proteasome is a large multi-subunit complex that is largely responsible for the degradation of targeted soluble proteins in the cytosol, nucleus, and endoplasmic reticulum. The 26S core proteasome is comprised of the catalytic 20S core, and two 19S regulatory complexes. The 19S regulator mediates the recognition of poly-ubiquinated proteins, and permits their access to the 20S core complex for degradation. In mammalian cells, the degradation of oxidized proteins is targeted by the smaller 20S proteasome. The free 20S core proteasome recognizes exposed hydrophobic patches, aromatic residues, and bulky aliphatic residues that are exposed during oxidative rearrangement of secondary and tertiary protein structure, which is a feature of proteins that have undergone oxidative modification. This selective recognition and removal of oxidatively damaged proteins is critical in minimizing protein aggregation, and the formation of cross-linked products, which are toxic to the cell.

The second major system is the mammalian Lon protease. Lon is primarily localized in mitochondria, with some data indicating that a Lon variant is transported to peroxisomes. Localization to an organelle such as the mitochondria is crucial, since the mitochondrial structure is enclosed by a double membrane system, making it impermeable to proteasome which is found throughout the rest of the cell. Mitochondria are a major source of free radical generation, and their macromolecules are highly susceptible to oxidative modification. The Lon protease is the only known system for the direct removal of oxidized proteins in mitochondria.

There is a growing body of evidence that suggests that aging and certain neurodegenerative diseases are a consequence of cumulative damage to macromolecules by free radicals [1]. The list ranges from heart attacks and strokes, to cancer, neurodegenerative diseases such as Alzheimer and Parkinson

Muscle Aging, Inclusion-Body Myositis and Myopathies, First Edition. Edited by Valerie Askanas and W. King Engel.
© 2012 Blackwell Publishing Ltd. Published 2012 by Blackwell Publishing Ltd.

disease, and inclusion-body myositis [2, 3]. Oxidatively modified proteins found in the cytoplasm, endoplasmic reticulum, and nucleus are rapidly degraded by the proteasome in younger individuals, but this rate of activity declines with age [4]. Carbonyl groups, one of the most abundant protein oxidation products, are commonly measured as a marker for aging [5–7]. Many independent studies have shown that protein carbonyl content increases with age in the tissues of various animals [8–12]. Also, there is an exponential increase in tissue carbonyl content during the last third of the lifespan of most individuals [13]. Although the mechanism causing this accumulation is not well established, the loss of proteasome activity probably contributes greatly to the increased level of protein aggregates found in older individuals, organs, and cells.

Protein maintenance in aging mitochondria

The mitochondrial electron transport chain is the primary machine of aerobic metabolism; however, its efficiency is not perfect. Some 1–5% (depending on physiological/pathological state) of electrons transferred through the chain actually leak, generating free radicals that can damage mitochondrial proteins, and other cellular macromolecules [14]. As a result, there are several layers of antioxidant defenses within the cell, as well as in the mitochondria itself, that ensure proper protein quality control. The initial line of protection against free radicals and other oxidants available within the mitochondria are detoxifying enzymes, such as manganese superoxide dismutase, glutathione peroxidase, and catalase. These enzymes intercept and scavenge reactive species, thus minimizing damage to mitochondrial macromolecules. However, reactive species can still bypass this initial line of defense, and cause damage to proteins, mitochondrial DNA (mtDNA), and lipids. Failure of proper protein maintenance has been implicated in the age-related accumulation of oxidized proteins. In this chapter, we will focus on protein damage.

Mitochondrial proteins are especially exposed to oxidative modification, and direct repair by

disulfide reducing enzymes, or removal of these damaged proteins by the Lon protease, is crucial in maintaining mitochondrial function and integrity. Oxidative modification of proteins can be reversible or irreversible. Reversible damage is limited to the repair of oxidation products of the sulfur containing amino acids such as cysteine and methionine [15]. Interestingly, sulfur-containing amino acids and aromatic amino acids are the most sensitive to oxidation. A number of reductase systems, available in both the cytosol and mitochondria, can repair these oxidative products and/or prevent the formation of disulfide bridges [16, 17]. These reductase systems include the thioredoxin/glutaredoxin system, the glutaredoxin/glutathione/glutathione reductase system [16], and finally, the methionine sulfoxide reductase enzymes, to name a few. These systems are present within mitochondria and have been implicated in longevity and resistance to oxidative stress [18–22].

Another form of reversible damage is the misfolding of previously functional proteins, or refolding of newly synthesized proteins. Chaperone and heat-shock proteins (HSPs) are present in the mitochondrial matrix where they assist in refolding, and/or the import of new proteins into the mitochondria. The majority of mitochondrial proteins are imported from the cytosol, and require the assistance of a variety of chaperone proteins from the HSP60, HSP70, and HSP100 families. These HSPs have also been implicated in protein folding, disaggregation, and degradation, and the prevention of aging [23, 24]. If mitochondrial oxidized proteins can no longer be repaired to their native and active conformation, they will be targeted to protein degradation pathways by ATP-stimulated proteases [25].

Irreversible protein damage includes the formation of hydroxyl and carbonyl groups and also the conjugation of lipid peroxidation products, or the formation of glycoxidation adducts [26]. Misfolded proteins are also prone to oxidation [27]. Such modified proteins are generally impaired or completely nonfunctional, and are prone to generate cross-links with one another, creating large protein aggregates if not promptly removed. Degradation pathways such as the proteasome in the cytosol, and the Lon protease in the mitochondria, serve as secondary lines of defense and are essential for the rapid and specific elimination of such damaged cellular constituents.

The Lon protein, like most other mitochondrial proteins, is encoded by the nuclear genome, and the protein is subsequently transported into mitochondria. Lon has a fascinating structure that encompasses all if its functional properties in one single peptide. Unlike the proteasome, and most other major catalytic proteases which are hetero-oligomeric, Lon is a homo-oligomeric complex that self associates from tetrameric ring structures, up to octomeric rings. The N-terminus of the mammalian Lon peptide contains a highly conserved ATPase and is involved in a number of important functions. It contains a "walker-type" motif that is involved in nucleotide binding and ATP hydrolysis [24]. This property is also important for Lon's suggested chaperone activity, as well as proteolysis, since both require ATP hydrolysis. In addition, Lon binds to mtDNA at promotor regions, which presumably may be occurring within this walker-type motif.

Towards the middle of the Lon peptide resides the substrate-recognition domain [28]. This area preferentially binds to specific proteins based on the amino acid sequence. In *Escherichia coli*, for example, a target protein is UmuD, but not UmuD′, which lacks the first 24 N-terminal amino acids of the UmuD sequence [28]. Whether the recognition domain prefers a specific sequence, or a certain property such as a charged environment, is not well understood; however, Lon proteolysis does have a preferential cleavage site. Lon has been shown to initiate cleavage between hydrophobic amino acids within a charged environment, with subsequent cleavage occurring sequentially along the primary polypeptide chain [29]. Increased surface hydrophobicity is a feature common to all oxidized proteins so far tested [7]. Similar to the 20S proteasome in the cytoplasm, the recognition of such (normally shielded) hydrophobic residues may be the mechanism by which Lon catalyzes the repair or removal of oxidatively modified proteins.

At the C-terminus of the Lon peptide resides Lon's proteolytic domain. Lon is a serine protease and requires a nucleophilic serine for hydrolysis and substrate proteolysis. In the majority of organisms, Lon proteolysis occurs via a conserved catalytic serine-dyad domain which interacts with the AAA+ module [30]. It is hypothesized that the binding of ATP to the AAA+ module translocates the N-terminus of a substrate protein through the ring structure of Lon, via hydrolysis energy, and progressive protein cleavage subsequently takes place [30].

The structure of Lon thus makes it a very important multi-functional protease for the mitochondria, and permits Lon to act as a chaperone, a mtDNA-binding protein, and a protease, which preferentially degrades exposed hydrophobic amino acids of a protein. All of these properties, built into one large complex, enable Lon to serve multiple purposes, as needed, as it comes across a damaged protein. So far, Lon seems to be an evolutionarily indispensable protein, and it has been found in almost every organism studied.

Relevance of proteolysis to the neuromuscular system

Oxidative damage to cells is a common phenomenon, and quality control of modified proteins is important to maintain normal cellular functions. In the cytoplasm, nucleus, and endoplasmic reticulum, the proteasome is involved in the removal of various types of proteins such as ubiquinated, misfolded, or unfolded proteins, and oxidized proteins. Abnormal inhibition of proteasome may contribute to neurodegenerative diseases such as Alzheimer disease, Parkinson disease, Lewy body dementia, and Huntington disease [31–40]. Neuromuscular diseases, such as sporadic inclusion-body myositis (s-IBM) share several phenotypes described in the brain tissues of Alzheimer and Parkinson disease patients [41]. One such similarity to Alzheimer disease is the accumulation of amyloid-β (Aβ), phosphorylated tau (p-tau), and ubiquitin, which are often found within these aggregates [42, 43]. In s-IBM patients, significant proteasome abnormalities were identified including, increased 26S proteasome expression and abnormal accumulation of 26S proteasome, but reduced proteasome activities [44]. The inverse relationship between increased expression and decreased activity may be an attempt to over-compensate for the loss of 26S function which these cells suffer. The overproduction of Aβ/Aβ precursor protein (AβPP) plays an important role in s-IBM pathogenesis [42, 43]. Supporting a possible link between Aβ accumulation and proteasome dysfuction, colocalization microscopy and immunoprecipitation assays have shown that Aβ does bind with proteasome [44]. In human muscle cells overexpressing Aβ/AβPP, proteasome activity was inhibited, suggesting that Aβ/AβPP overexpression may be causally involved in proteasome inhibition of s-IBM fibers [44]. Proteasome is responsible for the degradation of most proteins in the cell [36, 37]. The failure to remove damaged or surplus proteins, and the accumulation of ubiquinated, misfolded, or oxidized proteins can be detrimental to muscle fibers by creating toxic by-products while further inhibiting proteasome function [33, 45–48]. The vicious cycle of proteasome inhibition creating toxic by-products, which again further inhibits proteasome function, is extremely detrimental to the cell.

Oxidant damage incurred in mitochondria can lead to the progressive loss of ATP energy, cellular degeneration, and death, contributing greatly to the aging process [49–51]. The most dramatic age-related changes occur in post-mitotic cells, such as neurons, cardiac myocytes, and skeletal muscle cells, while proliferative cells such as bone marrow and epithelia exhibit seemingly mild changes [52]. This might be the result of the dilution in accumulated damage of older proliferative cells, as they undergo repetitive cell divisions [53]. In addition, the rate of replacement of long-lived post-mitotic cells is so slow that they accumulate lifetime damages much more dramatically [53].

There are different types of muscle cells, and the extent of damage in these cells actually correlates with their characteristic oxygen-consumption profiles. The highest degree of age-related changes occurs in cardiac myocytes [54, 55], which consume the highest amount of oxygen; followed by skeletal muscle cells [56, 57]; and finally, the least pronounced oxidative damage is observed in smooth muscles [58]. The aging of myocytes can lead to disorders that substantially decrease the quality of life such as sarcopenia, and various myopathies [59, 60], and may even result in fatal cardiac dysfunction [61].

Aging myocytes often display giant mitochondria [55, 56], typically much larger than mitochondria in younger cells. These enormous mitochondria are the result of swelling, loss of cristae, and the complete destruction of inner membranes, all of which result in the formation electron-dense waste material often observed in senescent mitochondria [62]. The progressive accumulation of mtDNA mutations and oxidative protein damage is common in these giant mitochondria and leads to impaired mitochondrial membrane potential [62] and energy production [63].

Impaired mitochondrial functionality in post-mitotic cells such as muscles, plays a major role in aging. Since we discovered that the Lon protease modulates oxidized protein levels in the mitochondria, we wondered about the cellular effects of Lon downregulation. Our initial experiments using RNA silencing in human fibroblasts indicate that the silencing of Lon expression led to the loss of mitochondrial function, decreased mitochondrial biogenesis, and cell death [64]. In a rhabdomyosarcoma (RD) muscle cell line, we further tested the effects of Lon downregulation and showed that Lon preserves mitochondrial function through protection against the accumulation of oxidized proteins during an oxidant stress. This type of protection is rapid, resulting up to an 8-fold surge of Lon protein levels upon initial exposure to multiple stressors [65]. The inducibility of Lon during such stressors led to protection against the production of protein carbonyls, preserved mitochondrial function and improved cell survival, until stress conditions subsided, after which Lon levels returned back toward initial basal levels [65]. These data suggest that overall mitochondrial functionality relies on the ability of the Lon protease to respond to stress, and maintain a protective environment, by keeping the level of toxic protein products to a minimum.

There are a number of studies that are beginning to reveal that Lon levels decrease with age. Lon was initially discovered by its dramatic 4-fold decrease in transcript levels in the leg muscle of old mice, and this difference was completely prevented in old calorie-restricted mice [66]. Our group conducted a follow-up study and found that there was more than a 5-fold reduction of Lon protein and activity in murine hindleg muscle, and this diminished Lon capacity contributed to the significantly higher levels of carbonylated aconitase exhibited in these animals [67]. In the same study, oxidatively challenged old mice, due to a heterozygous MnSOD$^{-/+}$ genotype, displayed significantly lower Lon levels than did wild-type MnSOD$^{+/+}$ old mice [67], further suggesting that there is an inverse correlation between Lon levels and age. In another aging study with rats, the total activity of Lon in old rat livers was about 2.5-fold lower, with a concomitant 52% higher content of ε-carboxymethyllysine (CML) protein in the matrix compared to young rats. These data suggests that the decline in Lon actually contributes to the observed increase in oxidative damage with age [68]. For a direct comparison of Lon downregulation, we used RNA silencing in human fibroblasts and observed that the cells which lack Lon expression not only suffered detrimental cellular defects, but also displayed giant mitochondria with empty giant vacuoles, filled with electron-dense inclusion bodies, loss of cristae, and miniature mitochondria. These pathological phenotypes resemble those of the aging myocytes described earlier [62].

We propose that the proteolytic degradation of damaged proteins is the major role for Lon in maintaining mitochondrial homeostasis. However, Lon is a multi-functional protein, with a unique protein structure, and it has chaperone activity and DNA-binding activity, in addition to proteolysis, and it may even regulate mtDNA replication or transcription. It has been shown that Lon-mediated protein degradation and Lon's chaperone ability to assemble electron transport chain complexes are functionally independent of one another [69]. How these different functions coexist *in vivo* is not well understood; however, we hypothesize that Lon may switch between roles depending on the condition of the mitochondria, and this might help mitochondria to sustain function during a stressful environment. For example, Lon would bind to mtDNA under normal conditions and help maintain genomic functions. In the event of a stress, mtDNA functions

are halted, and Lon will preferentially bind to its protein substrates instead, catalyzing proteolysis or protein refolding until stress conditions subside.

Conclusions

Proteases provide a secondary line of defense against a wide variety of oxidative protein modifications, which threaten the integrity of the cell. The selective degradation of oxidatively damaged proteins enables cells to restore vital protein functions on a continual basis during normal aerobic metabolism and through oxidant stress. A progressive decline in both proteasome [70] and Lon [67] occurs with age, and we propose that these phenomena contribute to the inverse relationship between decreased elimination of oxidized proteins, and the increase in the accumulation of free radical damage typically observed with age.

There is an intricate hierarchy of antioxidant defenses programmed into cells for protection against oxidative damage. Initial lines of defense are diverse and strong, but they are not sufficient for complete prevention against free radical reactions, including protein damage. The accumulation of abnormal proteins slows the rate of degradation of both normal and abnormal proteins, and also promotes cellular aging [71–75]. Numerous studies have reported that protein carbonyls increase with age and can be used as a rough index of oxidative protein damage. In a long-term study of human fibroblasts from 17–80-year-old donors, individuals between 60 and 80 years of age exhibited mitochondrial fraction carbonyls that were much higher than those seen in whole-cell lysates [76]. Several aspects of the aging process in human muscle fibers are related to mitochondrial abnormalities. In s-IBM muscle, common mitochondrial abnormalities include ragged-red fibers, cytochrome oxidase-negative muscle fibers, and mtDNA deletions [2, 77]. These age associated changes within muscles can lead to a predisposition to s-IBM abnormalities, creating a vicious cycle of mitochondrial impairment, creating oxidative stress and the accumulation of protein aggregation [77]. A better understanding of the regulation of both Lon and proteasome would be of great value, and would contribute to the study of aging, especially in the neuromuscular system. Interestingly, a promising study in *Podospora anserina* showed that the overexpression of Lon extends the lifespan of the fungus by 70%, with an associated increase in oxidative damage protection and a higher level of Lon proteolysis [78]. Future studies geared towards understanding how to manipulate Lon expression and activity in mammalian cells and animals may lead to the possibility of treatments that might improve protein quality control, and provide a better quality of life for those with myositis, sarcopenia, or other myopathies.

References

1 Harman D. (1956) Aging: a theory based on free radical and radiation chemistry. *J Gerontol* **11**(3), 298–300.

2 Oldfors A, Moslemi AR, Jonasson L et al. (2006) Mitochondrial abnormalities in inclusion-body myositis. *Neurology* **66** (2 Suppl 1), S49–S55.

3 Askanas V, McFerrin J, Baque S et al. (1996) Transfer of beta-amyloid precursor protein gene using adenovirus vector causes mitochondrial abnormalities in cultured normal human muscle. *Proc Natl Acad Sci USA* **93**(3), 1314–1319.

4 Shringarpure R, Davies K.J.A. (2002) Protein turnover by the proteasome in aging and disease. *Free Radic Biol Med* **32**(11), 1084–1089.

5 Berlett BS, Stadtman ER. (1997) Protein oxidation in aging, disease, and oxidative stress. *J Biol Chem* **272** (33), 20313–20316.

6 Stadtman ER. (1992) Protein oxidation and aging. *Science* **257**(5074), 1220–1224.

7 Grune T, Reinheckel T, Davies K.J.A. (1997) Degradation of oxidized proteins in mammalian cells. *FASEB J* **11**(7), 526–534.

8 Carney JM, Starke-Reed PE, Oliver CN et al. (1991) Reversal of age-related increase in brain protein oxidation, decrease in enzyme activity, and loss in temporal and spatial memory by chronic administration of the spin-trapping compound N-tert-butyl-alpha-phenylnitrone. *Proc Natl Acad Sci USA* **88**(9), 3633–3636.

9 Aksenova MV, Aksenov MY, Carney JM et al. (1998) Protein oxidation and enzyme activity decline in old brown Norway rats are reduced by dietary restriction. *Mech Aging Dev* **100**(2), 157–168.

10 Vittorini S, Paradiso C, Donati A et al. (1999) The age-related accumulation of protein carbonyl in rat liver correlates with the age-related decline in liver proteolytic activities. *J Gerontol A Biol Sci Med Sci* **54**(8), B318–B323.

11 Taylor A, Davies K.J.A. (1987) Protein oxidation and loss of protease activity may lead to cataract formation in the aged lens. *Free Radic Biol Med* **3**(6), 371–377.

12 Leeuwenburgh C, Hansen P, Shaish A et al. (1998) Markers of protein oxidation by hydroxyl radical and reactive nitrogen species in tissues of aging rats. *Am J Physiol Regul Integr Comp Physiol* **274**(2 Pt 2), R453–R461.

13 Stadtman ER, Levine RL. (2000) Protein oxidation. *Ann NY Acad Sci* **899**,191–208.

14 Cadenas E, Davies K.J.A. (2000) Mitochondrial free radical generation, oxidative stress, and aging. *Free Radic Biol Med* **29**(3–4) 222–230.

15 Petropoulos I, Friguet B. (2006) Maintenance of proteins and aging: the role of oxidized protein repair. *Free Radic Res* **40**(12), 1269–1276.

16 Holmgren A. (2000) Antioxidant function of thioredoxin and glutaredoxin systems. *Antioxid Redox Signal* **2** (4), 811–820.

17 Holmgren A, Johansson C, Berndt C et al. (2005) Thiol redox control via thioredoxin and glutaredoxin systems. *Biochem Soc Trans* **33**(6), 1375–1377.

18 Mary J, Vougier S, Picot CR et al. (2004) Enzymatic reactions involved in the repair of oxidized proteins. *Exp Gerontol* **39**(8), 1117–1123.

19 Moskovitz J. (2005) Roles of methionine sulfoxide reductases in antioxidant defense, protein regulation and survival. *Curr Pharm Des* **11**(11), 1451–1457.

20 Ugarte N, Petropoulos I, Friguet B. (2010) Oxidized mitochondrial protein degradation and repair in aging and oxidative stress. *Antioxid Redox Signal* **13**(4), 539–549.

21 Minniti AN, Cataldo R, Trigo C et al. (2009) Methionine sulfoxide reductase A expression is regulated by the DAF-16/FOXO pathway in *Caenorhabditis elegans*. *Aging Cell* **8**(6), 690–705.

22 Ruan H, Tang XD, Chen ML et al. (2002) High-quality life extension by the enzyme peptide methionine sulfoxide reductase. *Proc Natl Acad Sci USA* **99**(5), 2748–2753.

23 Morrow G, Tanguay RM. (2003) Heat shock proteins and aging in *Drosophila melanogaster*. *Semin Cell Dev Biol* **14**(5), 291–299.

24 Wiedemann N, Frazier AE, Pfanner N. (2004) The protein import machinery of mitochondria. *J Biol Chem* **279**(15), 14473–14476.

25 Wang N, Gottesman S, Willingham MC et al. (1993) A human mitochondrial ATP-dependent protease that is highly homologous to bacterial Lon protease. *Proc Natl Acad Sci USA* **90**(23), 11247–11251.

26 Beckman KB, Ames BN. (1998) The free radical theory of aging matures. *Physiol Rev* **78**(2), 547–581.

27 Dukan S, Farewell A, Ballesteros M et al. (2000) Protein oxidation in response to increased transcriptional or translational errors. *Proc Natl Acad Sci USA* **97**(11), 5746–5749.

28 Smith CK, Baker TA, Sauer RT. (1999) Lon and Clp family proteases and chaperones share homologous substrate-recognition domains. *Proc Natl Acad Sci USA* **96**(12), 6678–6682.

29 Ondrovicova G, Liu T, Singh K et al. (2005) Cleavage site selection within a folded substrate by the ATP-dependent lon protease. *J Biol Chem* **280**(26), 25103–25110.

30 Botos I, Melnikov EE, Cherry S et al. (2004) The catalytic domain of *Escherichia coli* Lon protease has a unique fold and a Ser-Lys dyad in the active site. *J Biol Chem* **279**(9), 8140–8148.

31 Keck S, Nitsch R, Grune T et al. (2003) Proteasome inhibition by paired helical filament-tau in brains of patients with Alzheimer's disease. *J Neurochem* **85**(1), 115–122.

32 Lam YA, Pickart CM, Alban A et al. (2000) Inhibition of the ubiquitin-proteasome system in Alzheimer's disease. *Proc Natl Acad Sci USA* **97**(18), 9902–9906.

33 Lindersson E, Beedholm R, Hojrup P et al. (2004) Proteasomal inhibition by alpha-synuclein filaments and oligomers. *J Biol Chem* **279**(13), 12924–34.

34 Lindsten K, de Vrij FM, Verhoef LG et al. (2002) Mutant ubiquitin found in neurodegenerative disorders is a ubiquitin fusion degradation substrate that blocks proteasomal degradation. *J Cell Biol* **157**(3), 417–427.

35 Lopez Salon M, Pasquini L, Besio Moreno M et al. (2003) Relationship between beta-amyloid degradation and the 26S proteasome in neural cells. *Exp Neurol* **180**(2), 131–143.

36 Voges D, Zwickl P, Baumeister W. (1999) The 26S proteasome: a molecular machine designed for controlled proteolysis. *Annu Rev Biochem* **68**, 1015–1068.

37 Sherman MY, Goldberg AL. (2001) Cellular defenses against unfolded proteins: a cell biologist thinks about neurodegenerative diseases. *Neuron* **29**(1), 15–32.

38 McNaught KS, Belizaire R, Isacson O et al. (2003) Altered proteasomal function in sporadic Parkinson's disease. *Exp Neurol* **179**(1), 38–46.

39 Schmidt T, Lindenberg KS, Krebs A et al. (2002) Protein surveillance machinery in brains with spinocerebellar ataxia type 3: redistribution and differential recruitment of 26S proteasome subunits and chaperones to neuronal intranuclear inclusions. *Ann Neurol* **51**(3), 302–310.

40 Keller JN, Hanni KB, Markesbery WR. (2000) Impaired proteasome function in Alzheimer's disease. *J Neurochem* **75**(1), 436–439.

41 Askanas V, Engel WK. (2008) Inclusion-body myositis: muscle-fiber molecular pathology and possible pathogenic significance of its similarity to Alzheimer's and Parkinson's disease brains. *Acta Neuropathol* **116**(6), 583–595.

42 Askanas V, Engel WK. (2003) Proposed pathogenetic cascade of inclusion-body myositis: importance of amyloid-beta, misfolded proteins, predisposing genes, and aging. *Curr Opin Rheumatol* **15**(6), 737–744.

43 Askanas V, Engel WK. (2001) Inclusion-body myositis: newest concepts of pathogenesis and relation to aging and Alzheimer disease. *J Neuropathol Exp Neurol* **60**(1), 1–14.

44 Fratta P, Engel WK, McFerrin J et al. (2005) Proteasome inhibition and aggresome formation in sporadic inclusion-body myositis and in amyloid-beta precursor protein-overexpressing cultured human muscle fibers. *Am J Pathol* **167**(2), 517–526.

45 Junn E, Lee SS, Suhr UT et al. (2002) Parkin accumulation in aggresomes due to proteasome impairment. *J Biol Chem* **277**(49), 47870–47877.

46 Bence NF, Sampat RM, Kopito RR. (2001) Impairment of the ubiquitin-proteasome system by protein aggregation. *Science* **292**(5521), 1552–1555.

47 Klein WL. (2002) ADDLs & protofibrils–the missing links? *Neurobiol Aging* **23**(2), 231–235.

48 Ellis RJ, Pinheiro TJ. (2002) Medicine: danger–misfolding proteins. *Nature* **416**(6880), 483–484.

49 Harman D. (1972) The biologic clock: the mitochondria? *J Am Geriatr Soc* **20**(4), 145–147.

50 Ames BN, Shigenaga MK, Hagen TM. (1995) Mitochondrial decay in aging. *Biochim Biophys Acta* **1271**(1), 165–170.

51 Brunk UT, Terman A. (2002) The mitochondrial-lysosomal axis theory of aging: accumulation of damaged mitochondria as a result of imperfect autophagocytosis. *Eur J Biochem* **269**(8), 1996–2002.

52 Strehler B. (1977) *Time, Cells, and Aging*, 2nd edn. Academic Press, New York.

53 Terman A, Brunk UT. (2004) Myocyte aging and mitochondrial turnover. *Exp Gerontol* **39**(5), 701–705.

54 Sachs HG, Colgan JA, Lazarus ML. (1977) Ultrastructure of the aging myocardium: a morphometric approach. *Am J Anat* **150**(1), 63–71.

55 Coleman R, Silbermann M, Gershon D et al. (1987) Giant mitochondria in the myocardium of aging and endurance-trained mice. *Gerontology* **33**(1), 34–39.

56 Beregi E, Regius O, Huttl T et al. (1988) Age-related changes in the skeletal muscle cells. *Z Gerontol* **21**(2), 83–86.

57 Carry MR, Horan SE, Reed SM et al. (1993) Structure, innervation, and age-associated changes of mouse forearm muscles. *Anat Rec* **237**(3), 345–357.

58 Lin AT, Hsu TH, Yang C et al. (2000) Effects of aging on mitochondrial enzyme activity of rat urinary bladder. *Urol Int* **65**(3), 144–147.

59 Marcell TJ. (2003) Sarcopenia: causes, consequences, and preventions. *J Gerontol A Biol Sci Med Sci* **58**(10), M911–6.

60 Askanas V, Engel WK. (1998) Sporadic inclusion-body myositis and hereditary inclusion-body myopathies: diseases of oxidative stress and aging? *Arch Neurol* **55**(7), 915–920.

61 Frolkis VV, Frolkis RA, Mkhitarian LS et al. (1988) Contractile function and Ca2 + transport system of myocardium in aging. *Gerontology* **34**(1–2) 64–74.

62 Terman A, Dalen H, Eaton JW et al. (2003) Mitochondrial recycling and aging of cardiac myocytes: the role of autophagocytosis. *Exp Gerontol* **38**(8), 863–876.

63 Ermini M. (1976) Aging changes in mammalian skeletal muscle: biochemical studies. *Gerontology* **22**(4), 301–316.

64 Bota DA, Ngo JK, Davies K.J.A. (2005) Downregulation of the human Lon protease impairs mitochondrial structure and function and causes cell death. *Free Radic Biol Med* **38**(5), 665–677.

65 Ngo JK, Davies K.J.A. (2009) Mitochondrial Lon protease is a human stress protein. *Free Radic Biol Med* **46**(8), 1042–1048.

66 Lee CK, Klopp RG, Weindruch R et al. (1999) Gene expression profile of aging and its retardation by caloric restriction. *Science* **285**(5432), 1390–1393.

67 Bota DA, Van Remmen H, Davies K.J.A. (2002) Modulation of Lon protease activity and aconitase turnover during aging and oxidative stress. *FEBS Lett* **532**(1–2) 103–106.

68 Bakala H, Delaval E, Hamelin M et al. (2003) Changes in rat liver mitochondria with aging. Lon protease-like reactivity and N(epsilon)-carboxymethyllysine accumulation in the matrix. *Eur J Biochem* **270**(10), 2295–2302.

69 Rep M, van Dijl JM, Suda K et al. (1996) Promotion of mitochondrial membrane complex assembly by a proteolytically inactive yeast Lon. *Science* **274**(5284), 103–106.

70 Shringarpure R, Grune T, Davies K.J.A. (2001) Protein oxidation and 20S proteasome-dependent proteolysis in mammalian cells. *Cell Mol Life Sci* **58**(10), 1442–1450.

71 Cuervo AM. (2008) Autophagy and aging: keeping that old broom working. *Trends Genet* **24**(12), 604–612.

72 Guarente L, Kenyon C. (2000) Genetic pathways that regulate aging in model organisms. *Nature* **408**(6809), 255–262.

73 Hekimi S, Guarente L. (2003) Genetics and the specificity of the aging process. *Science* **299**(5611), 1351–1354.

74 Kirkwood TB, Austad SN. (2000) Why do we age? *Nature* **408**(6809), 233–238.

75 Vellai T. (2009) Autophagy genes and aging. *Cell Death Differ* **16**(1), 94–102.

76 Miyoshi N, Oubrahim H, Chock PB et al. (2006) Age-dependent cell death and the role of ATP in hydrogen peroxide-induced apoptosis and necrosis. *Proc Natl Acad Sci USA* **103**(6), 1727–1731.

77 Santorelli FM, Sciacco M, Tanji K et al. (1996) Multiple mitochondrial DNA deletions in sporadic inclusion body myositis: a study of 56 patients. *Ann Neurol* **39**(6), 789–795.

78 Luce K, Osiewacz HD. (2009) Increasing organismal healthspan by enhancing mitochondrial protein quality control. *Nat Cell Biol* **11**(7), 852–858.

CHAPTER 6

Human muscle protein metabolism in relation to exercise and aging: potential therapeutic applications

Micah J. Drummond[1] *and Blake B. Rasmussen*[2]
[1]Department of Physical Therapy, University of Utah, Salt Lake City, UT, USA
[2]Department of Nutrition & Metabolism, Division of Rehabilitation Sciences, Sealy Center on Aging, University of Texas Medical Branch, Galveston, TX, USA

Introduction

Senescence is an inevitable process in humans. However, medical interventions, improvements in social and behavioral patterns, and renewed exercise and nutritional patterns have lengthened lifespan. As the aging population continues to increase, a consequence that will need to be attended to is age-related sarcopenia. A hallmark characterization of sarcopenia is a gradual loss in skeletal muscle mass and strength. However, identifying the sarcopenic process in a single person is more difficult since this would require decades of measurements. Clinically, sarcopenia is defined as an appendicular skeletal muscle mass/height^2 less than two standard deviations below the mean for populations of young, healthy adults [1]. Loss of skeletal muscle occurs at a rate of approximately 1–2% per year beyond the fifth decade of life [2] and, on average, approximately 35% of quadriceps cross-sectional area is reduced by the age of 70 [3, 4]. The prevalence of sarcopenia is about 10–24% in people aged 65 to 70 years while this value increases to 50% in people over the age of 80 [5, 6]. Since skeletal muscle contains the largest bulk of proteins in comparison to the existing cells in the human body (50–75%) [7] and is important for locomotion and performing daily tasks, significant reductions in skeletal muscle mass (sarcopenia) can reduce strength, increase falls and fractures, limit independence, and, ultimately, increase morbidity [8–11]. Therefore, it is of great value to reduce or restore the muscle loss that accompanies aging. Although great strides have been achieved, the mechanisms of aging skeletal muscle loss are still mostly unknown.

Muscle mass: a dynamic balancing act

Simply put, muscle size is determined by an intricate balance of muscle protein synthesis and breakdown (Figure 6.1). Both processes are critical: muscle protein synthesis makes new proteins while protein breakdown removes damaged ones. When synthesis of new proteins exceeds protein breakdown over time – due to increases in muscle protein synthesis, decreases in breakdown, or both – net protein balance is positive and muscle cell size increases. This is termed muscle hypertrophy. An increase in muscle cell size can easily be identified following a resistance exercise training paradigm complemented with adequate nutritional intake (e.g., essential amino acids). Alternatively, when protein breakdown

Muscle Aging, Inclusion-Body Myositis and Myopathies, First Edition. Edited by Valerie Askanas and W. King Engel.
© 2012 Blackwell Publishing Ltd. Published 2012 by Blackwell Publishing Ltd.

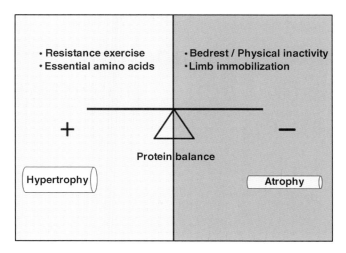

Figure 6.1 Simplified model of protein turnover represented by a plank resting on a fulcrum. Muscle protein balance tips in the positive direction (light shade) when protein synthesis is enhanced, breakdown is decreased, or both, resulting in muscle-mass increases (hypertrophy). This is commonly seen with resistance exercise and essential amino acid supplementation. Muscle protein balance tips toward the negative direction (dark shade) when protein breakdown is accelerated, synthesis is decreased, or both, resulting in muscle-mass decreases (atrophy). This can be seen in models of disuse such as bedrest/ physical inactivity and limb immobilization.

exceeds muscle protein synthesis – due to increases in protein breakdown, decreases in muscle protein synthesis, or both – net protein balance is negative and muscle cell size decreases. This is termed muscle atrophy. A decrease in muscle cell size can quickly be identified within days of bedrest or physical inactivity and limb immobilization but age-related sarcopenia, a much slower process, may take years or even decades for muscle loss to be recognized.

Muscle protein turnover: key intracellular signaling pathways

A series of peer-reviewed publications have emphasized that muscle protein synthesis (rather than breakdown) is primarily responsible for regulating muscle mass following various models of muscle atrophy [12] and possibly with sarcopenia. Therefore, research has focused on cellular mechanisms that control muscle protein synthesis, i.e., the regulation of mRNA translation initiation and elongation via the mammalian target of rapamycin (mTORC1) pathway. Many elegant reviews thoroughly detail this cellular sigaling cascade and discuss how essential amino acids, resistance exercise, and insulin feed in through this pathway at various points [13, 14]. However, other cellular pathways may also contribute to regulating muscle hypertrophy [15]. When

the mTORC1 pathway is upregulated, translation initiation and elongation is enhanced and muscle protein synthesis increased (Figure 6.2). mTORC1 has two primary targets that enhance translation initiation and elongation: ribosomal S6 kinase 1 (S6K1) and 4E-binding protein 1 (4E-BP1). Phosphorylation of 4E-BP1 releases its inhibition on eukaryotic initiation factor 4E while phosphorylation of S6K1 can target at least nine other proteins [16]. The two most studied are ribosomal S6 [17] and eukaryotic elongation factor 2 (eEF2) [18]. The contraction-induced mTORC1 activation was previously thought to occur via Akt [19]. However, recent evidence has linked muscle contraction to the activation of phospholipase D1 and D2 (PLD). PLD synthesizes phosphatidic acid which binds and activates mTORC1 [20–22]. Anabolic signals enter through another well-known signaling route, the extracellular signal-regulated kinase 1/2 (ERK1/2) pathway. In this circumstance, ERK signaling converges on the mTORC1 pathway through inhibition of tuberous sclerosis complex 2 (a negative regulator of mTORC1) [23, 24], activation of rpS6 by p90 ribosomal protein S6 kinase polypeptide 1 (RSK1) [17], and/or inhibition of eEF2 kinase (a negative regulator of eEF2) [18]. ERK signaling can also stimulate translation initiation independent of mTORC1 through mitogen-activating protein kinase-interacting kinase 1 (MNK1) [25].

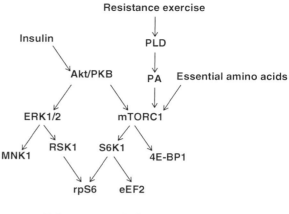

Figure 6.2 Essential amino acids, resistance exercise, and insulin activate the mammalian target of rapamycin (mTORC1) pathway and enhance translation initiation and elongation, therefore increasing muscle protein synthesis. 4E-BP1, 4E 4E-binding protein 1; Akt/PKB, protein kinase B; eEF2, eukaryotic elongation factor 2; ERK1/2, extracellular signal-regulated kinase 1/2; MNK1, mitogen-activating protein kinase-interacting kinase 1; PA, phosphatidic acid; PLD, phospholipase D1 and D2; rpS6, ribosomal protein S6; RSK1, p90 ribosomal protein S6 kinase polypeptide 1; mTORC1, mammalian target of rapamycin; S6K1, ribosomal S6 kinase 1.

Most cellular signaling data associated with protein turnover have been collected in *Drosophila*, cell lines, and rodents. In the forthcoming paragraphs we will briefly summarize the literature with the latest understanding of the cellular and molecular mechanisms associated with human age-related muscle wasting in response to nutrition and exercise, then detail potential therapeutic interventions that may counteract age-related muscle loss.

Contributions of muscle wasting

Dysregulated protein turnover rates at rest?

Overwhelming data indicate altered basal gene and protein expression levels of molecules associated with protein anabolism and catabolism in older subjects [26–30] and it seems likely that basal protein turnover would likewise be affected. Although some report slower muscle protein synthesis rates in older human skeletal muscle [31, 32] and different rates between older men and women [33], our research group [34] and others [35] have found no detectable differences in muscle protein synthesis compared to the young. Similarly, the rate of breakdown also appears to be the same between age groups [34, 36–39]. The fact that differences in protein synthesis and breakdown are not detectable

at rest between the age groups is not surprising. For instance, using a similar example as presented in Volpi et al. [34], if a difference as little as 10% in basal protein synthesis were detected between young and old subjects (assuming that an individual is in the basal state for approximately 16 h/day and that the response to feeding and other stimuli are constant with aging), this would result in a 17% loss of skeletal muscle in 1 year. Realistically, sarcopenia is a gradual loss in skeletal muscle occurring over decades and any changes in protein turnover (protein synthesis or breakdown) from day to day would be too small to detect even with the most advanced technologies. Therefore, a probable hypothesis to the gradual loss of muscle mass in older adults is that aged skeletal muscle has a reduced acute response to anabolic stimuli (i.e., resistance exercise, feeding).

Anabolic resistance to insulin and amino acids

Essential amino acids (in particular leucine) and insulin are powerful stimulators of muscle anabolism in young, healthy muscle [40–42]. Although the old are capable of responding positively to anabolic nutrients, numerous studies have indicated that when insulin is infused alone or amino acids and carbohydrate are co-ingested, the anabolic response is attenuated or blunted in comparison to the young [38, 43–45]. For instance, Guillet et al. reported that, following an insulin and amino acid intravenous infusion, older subjects had a reduced muscle protein synthesis response and mTORC1 signaling (e.g., S6K1 phosphorylation) compared to younger individuals [44]. It has been suggested that this anabolic resistance may be partially attributed to a reduced ability of insulin to vasodilate the endothelium and deliver nutrients to the muscle [42, 43, 46]. Fujita et al. showed a nice relationship between muscle protein synthesis and blood flow following a supraphysiological insulin infusion in older adults [46]. In this study, a high insulin infusion stimulated muscle protein synthesis, mTORC1 signaling and muscle blood flow but a normal increase in insulin did not [46]. Interestingly, this insulin resistance can be counteracted with an acute bout of aerobic exercise [47]. Anabolic resistance can also be identified in older persons following ingestion of amino acids [45, 48]. The mechanism of resistance to amino acids is unclear, but since amino acids can increase insulin levels, the level of dysfunction may also be at the endothelium. However, amino acids can activate mTORC1 independent of insulin (Figure 6.2) [49, 50]. It is unknown whether impairment may also occur along this nutrient-sensitive pathway.

Anabolic resistance to exercise

Physical activity is a key factor in reducing physical disability [9–11]. The best known protection against the effects of age-related muscle loss is the use of resistance exercise training. Resistance exercise training is well known to increase muscle protein synthesis [36, 51], skeletal muscle mass [37, 52–54], and strength [55–57] in older adults and even in frail elders [57]. However, resistance exercise training studies typically show an attenuated muscle anabolic response in older compared to younger adults [37, 54, 58] or, in the case of older women (>85 years), anabolic responses are blunted [59]. Furthermore, many researchers have repeatedly indicated that older adults have an altered anabolic response at the gene and protein level during the early recovery hours following a single bout of resistance exercise [26, 27, 60–64]. In a recent study, Sheffield-Moore and coworkers showed unchanged muscle protein synthesis 3 h after a single bout of resistance exercise in older

adults [65]. This was later confirmed in a study by Kumar and colleagues that found blunted muscle protein synthesis and cellular signaling (identified by S6K1 and 4E-BP1 phosphorylation) in older adults (versus younger adults) following a single bout of resistance exercise at intensities of 60–90% of the individual's one repetition maximum (1RM) [66]. In another study by Mayhew et al. older adults had an unresponsive muscle protein synthesis response while mTORC1 signaling was dysregulated 24 h following a single bout of resistance exercise [67]. These data are in stark contrast to young muscle, which responds robustly with an increase in muscle protein synthesis and mTORC1 signaling 1–48 h following an acute bout of resistance exercise [66–68]. In previous work, we suggested that the impaired anabolic response (either acutely or with repeated bouts of exercise) in older adults may be due (in part) to not being able to generate the same level of muscular tension (in spite of exercising at the same relative intensity) as the young during a bout of heavy resistance exercise [62]. In support, phosphorylation of ERK1/2 and MNK1 were increased in the young but unchanged in older subjects [62]. A purported hypothesis is that older adults have an increase in markers of cellular stress that may affect the remodeling response following resistance exercise [62, 69, 70]. Perhaps AMP-activated protein kinase, a negative regulator of muscle protein synthesis, plays a role as it was seen to be elevated in older (but not in the young) subjects following resistance exercise [62]. Although older adults do experience improvement in muscle mass and strength following resistance exercise training [37, 54, 71], these responses are less than those seen in young healthy subjects. Together, these data suggest that older adults have an impaired anabolic response to both acute and chronic resistance exercise training as compared to their younger counterparts.

Summary

It is very probable that anabolic resistance to nutrition and/or exercise contributes to age-related muscle loss. More likely, sarcopenia is a very complex process caused by a multiplicity of events, some of which have been mentioned above. However, other contributors of sarcopenia that are beyond the scope of this chapter include neuromuscular impairments, hormonal deficiencies, low-grade chronic inflammation, and apoptosis. We recommend the following review articles for insight into these areas: [72–75].

Therapeutic interventions to prevent/restore muscle wasting

Nutritional supplementation

Inadequate protein intake and a reduced anabolic response to nutrients may be contributing factors to age-related loss in skeletal muscle [76, 77]. Therefore, protein quantity must be considered to maximize muscle protein anabolic responses. Reports have uncovered that the muscle protein synthesis response is the same between young and older adults when the amino acid or protein dosage is of sufficient amount (10–15 g of essential amino acids) [35, 78]. For this reason, some have suggested that the protein intake for older adults be increased from the recommended daily allowance of 0.8 g/kg/day [79, 80]. Another useful strategy may be to optimize the specific amino acid profile, such as increasing the amount of leucine. Katsanos et al. showed that an amino acid mixture containing 41% leucine (2.79 g) was more effective at eliciting an increase in muscle protein synthesis than about half the dose (26%) in older subjects [81]. Leucine is a key branched-chain amino acid that stimulates muscle protein synthesis through the mTORC1 pathway [41] while simultaneously slightly reducing muscle protein breakdown [82], with the overall effect of improving muscle protein turnover. There also appears to be a maximal muscle protein synthesis response to a given amount of ingested protein. Symons et al. indicated that 30 g of protein was sufficient to stimulate muscle protein synthesis in older subjects, but a dosage of 90 g did not increase muscle protein synthesis [78]. Therefore, utilizing the correct amino acid or protein dose ($\approx$30 g of protein; 10–15 g of essential amino acids) and supplementing meals with extra leucine may stimulate muscle protein synthesis and intracellular signaling in older human skeletal muscle.

Few data are available on chronic protein supplementation to improve the muscle protein synthesis response in older adults. Rieu et al. showed that when meals are supplemented with leucine over a single day, the protein anabolic response to feeding is improved in older adults [83]. However, the therapeutic potential of supplementing with leucine is suspect. Recently, Verhoeven and colleagues performed a 12-week intervention in older adults in which they supplemented leucine (2.5 g) with each meal (7.5 g/day) [84]. Unfortunately, muscle mass or strength was not improved [84] over that of a group receiving a placebo. It is unclear if a longer period of leucine supplementation (i.e., 1 year) is needed or perhaps in persons such as the frail elderly or those with other muscle wasting conditions chronic leucine supplementation would be of significant benefit. Furthermore, supplementing with high quantities of protein in older adults may impair renal function [85]. Leucine supplementation may be less of a physiological concern in older adults [85] if supplementation was intermittent (i.e., 1 day on, 1 day off). Whatever the case, supplementation with leucine may prove to be a noteworthy intervention for age-related muscle loss.

Resistance exercise and nutritional supplementation

As mentioned previously, following an acute bout of resistance exercise, muscle protein synthesis rapidly increases within 1 h [68] and can remain elevated up to 24–48 h post-exercise in young, healthy participants [86, 87]. When resistance exercise is performed independently of nutrient intake, protein breakdown exceeds synthesis and protein balance is negative [88, 89]. However, when nutrients in the form of amino acids or protein are given shortly after a bout of resistance exercise, muscle protein balance is positive [41, 90]. Research from our laboratory and others have shown that nutrition, whether in the form of amino acids or protein, given after exercise augments the acute muscle protein synthesis response [41, 91–93]. Furthermore, resistance exercise training combined with protein supplementation has been shown to increase muscle mass [52, 94–99] and muscle growth markers [98, 99] beyond that of resistance exercise alone.

When nutrition in the form of amino acids is given to older adults after a heavy bout of resistance exercise, muscle protein synthesis increases to a similar extent, albeit delayed, compared to young adults [62]. However, if muscle protein synthesis is calculated over the entire 6 h post-resistance exercise period, the response was similar between age groups [62]. This result has also been supported by Koopman et al. [100]. It remains unknown if muscle protein synthesis in the old continues to be elevated beyond 6 h post-resistance exercise and protein ingestion, or diverges from the anabolic response found in young subjects. There also appears to be a critical time period in which to ingest amino acids following a resistance-exercise bout. After a 12-week resistance-exercise training program, older subjects who consumed a 10 g protein mixture immediately after the exercise bout experienced muscle hypertrophy while this was not the case in another group of older adults that consumed protein 2 h later [52]. Therefore, providing nutritional supplementation (e.g., essential amino acids, protein) in combination with each resistance exercise session may maximize muscle size following a resistance-exercise training program in older adults [101]. There is some disagreement on the effectiveness of combining protein supplementation with resistance exercise. Verdijk et al. found that protein supplementation taken before and after each resistance exercise session during a 12-week resistance-exercise training program in healthy, older adults did not further enhance muscle anabolic responses in comparison to a placebo group [102]. However, the authors may not have seen an effect since the total amount of essential amino acids consumed was rather low and protein synthesis is not enhanced when amino acids are consumed prior to resistance exercise [103]. Future interventions in sarcopenic populations should utilize a larger amount of essential amino acids consumed during the post-exercise recovery period. We have recently shown that this approach is successful in older men following an acute bout of exercise [62].

Blood-flow restriction exercise

It is generally accepted that a resistance exercise program must be of sufficient intensity to increase muscle mass. The American College of Sports Medicine recommends that exercise intensity be at least 70% of the 1RM to achieve maximum muscle hypertrophy [104]. However, for most older individuals, such resistance-exercise intensity is too great to complete or perform, especially in those with osteoarthritis, frailty, or following surgery undergoing a rehabilitation program. Recent attention has focused on resistance exercise that requires intensities ranging around 20–50% 1RM. In normal circumstances, resistance exercise at a low load is more useful for improving muscular endurance [104] with little improvement in muscle size [105]. Initially popularized in Japan, when low-intensity resistance exercise (20–50% 1RM) is combined with moderate blood-flow restriction (BFR), muscle mass and strength increase, even to a similar extent as traditional resistance exercise [106–111]. Low-intensity BFR is characterized by a high number of repetitions (15–45) of each set performed to fatigue, while blood flow is restricted (predominately venous blood flow) typically through a pressurized cuff around the proximal thigh. It is only after completion of several sets that the pressure is released from the cuff. Manini et al. provide a recent review of the topic of BFR exercise [112].

Several laboratories have taken steps to understand the metabolic and molecular mechanisms of BFR. Evidence from our laboratory suggests that translation initiation through the mTORC1 pathway is acutely enhanced following BFR [113], while gene transcription is unaffected [114]. In our study, phosphorylation of S6K1 and muscle protein synthesis were increased within hours of a single bout of BFR exercise (20% 1RM), while these changes were not observed following low-intensity resistance exercise without BFR in young, healthy adults [113]. Interestingly, we have also observed these results in healthy older men following BFR exercise. Perhaps BFR causes type 2 muscle fibers to be recruited [115] through a premature fatigue of active fibers. This would seem logical, since type 2 muscle fibers express more S6K1 than do type 1 muscle fibers [116]. Another possible mechanism would be through hormonal regulation. The most common hormonal feature following a bout of BFR exercise is an increase in growth hormone and cortisol [110, 113] similar to that found in high-intensity resistance-exercise paradigms [117]. The role of these hormones is unclear, other than as an acute cellular "stress" mechanism since, at least in the case of growth hormone, muscle hypertrophy can occur in the absence of anabolic hormones [118].

Of immediate concern is the safety of performing BFR, especially in older, diseased, and physically limited populations. Few studies on safety measures have been done following acute [119] and chronic [120–122] bouts of BFR exercise. Recent reports suggest that BFR exercise training produces minor adverse advents in healthy, young adults. Nakajima et al. conducted a national study in Japan to determine the effects of BFR during exercise training [120]. The most common side effect was localized bruising while smaller incidents of numbness and lightheadedness were reported [120]. Others have reported no effect on prothrombin time or markers of coagulation [122], while only a few cases of venous thrombosis were indicated [121]. Although the concern of BFR is far from exhaustive, data on the relative safety of BFR in older persons are limited. The only information available at this time is from a small pilot study conducted by our research group in which we recruited seven healthy, older men to perform a single bout of low-intensity resistance exercise with BFR. In this instance, a D-dimer test (a fibrin-degradation product) showed no change immediately following BFR exercise in comparison to before exercise. While more confidence will need to be accumulated, particularly in the healthcare setting, before BFR can become a rehabilitative tool in older persons, the data so far are promising.

Summary

Interventions such as leucine supplementation, ingestion of an adequate amount of essential amino acids or protein following traditional resistance exercise, and low-load BFR to prevent and reverse muscle loss with aging seem hopeful. The key to all of these therapeutic techniques is in their ability to overcome anabolic resistance to exercise and nutrients by stimulating muscle protein synthesis and translation initiation through the mTORC1 pathway.

Conclusion

Human sarcopenia, characterized by a gradual loss in muscle mass and strength, can be partly attributed to reductions in sensitivity to anabolic stimuli such as essential amino acids, insulin, and resistance exercise. Overcoming anabolic resistance in older muscle is the focus of our proposed therapeutic interventions. Appropriate protein amounts and quality, combining resistance exercise with protein/essential amino acid ingestion following exercise, and the implementation of BFR, are cost-effective and practical measures by which to reverse or attenuate the muscular decline due to aging.

References

1 Iannuzzi-Sucich M, Prestwood KM, Kenny AM. (2002) Prevalence of sarcopenia and predictors of skeletal muscle mass in healthy, older men and women. *J Gerontol A Biol Sci Med Sci* **57**, M772–M777.

2 Hughes VA, Frontera WR, Roubenoff R et al. (2002) Longitudinal changes in body composition in older men and women: role of body weight change and physical activity. *Am J Clin Nutr* **76**, 473–481.

3 Young A, Stokes M, Crowe M. (1985) The size and strength of the quadriceps muscles of old and young men. *Clin Physiol* **5**, 145–154.

4 Young A, Stokes M, Crowe M. (1984) Size and strength of the quadriceps muscles of old and young women. *Eur J Clin Invest* **14**, 282–287.

5 Melton 3rd LJ, Khosla S, Riggs BL. (2000) Epidemiology of sarcopenia. *Mayo Clin Proc* **75** (Suppl), S10–S12; discussion S12–S13.

6 Janssen I, Heymsfield SB, Ross R. (2002) Low relative skeletal muscle mass (sarcopenia) in older persons is associated with functional impairment and physical disability. *J Am Geriatr Soc* **50**, 889–896.

7 Matthews DE. (1999) *Proteins and amino acids*. In: Shils ME, Olson JA, Shike M, Ross AC (eds), *Modern Nutrition and Health and Disease*. Williams and Wilkins, Baltimore, MD pp. 11–48.

8 Fried LP, Hadley EC, Walston JD et al. (2005) From bedside to bench: research agenda for frailty. *Sci Aging Knowledge Environ* **2005**, pe24.

9 Ferrucci L, Izmirlian G, Leveille S et al. (1999) Smoking, physical activity, and active life expectancy. *Am J Epidemiol* **149**, 645–653.

10 Leveille SG, Guralnik JM, Ferrucci L et al. (1999) Aging successfully until death in old age: opportunities for increasing active life expectancy. *Am J Epidemiol* **149**, 654–664.

11 Ruiz JR, Sui X, Lobelo F et al. (2008) Association between muscular strength and mortality in men: prospective cohort study. *BMJ* **337**, a439.

12 Phillips SM, Glover EI, Rennie MJ. (2009) Alterations of protein turnover underlying disuse atrophy in human skeletal muscle. *J Appl Physiol* **107**, 645–654.

13 Drummond MJ, Dreyer HC, Fry CS et al. (2009) Nutritional and contractile regulation of human skeletal muscle protein synthesis and mTORC1 signaling. *J Appl Physiol* **106**, 1374–1384.

14 Wang X, Proud CG. (2006) The mTOR pathway in the control of protein synthesis. *Physiology (Bethesda)* **21**, 362–369.

15 Glass DJ. (2003) Signalling pathways that mediate skeletal muscle hypertrophy and atrophy. *Nat Cell Biol* **5**, 87–90.

16 Ruvinsky I, Meyuhas O. (2006) Ribosomal protein S6 phosphorylation: from protein synthesis to cell size. *Trends Biochem Sci* **31**, 342–348.

17 Roux PP, Shahbazian D, Vu H et al. (2007) RAS/ERK signaling promotes site-specific ribosomal protein S6 phosphorylation via RSK and stimulates cap-dependent translation. *J Biol Chem* **282**, 14056–14064.

18 Wang X, Li W, Williams M et al. (2001) Regulation of elongation factor 2 kinase by p90(RSK1) and p70 S6 kinase. *EMBO J.* **20**, 4370–4379.

19 Sakamoto K, Hirshman MF, Aschenbach WG et al. (2002) Contraction regulation of Akt in rat skeletal muscle. *J Biol Chem* **277**, 11910–11917.

20 Hornberger TA, Chien S. (2006) Mechanical stimuli and nutrients regulate rapamycin-sensitive signaling through distinct mechanisms in skeletal muscle. *J Cell Biochem* **97**, 1207–1216.

21 O'Neil TK, Duffy LR, Frey JW et al. (2009) The role of phosphoinositide 3-kinase and phosphatidic acid in the regulation of mammalian target of rapamycin following eccentric contractions. *J Physiol* **587**, 3691–3701.

22 Hornberger TA, Chu WK, Mak YW et al. (2006) The role of phospholipase D and phosphatidic acid in the mechanical activation of mTOR signaling in skeletal muscle. *Proc Natl Acad Sci USA* **103**, 4741–4746.

23 Ma L, Chen Z, Erdjument-Bromage H et al. (2005) Phosphorylation and functional inactivation of TSC2 by Erk implications for tuberous sclerosis and cancer pathogenesis. *Cell* **121**, 179–193.

24 Rolfe M, McLeod LE, Pratt PF et al. (2005) Activation of protein synthesis in cardiomyocytes by the hypertrophic agent phenylephrine requires the activation of ERK and involves phosphorylation of tuberous sclerosis complex 2 (TSC2). *Biochem J.* **388**, 973–984.

25 Wang X, Yue P, Chan CB et al. (2007) Inhibition of mammalian target of rapamycin induces phosphatidylinositol 3-kinase-dependent and Mnk-mediated eukaryotic translation initiation factor 4E phosphorylation. *Mol Cell Biol* **27**, 7405–7413.

26 Jozsi AC, Dupont-Versteegden EE, Taylor-Jones JM et al. (2000) Aged human muscle demonstrates an altered gene expression profile consistent with an impaired response to exercise. *Mech Ageing Dev* **120**, 45–56.

27 Drummond MJ, Miyazaki M, Dreyer HC et al. (2009) Expression of growth-related genes in young and older human skeletal muscle following an acute stimulation of protein synthesis. *J Appl Physiol* **106**, 1403–1411.

28 Raue U, Slivka D, Jemiolo B et al. (2006) Myogenic gene expression at rest and after a bout of resistance exercise in young (18–30 yr) and old (80–89 yr) women. *J Appl Physiol* **101**, 53–59.

29 Welle S, Brooks AI, Delehanty JM et al. (2004) Skeletal muscle gene expression profiles in 20–29 year old and 65–71 year old women. *Exp Gerontol* **39**, 369–377.

30 Welle S, Brooks AI, Delehanty JM et al. (2003) Gene expression profile of aging in human muscle. *Physiol Genomics* **14**, 149–159.

31 Welle S, Thornton C, Statt M et al. (1994) Postprandial myofibrillar and whole body protein synthesis in young and old human subjects. *Am J Physiol Endocrinol Metab* **267**, E599–E604.

32 Balagopal P, Rooyackers OE, Adey DB et al. (1997) Effects of aging on in vivo synthesis of skeletal muscle myosin heavy-chain and sarcoplasmic protein in humans. *Am J Physiol Endocrinol Metab* **273**, E790–E800.

33 Smith GI, Atherton P, Villareal DT et al. (2008) Differences in muscle protein synthesis and anabolic signaling in the postabsorptive state and in response to food in 65–80 year old men and women. *PLoS One* **3**, e1875.

34 Volpi E, Sheffield-Moore M, Rasmussen BB et al. (2001) Basal muscle amino acid kinetics and protein synthesis in healthy young and older men. *JAMA* **286**, 1206–1212.

35 Paddon-Jones D, Sheffield-Moore M, Zhang XJ et al. (2004) Amino acid ingestion improves muscle

protein synthesis in the young and elderly. *Am J Physiol Endocrinol Metab* **286**, E321–E328.

36 Yarasheski KE, Zachwieja JJ, Bier DM. (1993) Acute effects of resistance exercise on muscle protein synthesis rate in young and elderly men and women. *Am J Physiol Endocrinol Metab* **265**, E210–E214.

37 Welle S, Thornton C, Statt M. (1995) Myofibrillar protein synthesis in young and old human subjects after three months of resistance training. *Am J Physiol Endocrinol Metab* **268**, E422–E427.

38 Volpi E, Mittendorfer B, Rasmussen BB et al. (2000) The response of muscle protein anabolism to combined hyperaminoacidemia and glucose-induced hyperinsulinemia is impaired in the elderly. *J Clin Endocrinol Metab* **85**, 4481–4490.

39 Hasten DL, Pak-Loduca J, Obert KA et al. (2000) Resistance exercise acutely increases MHC and mixed muscle protein synthesis rates in 78–84 and 23–32 yr olds. *Am J Physiol Endocrinol Metab* **278**, E620–E626.

40 Fujita S, Dreyer HC, Drummond MJ et al. (2007) Nutrient signalling in the regulation of human muscle protein synthesis. *J Physiol* **582**, 813–823.

41 Dreyer HC, Drummond MJ, Pennings B et al. (2008) Leucine-enriched essential amino acid and carbohydrate ingestion following resistance exercise enhances mTOR signaling and protein synthesis in human muscle. *Am J Physiol Endocrinol Metab* **294**, E392–E400.

42 Fujita S, Rasmussen BB, Cadenas JG et al. (2006) Effect of insulin on human skeletal muscle protein synthesis is modulated by insulin-induced changes in muscle blood flow and amino acid availability. *Am J Physiol Endocrinol Metab* **291**, E745–E754.

43 Rasmussen BB, Fujita S, Wolfe RR et al. (2006) Insulin resistance of muscle protein metabolism in aging. *FASEB J.* **20**, 768–769.

44 Guillet C, Prod'homme M, Balage M et al. (2004) Impaired anabolic response of muscle protein synthesis is associated with S6K1 dysregulation in elderly humans. *FASEB J.* **18**, 1586–1587.

45 Cuthbertson D, Smith K, Babraj J et al. (2005) Anabolic signaling deficits underlie amino acid resistance of wasting, aging muscle. *FASEB J.* **19**, 422–424.

46 Fujita S, Glynn EL, Timmerman KL et al. (2009) Supraphysiological hyperinsulinaemia is necessary to stimulate skeletal muscle protein anabolism in older adults: evidence of a true age-related insulin resistance of muscle protein metabolism. *Diabetologia* **52**, 1889–1898.

47 Fujita S, Rasmussen BB, Cadenas JG et al. (2007) Aerobic exercise overcomes the age-related insulin resistance of muscle protein metabolism by improving endothelial function and Akt/mammalian target of rapamycin signaling. *Diabetes* **56**, 1615–1622.

48 Katsanos CS, Kobayashi H, Sheffield-Moore M et al. (2005) Aging is associated with diminished accretion of muscle proteins after the ingestion of a small bolus of essential amino acids. *Am J Clin Nutr* **82**, 1065–1073.

49 Byfield MP, Murray JT, Backer JM. (2005) hVps34 is a nutrient-regulated lipid kinase required for activation of p70 S6 kinase. *J Biol Chem* **280**, 33076–33082.

50 Nobukuni T, Joaquin M, Roccio M et al. (2005) Amino acids mediate mTOR/raptor signaling through activation of class 3 phosphatidylinositol 3OH-kinase. *Proc Natl Acad Sci USA* **102**, 14238–14243.

51 Yarasheski KE, Pak-Loduca J, Hasten DL et al. (1999) Resistance exercise training increases mixed muscle protein synthesis rate in frail women and men >/=76 yr old. *Am J Physiol Endocrinol Metab* **277**, E118–E125.

52 Esmarck B, Andersen JL, Olsen S et al. (2001) Timing of postexercise protein intake is important for muscle hypertrophy with resistance training in elderly humans. *J Physiol* **535**, 301–311.

53 Frontera WR, Meredith CN, O'Reilly KP et al. (1988) Strength conditioning in older men: skeletal muscle hypertrophy and improved function. *J Appl Physiol* **64**, 1038–1044.

54 Kosek DJ, Kim JS, Petrella JK et al. (2006) Efficacy of 3 days/wk resistance training on myofiber hypertrophy and myogenic mechanisms in young vs. older adults. *J Appl Physiol* **101**, 531–544.

55 Brown AB, McCartney N, Sale DG. (1990) Positive adaptations to weight-lifting training in the elderly. *J Appl Physiol* **69**, 1725–1733.

56 McCartney N, Hicks AL, Martin J et al. (1996) A longitudinal trial of weight training in the elderly: continued improvements in year 2. *J Gerontol A Biol Sci Med Sci* **51**, B425–B433.

57 Fiatarone MA, Marks EC, Ryan ND et al. (1990) High-intensity strength training in nonagenarians. Effects on skeletal muscle. *JAMA* **263**, 3029–3034.

58 Slivka D, Raue U, Hollon C et al. (2008) Single muscle fiber adaptations to resistance training in old (>80 yr) men: evidence for limited skeletal muscle plasticity. *Am J Physiol Regul Integr Comp Physiol* **295**, R273–R280.

59 Raue U, Slivka D, Minchev K et al. (2009) Improvements in whole muscle and myocellular function are limited with high-intensity resistance training in octogenarian women. *J Appl Physiol* **106**, 1611–1617.

60 Carey KA, Farnfield MM, Tarquinio SD et al. (2007) Impaired expression of Notch signaling genes in aged human skeletal muscle. *J Gerontol A Biol Sci Med Sci* **62**, 9–17.

61 Dennis RA, Przybyla B, Gurley C et al. (2008) Aging alters gene expression of growth and remodeling factors in human skeletal muscle both at rest and in response to acute resistance exercise. *Physiol Genomics* **32**, 393–400.

62 Drummond MJ, Dreyer HC, Pennings B et al. (2008) Skeletal muscle protein anabolic response to resistance exercise and essential amino acids is delayed with aging. *J Appl Physiol* **104**, 1452–1461.

63 Kim JS, Cross JM, Bamman MM. (2005) Impact of resistance loading on myostatin expression and cell cycle regulation in young and older men and women. *Am J Physiol Endocrinol Metab* **288**, E1110–E1119.

64 Williamson D, Gallagher P, Harber M et al. (2003) Mitogen-activated protein kinase (MAPK) pathway activation: effects of age and acute exercise on human skeletal muscle. *J Physiol* **547**, 977–987.

65 Sheffield-Moore M, Paddon-Jones D, Sanford AP et al. (2005) Mixed muscle and hepatic derived plasma protein metabolism is differentially regulated in older and younger men following resistance exercise. *Am J Physiol Endocrinol Metab* **288**, E922–E929.

66 Kumar V, Selby A, Rankin D et al. (2008) *Age-related differences in the dose-response of muscle protein synthesis to resistance exercise in young and old men. J Physiol.*

67 Mayhew DL, Kim JS, Cross JM et al. (2009) Translational signaling responses preceding resistance training-mediated myofiber hypertrophy in young and old humans. *J Appl Physiol* **107**, 1655–1662.

68 Dreyer HC, Fujita S, Cadenas JG et al. (2006) Resistance exercise increases AMPK activity and reduces 4E-BP1 phosphorylation and protein synthesis in human skeletal muscle. *J Physiol* **576**, 613–624.

69 Thalacker-Mercer A, Dell'italia LJ, Cui X et al. (2010) Differential genomic responses in old vs. young humans despite similar levels of modest muscle damage after resistance loading. *Physiol Genomics* **40**, 141–149.

70 Kim JS, Kosek DJ, Petrella JK et al. (2005) Resting and load-induced levels of myogenic gene transcripts differ between older adults with demonstrable sarcopenia and young men and women. *J Appl Physiol* **99**, 2149–2158.

71 Melov S, Tarnopolsky MA, Beckman K et al. (2007) Resistance exercise reverses aging in human skeletal muscle. *PLoS One* **2**, e465.

72 Alway SE, Siu PM. (2008) Nuclear apoptosis contributes to sarcopenia. *Exerc Sport Sci Rev* **36**, 51–57.

73 Giovannini S, Marzetti E, Borst SE et al. (2008) Modulation of GH/IGF-1 axis: potential strategies to counteract sarcopenia in older adults. *Mech Ageing Dev* **129**, 593–601.

74 Edstrom E, Altun M, Bergman E et al. (2007) Factors contributing to neuromuscular impairment and sarcopenia during aging. *Physiol Behav* **92**, 129–135.

75 Jensen GL. (2008) Inflammation: roles in aging and sarcopenia. *JPEN J Parenter Enteral Nutr* **32**, 656–659.

76 Thalacker-Mercer AE, Fleet JC, Craig BA et al. (2007) Inadequate protein intake affects skeletal muscle transcript profiles in older humans. *Am J Clin Nutr* **85**, 1344–1352.

77 Houston DK, Nicklas BJ, Ding J et al. (2008) Dietary protein intake is associated with lean mass change in older, community-dwelling adults: the Health, Aging, and Body Composition (Health ABC) Study. *Am J Clin Nutr* **87**, 150–155.

78 Symons TB, Schutzler SE, Cocke TL et al. (2007) Aging does not impair the anabolic response to a protein-rich meal. *Am J Clin Nutr* **86**, 451–456.

79 Campbell WW, Trappe TA, Wolfe RR et al. (2001) The recommended dietary allowance for protein may not be adequate for older people to maintain skeletal muscle. *J Gerontol A Biol Sci Med Sci* **56**, M373–M380.

80 Wolfe RR, Miller SL. (2008) The recommended dietary allowance of protein: a misunderstood concept. *JAMA* **299**, 2891–2893.

81 Katsanos CS, Kobayashi H, Sheffield-Moore M et al. (2006) A high proportion of leucine is required for optimal stimulation of the rate of muscle protein synthesis by essential amino acids in the elderly. *Am J Physiol Endocrinol Metab* **291**, E381–E387.

82 Louard RJ, Barrett EJ, Gelfand RA. (1995) Overnight branched-chain amino acid infusion causes sustained suppression of muscle proteolysis. *Metabolism* **44**, 424–429.

83 Rieu I, Balage M, Sornet C et al. (2006) Leucine supplementation improves muscle protein synthesis in elderly men independently of hyperaminoacidaemia. *J Physiol* **575**, 305–315.

84 Verhoeven S, Vanschoonbeek K, Verdijk LB et al. (2009) Long-term leucine supplementation does not increase muscle mass or strength in healthy elderly men. *Am J Clin Nutr* **89**, 1468–1475.

85 Walrand S, Short KR, Bigelow ML et al. (2008) Functional impact of high protein intake on healthy elderly people. *Am J Physiol Endocrinol Metab* **295**, E921–E928.

86 Phillips SM, Tipton KD, Ferrando AA et al. (1999) Resistance training reduces the acute exercise-induced

increase in muscle protein turnover. *Am J Physiol Endocrinol Metab* **276**, E118–E124.

87 MacDougall JD, Gibala MJ, Tarnopolsky MA et al. (1995) The time course for elevated muscle protein synthesis following heavy resistance exercise. *Can J Appl Physiol* **20**, 480–486.

88 Phillips SM, Tipton KD, Aarsland A et al. (1997) Mixed muscle protein synthesis and breakdown after resistance exercise in humans. *Am J Physiol Endocrinol Metab* **273**, E99–E107.

89 Biolo G, Maggi SP, Williams BD et al. (1995) Increased rates of muscle protein turnover and amino acid transport after resistance exercise in humans. *Am J Physiol Endocrinol Metab* **268**, E514–E520.

90 Borsheim E, Aarsland A, Wolfe RR. (2004) Effect of an amino acid, protein, and carbohydrate mixture on net muscle protein balance after resistance exercise. *Int J Sport Nutr Exerc Metab* **14**, 255–271.

91 Biolo G, Tipton KD, Klein S et al. (1997) An abundant supply of amino acids enhances the metabolic effect of exercise on muscle protein. *Am J Physiol Endocrinol Metab* **273**, E122–E129.

92 Tipton KD, Ferrando AA, Phillips SM et al. (1999) Postexercise net protein synthesis in human muscle from orally administered amino acids. *Am J Physiol Endocrinol Metab* **276**, E628–E634.

93 Rasmussen BB, Tipton KD, Miller SL et al. (2000) An oral essential amino acid-carbohydrate supplement enhances muscle protein anabolism after resistance exercise. *J Appl Physiol* **88**, 386–392.

94 Andersen LL, Tufekovic G, Zebis MK et al. (2005) The effect of resistance training combined with timed ingestion of protein on muscle fiber size and muscle strength. *Metabolism* **54**, 151–156.

95 Bird SP, Tarpenning KM, Marino FE. (2006) Independent and combined effects of liquid carbohydrate/essential amino acid ingestion on hormonal and muscular adaptations following resistance training in untrained men. *Eur J Appl Physiol* **97**, 225–238.

96 Rankin JW, Goldman LP, Puglisi MJ et al. (2004) Effect of post-exercise supplement consumption on adaptations to resistance training. *J Am Coll Nutr* **23**, 322–330.

97 Ballard TL, Clapper JA, Specker BL et al. (2005) Effect of protein supplementation during a 6-mo strength and conditioning program on insulin-like growth factor I and markers of bone turnover in young adults. *Am J Clin Nutr* **81**, 1442–1448.

98 Hulmi JJ, Tannerstedt J, Selanne H et al. (2009) Resistance exercise with whey protein ingestion affects mTOR signaling pathway and myostatin in men. *J Appl Physiol* **106**, 1720–1729.

99 Willoughby DS, Stout JR, Wilborn CD. (2007) Effects of resistance training and protein plus amino acid supplementation on muscle anabolism, mass, and strength. *Amino Acids* **32**, 467–477.

100 Koopman R, Verdijk L, Manders RJ et al. (2006) Co-ingestion of protein and leucine stimulates muscle protein synthesis rates to the same extent in young and elderly lean men. *Am J Clin Nutr* **84**, 623–632.

101 Campbell WW, Leidy HJ. (2007) Dietary protein and resistance training effects on muscle and body composition in older persons. *J Am Coll Nutr* **26**, 696S–703S.

102 Verdijk LB, Jonkers RA, Gleeson BG et al. (2009) Protein supplementation before and after exercise does not further augment skeletal muscle hypertrophy after resistance training in elderly men. *Am J Clin Nutr* **89**, 608–616.

103 Fujita S, Dreyer HC, Drummond MJ et al. (2009) Essential amino acid and carbohydrate ingestion before resistance exercise does not enhance postexercise muscle protein synthesis. *J Appl Physiol* **106**, 1730–1739.

104 Kraemer WJ, Adams K, Cafarelli E et al. (2002) American College of Sports Medicine position stand. Progression models in resistance training for healthy adults. *Med Sci Sports Exerc* **34**, 364–380.

105 Holm L, Reitelseder S, Pedersen TG et al. (2008) Changes in muscle size and MHC composition in response to resistance exercise with heavy and light loading intensity. *J Appl Physiol* **105**, 1454–1461.

106 Abe T, Kearns CF, Sato Y. (2006) Muscle size and strength are increased following walk training with restricted venous blood flow from the leg muscle, Kaatsu-walk training. *J Appl Physiol* **100**, 1460–1466.

107 Shinohara M, Kouzaki M, Yoshihisa T et al. (1998) Efficacy of tourniquet ischemia for strength training with low resistance. *Eur J Appl Physiol Occup Physiol* **77**, 189–191.

108 Takarada Y, Sato Y, Ishii N. (2002) Effects of resistance exercise combined with vascular occlusion on muscle function in athletes. *Eur J Appl Physiol* **86**, 308–314.

109 Takarada Y, Takazawa H, Sato Y et al. (2000) Effects of resistance exercise combined with moderate vascular occlusion on muscular function in humans. *J Appl Physiol* **88**, 2097–2106.

110 Takarada Y, Tsuruta T, Ishii N. (2004) Cooperative effects of exercise and occlusive stimuli on muscular function in low-intensity resistance exercise with

moderate vascular occlusion. *Jpn J Physiol* **54**, 585–592.

111 Abe T, Yasuda T, Midorikawa T et al. (2005) Skeletal muscle size and circulating IGF-1 are increased after two weeks of twice daily KAATSU resistance training. *Int J Kaatsu Training Res* **1**, 6–12.

112 Manini TM, Clark BC. (2009) Blood flow restricted exercise and skeletal muscle health. *Exerc Sport Sci Rev* **37**, 78–85.

113 Fujita S, Abe T, Drummond MJ et al. (2007) Blood flow restriction during low-intensity resistance exercise increases S6K1 phosphorylation and muscle protein synthesis. *J Appl Physiol* **103**, 903–910.

114 Drummond MJ, Fujita S, Takashi A et al. (2008) Human muscle gene expression following resistance exercise and blood flow restriction. *Med Sci Sports Exerc* **40**, 691–698.

115 Kinugasa R, Watanabe T, Ijima H et al. (2006) Effects of vascular occlusion on maximal force, exercise-induced T2 changes, and EMG activities of quadriceps femoris muscles. *Int J Sports Med* **27**, 511–516.

116 Koopman R, Zorenc AH, Gransier RJ et al. (2006) Increase in S6K1 phosphorylation in human skeletal muscle following resistance exercise occurs mainly in type II muscle fibers. *Am J Physiol Endocrinol Metab* **290**, E1245–E1252.

117 Kraemer WJ, Hakkinen K, Newton RU et al. (1998) Acute hormonal responses to heavy resistance exercise in younger and older men. *Eur J Appl Physiol Occup Physiol* **77**, 206–211.

118 West DW, Kujbida GW, Moore DR et al. (2009) Resistance exercise-induced increases in putative anabolic hormones do not enhance muscle protein synthesis or intracellular signalling in young men. *J Physiol* **587**, 5239–5247.

119 Takano H, Morita T, Iida H et al. (2005) Hemodynamic and hormonal responses to a short-term low-intensity resistance exercise with the reduction of muscle blood flow. *Eur J Appl Physiol* **95**, 65–73.

120 Nakajima T, Kurano M, Iida H et al. (2006) Use and safety of KAATSU training: Results of a national survey. *Int J KAATSU Training Res* **2**, 5–13.

121 Klatsky AL, Armstrong MA, Poggi J. (2000) Risk of pulmonary embolism and/or deep venous thrombosis in Asian-Americans. *Am J Cardiol* **85**, 1334–1337.

122 Nakajima T, Takano H, Kurano M et al. (2007) Effects of KAATSU training on haemostasis in healthy subjects. *Int J KAATSU Training Res* **3**, 11–20.

PART 2

Sporadic Inclusion-Body Myositis

Pathogenesis of sporadic inclusion-body myositis: role of aging and muscle-fiber degeneration, and accumulation of the same proteins as in Alzheimer and Parkinson brains

Valerie Askanas, W. King Engel, and Anna Nogalska

Departments of Neurology and Pathology, University of Southern California Neuromuscular Center, University of Southern California Keck School of Medicine, Good Samaritan Hospital, Los Angeles, CA, USA

Introduction

Sporadic inclusion-body myositis (s-IBM) is pathogenically a complex, multi-factorial muscle disease associated with aging. The s-IBM muscle biopsy exhibits an unusual, specific pathologic phenotype, which combines multi-faceted muscle-fiber degeneration with extracellular T-cell inflammation. s-IBM muscle-fiber degeneration is characterized by vacuolization and intracellular accumulation of ubiquitinated multiple-protein aggregates (inclusions) [1–3]. Although it is yet not known whether (a) mononuclear cell inflammation precedes muscle-fiber degeneration, or (b) abnormal metabolically modified proteins accumulated within the muscle fibers provoke an inflammatory response, it is becoming more apparent that s-IBM is a unique type of muscle-fiber degeneration leading to muscle-fiber atrophy. The result is muscle-fiber death and relentlessly progressive clinical muscle weakness [1–7]. This proposal is supported by the observations that s-IBM patients do not satisfactorily respond to various anti-dysimmune/anti-inflammatory treatments (see below). Therefore, we have proposed that in s-IBM the prominent "degenerative" component, including accumulation of misfolded proteins within muscle fibers (see below), is eliciting the T-cell inflammatory reaction [1, 3]. We have also postulated for several years that the aging milieu of the s-IBM muscle fiber and of the total patient may be facilitating the lymphocytic inflammation. Interestingly, some of the older patients with hereditary inclusion-body myopathy (h-IBM), caused by missense mutations in the UDP-N-acetylglucosamine-2 epimerase/N-acetylmannosamine kinase (*GNE*) gene, have various degrees of lymphocytic inflammation [8–10], even though that form of h-IBM is not considered immune-mediated. The reason is not understood, but we postulate that the aging cellular environment, and perhaps other individual intrinsic muscle-fiber abnormalities might, in older h-IBM patients, make some of the accumulated proteins appear "foreign" to the immune system and induce the lymphocytic inflammation.

Clinically, s-IBM leads to pronounced patient frailty and disability. Walking becomes precarious.

Muscle Aging, Inclusion-Body Myositis and Myopathies, First Edition. Edited by Valerie Askanas and W. King Engel.
© 2012 Blackwell Publishing Ltd. Published 2012 by Blackwell Publishing Ltd.

Sudden falls, sometimes resulting in major injury to the skull or other bones, can occur, even from walking on minimally irregular ground or from other minor imbalances outside or within the home, due to weakness of quadriceps and gluteal muscles, depriving the patient of automatic posture maintenance ([7], also see Chapter 9 in this volume). A foot-drop can increase the likelihood of tripping and falling [7]. There is currently no enduring treatment available for this devastating muscle disease (see below).

Very intriguing is the multi-faceted muscle degeneration in s-IBM and its many similarities to the complex neuronal degenerations occurring both in Alzheimer and Parkinson disease brains. The similarities include (a) abnormal accumulations of many of the same putatively pathogenic proteins, (b) their similar posttranslational modifications, and (c) similar defective mechanisms of protein disposal: those contribute to the observed abnormal protein aggregations, β-pleated sheet amyloid accumulation, and cytoplasmic vacuolization.

Because the same proteins accumulate within IBM muscle fibers that accumulate in the brain of Alzheimer and Parkinson disease patients, the muscle and the brain diseases might share certain pathogenic steps, and knowledge of one disease might help elucidate the other. All those diseases include sporadic and hereditary forms, and all are multi-factorial and polygenetic.

Cellular aging, endoplasmic reticulum and oxidative stresses, and abnormalities of both the 26S proteasome and autophagy have been proposed to contribute to the s-IBM [1, 2, 11–15] and to the Alzheimer and Parkinson disease pathogenesis [16–20]. Yet each disease category remains organ-specific, involving postmitotic muscle fibers or postmitotic neurons. s-IBM patients do not develop dementia, and Alzheimer and Parkinson disease patients do not have the muscle weakness characteristic of IBM, indicating that the mechanism of *organ targeting* is different in those diseases. The tissue affected, muscle versus brain, may be influenced by various epigenetic and/or genetic factors, such as: (a) etiologic agent (a virus?), (b) previous exposure to a specific environmental factor(s), and (c) the patient's genetic predisposition (the cellular microclimate).

Abnormal accumulation of ubiquitinated intracellular proteinacious inclusions is characteristic of the s-IBM phenotype, thus s-IBM, similarly to Alzheimer and Parkinson disease, is considered a "conformational disorder," caused by protein unfolding/misfolding and associated with formation of proteinacious inclusion bodies (reviewed in [1–4]). Similarly to Alzheimer and Parkinson brains, the sequence of the detrimental pathologic events comprising cellular degeneration in s-IBM muscle fibers is not yet well delineated. However, several aspects of the s-IBM intra-muscle-fiber pathogenic cascade are being uncovered and their causative mechanisms elucidated.

Here we describe the multiple proteins that are accumulated in the form of aggregates within s-IBM muscle fibers, and discuss their possible causes and consequences. We also emphasize the most recent research advances directed toward understanding the underlying mechanisms causing impaired protein degradation, their molecular modifications and abnormal aggregation. These aspects are important because in s-IBM muscle fibers the abnormal misfolding, accumulation, and aggregation of proteins are associated with their inadequate disposal, both through impaired autophagy and inhibited function of the 26S proteasome. We propose that these factors are combined with, and perhaps provoked by, an aging intracellular milieu. The importance of the identified endoplasmic reticulum stress in causing abnormal autophagy, impaired SIRT1 deacetylase activity, and subsequent increase of nuclear factor κB (NFκB) activity, are also discussed.

We summarize various experimental IBM models that are intended to help elucidate the s-IBM pathogenesis and, if successful, might be useful in developing treatment approaches to benefit s-IBM patients.

Vacuoles, protein accumulation, and their putative pathogenic role

General considerations
The IBM autophagic vacuoles, which typically contain membranous debris, appear to be lysosomal, and to be a result of muscle-fiber destruction [2, 7]

(Plate 7.1). While some of the vacuoles appear "rimmed" by a trichrome reddish material (that color indicating lipoprotein membranous material [21]), often the vacuoles do not have an obvious rim and appear "empty" (those sometimes must be differentiated from freezing artifact holes, detailed in Chapter 10).

Normal human multi-nucleated skeletal muscle fibers are usually several centimeters long. On a given 10 μm transverse section of an s-IBM muscle biopsy, the aggregates are present mainly in vacuole-free regions of vacuolated muscle-fiber cytoplasm and in cytoplasm of "non-vacuolated" fibers: the latter can have vacuoles located in sections cut further along the fiber. Thus in a given region of a fiber, aggregates seem to precede formation of the vacuoles, or possibly are not related to them. The vacuoles themselves usually do not contain the IBM-characteristic inclusions. Intra-muscle-fiber protein aggregates, identified by immunocytochemical staining with an antibody recognizing a specific protein accumulated within a given aggregate, are of two major types: (a) larger rounded "plaque-like" inclusions, containing amyloid-β (Aβ), α-synuclein (α-syn), cellular prion protein (PrPᶜ), and other proteins (referenced in Table 7.1 [4–6, 11, 13–15, 22–72]; Plate 7.2a–c);); and (b) delicate squiggly and skein-like inclusions containing phosphorylated tau (p-tau), and other proteins (referenced in Table 7.1; Plate 7.2d). Several of those proteins are capable of forming β-pleated-sheet amyloid. Accumulations of that amyloidic structures are identifiable by fluorescence-enhanced Congo red staining visualized through Texas Red filters [1, 2, 26] and also, but less abundantly, by crystal violet: those amyloidic positivities typically have patterns similar to the inclusions formed by Aβ and p-tau [1, 2, 5] (Plate 7.3a–d). (Note: "amyloid-β" refers to one specific protein, whereas "amyloid" designates congophilic β-pleated-sheet configuration of any one of various proteins that can pathologically aggregate into this rather insoluble, three-dimensional shape configuration; these similar terms are sometimes confused in the literature.). Intra-muscle-fiber β-pleated-sheet amyloid inclusions in s-IBM muscle fibers were first identified in 1991 [27]. Now, for an experienced muscle pathologist using

our recommended fluorescence-enhanced Congo red technique [26], multiple or single foci of amyloid are easily recognizable within the s-IBM abnormal muscle fibers in a given transverse section. Both the plaque-like and squiggly aggregates contain many other proteins that are listed in Table 7.1. They include Aβ precursor protein (AβPP), Aβ40 and Aβ42 oligomers, as well as proteins participating in AβPP proteolysis, such as β-secretase (β-site AβPP-cleaving enzyme 1, BACE1) and the γ-secretase complex (containing presenilin 1 and nicastrin). Also accumulated within some of those aggregates are α-syn and cellular prion protein, and a number of other proteins having various functions and significance including: (a) markers of oxidative stress; (b) endoplasmic reticulum (ER) chaperones indicative of the unfolded protein response (UPR); (c) 26S proteasome components, and the proteasome shuttle protein p62; (d) autophagosome-related protein LC3; (e) mutated ubiquitin (UBB⁺¹); (f) various transduction and transcription factors; and (g) several other proteins (Table 7.1 and references therein, and reviewed in [1–5]). Immunohistochemically identified accumulated protein within an aggregate could accumulate due to its (a) impaired catabolism (related to lysosome or proteasome inadequacy), (b) overproduction, or (c) being "stuck" to other accumulated proteins. Accumulated proteins might or might not have their normal cellular function and/or structure.

Below we describe properties of some of the major proteins that accumulate, emphasizing their possible pathogenic roles. Details of other accumulated proteins are available in the references cited in Table 7.1.

Increased synthesis of AβPP and abnormalities of AβPP processing

s-IBM muscle fibers have increased mRNA signal for AβPP-751, which contains the Kunitz-type protease inhibitor motif [73]. The mechanism of this apparent AβPP overproduction in s-IBM is not yet clarified, but the AP-1 transcription complex, Redox-factor-1 [1], and transcription factor NFκB (reviewed in [4, 5, 74]) might contribute to its increased synthesis. Our recent studies have shown that NFκB binding to DNA is increased in s-IBM muscle fibers [75].

Table 7.1 Molecules accumulated within the Aβ and p-tau intracellular multi-protein aggregates in s-IBM muscle fibers.

	Aβ aggregates		p-Tau aggregates		References
	Light microscopy	Electron microscopy	Light microscopy	Electron microscopy	
Morphology, typical	Plaque-like, rounded, various-sized inclusions	6–10 nm filaments, floccular and amorphous material	Squiggly	15–21 nm paired helical filaments	[22–25]
β-pleated sheet amyloid (Congo red +, crystal violet +)	+		+		[4–6, 26, 27]
Proteins, various					
Aggregate-prone proteins					
Aβ42/40	+	+	−	−	[22, 23, 28]
α-Synuclein	+	+	−	−	[29–31]
Phosphorylated tau	−	−	+	+	[24, 25]
Prion protein, cellular	+	+	+	+	[32]
Myostatin	+	+	−	−	[33]
AβPP/AβPP processing/Aβ deposition					
AβPP/ phosphorylated AβPP	+	+			[22, 34]
BACE1 and BACE2	+	+	−	−	[35, 36]
Nicastrin	+	+	+	+	[37]
Presenilin 1	+	+	+	+	[38]
Neprilysin	+	+	NK	NK	[39]
NOGO-B	+	+	−	−	[40]
Cystatin C	+	+	−	−	[41]
Transglutaminase 1 and 2	+	NK	NK	NK	[42]
Protein degradation systems					
Ubiquitin-proteasome system					
Ubiquitin	+	+	+	+	[43, 44]
Proteasome subunits	+	+	+	+	[11]
Parkin	+	+	NK	NK	[31]
UbcH7	+	+	−	−	[35]
UBB^{+1}	+	+	+	+	[45]
RNF5	+	NK	−	NK	[46]
Autophagy					
LC3	+	−	−	−	[13, 47]
Both					
p62	−	−	+	+	[48]
VCP	NK	NK	NK	NK	[49]

Table 7.1 (*Continued*)

	Aβ aggregates		p-Tau aggregates		References
	Light microscopy	Electron microscopy	Light microscopy	Electron microscopy	
Heat-shock proteins					
Hsp70 and its cofactors	+	+	+	+	[50]
Hsp40	+	+	+	+	[50]
CHIP	+	+	+	+	Paciello and Askanas, unpublished results (2006)
Endoplasmic reticulum chaperones					
BiP/GRP78	+	+	−	−	[15]
GRP94	+	+	−	−	[15]
Calnexin	+	+	−	−	[15]
Calreticulin	+	+	−	−	[15]
ERP72	+	+	−	−	[15]
HERP	+	+	−	−	[14]
Tau protein kinases					
ERK	−	−	+	+	[51]
CDK5	−	−	+	+	[52]
GSK-3β	NK	NK	+	+	[53]
Casein kinase 1α	NK	NK	+	NK	[54]
Markers of oxidative stress					
Nitrotyrosine	+	+	+	+	[55]
SOD1	NK	NK	NK	NK	[56]
Malondialdehyde	+	+	+	+	[57]
α1-Antichymotrypsin	+	NK	NK	NK	[58]
NFκB	NK	NK	+	+	[59]
Seleno-gluththione peroxidase-1	NK	NK	NK	NK	[60]
Catalase	NK	NK	NK	NK	[60]
Ref-1	+	+	+	+	[64]
iNOS, eNOS	−	−	+	+	[65]
Transcription/RNA metabolism					
RNA polymerase II	−	−	+	+	[61]
RNA	−	NK	+	NK	[62]
SMN	−	−	+	+	[62]
c-Jun	+	+	+	+	[65]
NFκB	NK	NK	+	+	[59]
PPARγ	+	−	NK	−	[63]
Ref-1	+	+	+	+	[64]
TDP-43	NK	+	−	+	[66–70]
Cholesterol metabolism					
Apolipoprotein E	+	+	+	+	[71]
LDLR	+	+	+	+	[72]
VLDL	+	+		−	[72]
Cholesterol	+		+		[72]

In addition to the apparently increased synthesis of AβPP in s-IBM muscle fibers, there are distinct abnormalities in AβPP processing. Evidence is as follows.

First, BACE1 is increased in s-IBM muscle fibers on both the mRNA and protein levels [35, 36, 40, 76]. BACE1, a transmembrane protein and a member of the aspartyl-protease family, cleaves AβPP at the N-terminus of Aβ [77, 78], and it is a major β-*secretase* participating in Aβ generation. Increase of BACE1 leads to overproduction of toxic Aβ42 [77, 79]. Recently, a novel regulation of BACE1 mRNA and protein expression involving a conserved non-coding BACE1-antisense transcript (BACE1-AS) was described *in vivo* and *in vitro* [80]. Increased levels of BACE1-AS transcript were reported in brains of Alzheimer disease patients and of Alzheimer transgenic mice models [80]. Increased BACE1-AS transcript was also demonstrated in s-IBM muscle fibers, providing another similarity to Alzheimer disease brain [76].

Second, *nicastrin* and the *presenilins*, which are components of the γ-*secretase system* that cleaves AβPP at the C-terminus of Aβ to generate either Aβ40 or Aβ42 (reviewed in [78, 81]), are also strongly overexpressed in s-IBM muscle fibers. There they (a) colocalize with each other and with Aβ, [5, 6, 37], and (b) are physically associated with AβPP in s-IBM and in experimentally AβPP-over-expressing cultured muscle fibers (Vattemi and Askanas, unpublished observation, 2003). Accordingly, both β- and γ-secretases appear to participate in Aβ production within s-IBM muscle fibers.

Finally, other factors contributing to Aβ production, deposition, and oligomerization, are also increased in s-IBM muscle fibers. These include: (a) *transglutaminases 1a* and *2*, which can contribute to Aβ pathologic aggregation and insolubility by cross-linking Aβ molecules, are present in s-IBM muscle [42]; (b) *cystatin C*, an endogenous cysteine-protease inhibitor, was previously proposed to participate in Aβ deposition within amyloid plaques of Alzheimer disease brain [82], is also increased in s-IBM muscle fibers [41]; (c) *free cholesterol*, which in various non-muscle cells increases Aβ production and amyloidogenesis (referenced in [72]

and reviewed in [83]), is abnormally accumulated in s-IBM muscle fibers [72]. It colocalizes with the abnormally accumulated Aβ and caveolin-1 [72, 84]; and (d) *caveolin-1*, a major protein of plasma-lemmal microdomain caveolae, an intracellular transporter of cholesterol [83], is abnormally accumulated within s-IBM muscle fibers. We therefore propose that within s-IBM muscle fibers cholesterol, instead of being properly metabolized or cleared, is deposited with caveolin-1 inside the IBM muscle fibers at sites of Aβ accumulation and possibly AβPP processing, and that it might be influencing Aβ deposition there.

Putatively protective mechanisms that have been shown to prevent abnormal AβPP processing are also concurrently expressed in s-IBM muscle fibers, including: (a) *neprilysin*, which participates in Aβ degradation [39]; (b) *insulin-like-growth factor 1* (IGF1), which protects against Aβ toxicity [85]; and (c) *NOGO-B*, which prevents binding of BACE1 to AβPP, thereby inhibiting Aβ production [40]. Those data together support our hypothesis that both cytotoxic and protective mechanisms are concurrently operating in s-IBM muscle fibers; however, the protective mechanisms seem insufficient because the disease is relentlessly progressive.

Phosphorylated AβPP and activated GSK-3β

Increased phosphorylation of neuronal AβPP[695] on Thr-668 has been demonstrated in Alzheimer disease brain and in brains of Alzheimer mouse models, and it was considered to be detrimental by increasing generation of Aβ and inducing tau phosphorylation [34, 86, 87]. Active glycogen synthase kinase 3β (GSK-3β) was proposed to have an important role in Alzheimer disease pathogenesis because it was shown to modulate both phosphorylation of tau, and of AβPP on Thr-668 [88]. GSK-3β has been considered a link between AβPP and phosphorylation of tau [89].

While AβPP[695] is preferentially present in neuronal cells, the AβPP[751] isoform is more abundant in peripheral tissues [90], and is the isoform overproduced and accumulated as aggregates in s-IBM muscle fibers [22, 73, 91]. Phosphorylation of AβPP is considered a regulatory mechanism of AβPP metabolism. Phosphorylation on Thr-668 of neuronal isoform AβPP^{695} (equivalent to Thr-724 of AβPP^{751}) was reported to be associated with increased Aβ production [87, 88], and to mediate pathological interaction between Aβ and tau [86].

Phosphorylated (p-) GSK-3β^{Y216}, the active form, has been shown increased in the frontal cortex of Alzheimer disease patients [92] and proposed to be a component of Alzheimer disease pathogenesis [93]. Active p-GSK-3β^{Y216} was also shown to phosphorylate both AβPP on Thr-688 [88] and tau protein [89].

Recently, we demonstrated for the first time that (a) in biopsied s-IBM muscle fibers and in the AβPP-overexpressing cultured human muscle fibers, AβPP is phosphorylated on Thr-724, and (b) in s-IBM patients active GSK-3β is significantly increased as compared to the normal aged-matched control muscle biopsies [34]. In addition, in cultured human muscle fibers, proteasome inhibition significantly contributed to the increase of active GSK-3β, which corresponded to the increase of phosphorylated AβPP. Accordingly, we have postulated that in s-IBM the pathologic phosphorylation of AβPP is increased by proteasome inhibition, possibly via activation of GSK-3β [34]. The increase of total AβPP after proteasome inhibition also suggests that in this culture system, and also possibly in s-IBM muscle, the ubiquitin-proteasome system (UPS) is involved in the degradation of AβPP ([34], and see below).

Increased accumulation of Aβ42 and Aβ42 oligomers

Our s-IBM studies from about two decades ago were the first to identify an *intra*cellular accumulation of Aβ in any disease [22, 23, 29, 94]. They were the basis for our proposal of an important cytotoxic role of *intra*cellular Aβ, not only for s-IBM muscle fibers but also for Alzheimer neurons [95].

In Alzheimer disease it has been suggested that abnormal proteolytic processing of AβPP leads to extracellular liberation of free Aβ, which then aggregates into extracellular congophilic β-pleated sheets composed of 6–10 nm amyloid-like fibrils, which themselves are clustered as extracellular amyloid plaques (reviewed in [96]). For years it has been considered that it is the *extra*cellular Aβ that is exerting a detrimental role in Alzheimer disease brain [96]. However, our proposal regarding the importance of intracellular Aβ in Alzheimer disease [95] seems now to be gaining traction, because now the presence of intraneuronal Aβ is well established and its possible toxicity and importance in the Alzheimer pathogenesis is being considered [78, 97].

s-IBM, and more recently h-IBM due to *GNE* mutation (see Chapters 11 and 13 in this volume) are the only muscle diseases in which accumulation of Aβ in abnormal muscle fibers appears to play a key pathogenic role. Based on *in vitro* human muscle tissue culture and *in vivo* animal models, increased AβPP and Aβ accumulation are upstream steps in the development of the s-IBM pathologic phenotype (details below in the section entitled Experimental models designed to elucidate the IBM pathogenesis). Aβ is released from AβPP as a 40- or 42-amino acid peptide. Aβ42 is considered more cytotoxic than Aβ40, and it has a higher propensity to aggregate and form amyloid fibrils (reviewed in [97–99]). The cytotoxic, more prone to self-associate and oligomerize Aβ42 [97–99], is much more increased in s-IBM muscle fibers than Aβ40, by both quantative immunohistochemistry and ELISA [28]. By contrast, Aβ42 was not detectable in polymyositis or any other disease control, or in normal muscle biopsies [28]. Only Aβ42, and not Aβ40, was associated with the Congo-red-positive amyloid inclusions, which corresponded to Aβ42 immuno-electron-microscopic localization to 6–10 nm amyloid-like fibrils [28] (see Figure 7.3a, below). By ELISA, in s-IBM muscle biopsies Aβ42 was present and Aβ40 was not detectable, while normal age-matched control biopsies did not have any detectable Aβ42 or Aβ40 [28].

Recently, the putative importance of Aβ42 cytotoxicity in s-IBM muscle fibers was strengthened by the novel demonstration of Aβ42 oligomers [100].

Cytotoxicity of Aβ is considered to depend on its initial assembly into oligomers. In contrast to Aβ monomers, which in other systems are considered not cytotoxic (reviewed in [78, 97]), small oligomers and protofibrils are thought to be the most cytotoxic forms of Aβ42 [78, 97, 101].

Nonfibrillar, cytotoxic "Aβ-derived diffusible ligands" (ADDLs), originally derived from Aβ42 [102], are mainly trimeric to 12-meric, or higher, Aβ oligomers. They are increased in Alzheimer disease brain and were proposed in Alzheimer disease to play an important pathogenic role [101]. In s-IBM muscle biopsies, Aβ dimers, trimers, and tetramers were evident by immunoblots [100]. None of the control muscle biopsies had Aβ oligomers. Dot-immunoblots using highly specific anti-ADDL monoclonal antibodies also showed prominently increased ADDLs in all s-IBM biopsies studied, while controls were negative. By immuno-fluorescence, in some of the abnormal s-IBM muscle fibers, ADDLs were accumulated in the form of plaque-like inclusions, and in very small fibers were often increased diffusely. Normal and disease controls were negative [100]. This novel demonstration of Aβ42 oligomers in s-IBM muscle biopsies provides additional evidence that intra-muscle-fiber accu-mulation of Aβ42 oligomers in s-IBM may contrib-ute importantly to the s-IBM pathogenic cascade. (Experimental evidence of AβPP/Aβ contribution to various aspects of the s-IBM phenotype is described below under Experimental models designed to elu-cidate the IBM pathogenesis).

Phosphorylated tau

In s-IBM muscle fibers as in Alzheimer disease brain [103–105], p-tau is accumulated intracellular-ly in the form of congophilic delicate squiggly or linear inclusions [24, 25] (Plates 7.2d and 7.3c, d), which by electron microscopy appear as paired helical filaments (PHFs) (Figure 7.1a–d). Various antibodies recognizing several epitopes of p-tau present in Alzheimer disease brain, including ones specifically recognizing Alzheimer disease-specific conformational tau [106], and described in detail previously, exclusively associate with s-IBM PHFs by both the light- and electron-microscopic immu-nohistochemistry (Figure 7.1b–d) [24, 25]. A well-characterized AT-100 antibody, which recognizes p-tau on Ser-212/Thr-214 [107], was shown to be immunopositive in s-IBM [48] (Plate 7.4b).

Occasionally accumulations of p-tau occur on PHFs within s-IBM muscle-fiber nuclei (Figure 7.1e, f).

Several kinases known to phosphorylate tau [104, 107, 108] are also accumulated within s-IBM muscle fibers, where they colocalize with p-tau-positive inclusions. These include extracel-lular signal-regulated kinase (ERK) [51], CDK5 [52], GSK-3β [53], and casein kinase 1 (Table 7.1) [54]. Also, GSK-3β is hyperphosphorylated and activated in s-IBM muscle fibers [34].

s-IBM PHFs additionally contain RNA and the RNA-binding protein survival motor neuron (SMN), both of which were proposed to contribute to PHF formation [62]. New studies related to neurodegeneration strongly suggest that accumu-lations of p-tau could be cytotoxic to neurons (reviewed in [104, 109]). In contrast to Aβ exerting an intra-muscle-fiber cytotoxicity, there is no di-rect evidence yet that p-tau might be toxic to s-IBM muscle fibers; however, this possibility should be explored.

Masses of PHFs accumulated in the form of p-tau-containing aggregates, which are visible in many muscle fibers on a given transverse section, and are known to be present in various places along the muscle fibers, could severely impair muscle-fiber integrity and function. Several other proteins are also accumulated within the bundles of p-tau-containing PHFs (referenced in Table 7.1). Hypothet-ically, those proteins might be either passively captured within the p-tau-containing PHFs and thereby be removed from their normal locale, which might impair their normal physiological functions, or they might be "actively," and disruptively, bound to tau or other proteins there by the interaction with the exposed hydrophobic surfaces of misfolded proteins associated with the PHF. Large clusters of PHFs can physically displace and impair the function of other cytoplasmic proteins and organelles, such as mitochondria and endoplasmic reticulum. Proteins that accumulate within the aggregates are suscepti-ble to oxidative damage [110]. Oxidative and nitrotyrosine stress is known to occur in s-IBM mus-cle fibers ([12, 55] and below), and nitration and oxidative stress affect tau assembly and phosphorylation [111, 112].

Figure 7.1 Electron microscopy of paired helical filaments and of p-tau in s-IBM muscle fibers. (a) Transmission electron microscopy (EM) of a cluster of typical paired helical filaments (PHFs). (b–d) Gold immuno-electron microscopy of p-tau protein on clusters of PHFs. (b) Immunostaining with Alz-50 antibody (which also recognizes conformational p-tau of PHFs in Alzheimer disease brain); (c) immunostaining with PHF-1 antibody (which also recognizes p-tau of PHFs in Alzheimer disease brain); (d) immunostaining with SMI-31 antibody (which is also able to recognize p-tau of PHFs in Alzheimer disease brain and in s-IBM muscle). (e) A low-power electron micrograph demonstrates a nuclear inclusion composed of PHFs and gold immunostained with SMI-31 antibody. (f) Higher magnification of the area indicated by the square shown in (e) clearly demonstrates that the nuclear inclusion is composed of PHF-associated p-tau (10 nm gold particles). Magnification: (a) ×21,000; (b) ×48,000 (5 nm gold); (c) ×24,000 (10 nm gold); (d) ×12,000 (10 nm gold); (e) ×6000; F ×30,000. Antibodies Alz-50 and PHF-1 were generously provided by Dr Peter Davies.

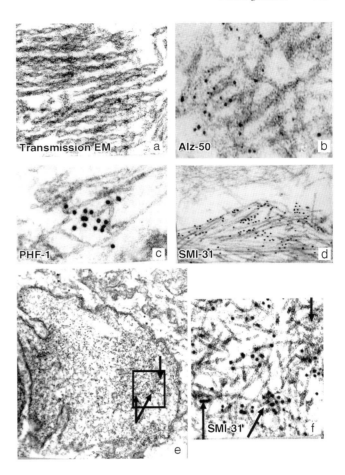

The mechanisms leading to the abnormal phosphorylation and accumulation of tau in s-IBM are not well understood. In addition to the overexpression of various kinases that participate in tau phosphorylation (see above), it has been recently reported that Aβ42 oligomers induce tau phosphorylation in various experimental models, including an AβPP-overexpressing IBM mouse model [97, 113]. Tau is known to be ubiquitinated and its accumulation has been at least partially attributed to inhibition of the 26S proteasome (reviewed in [114]). Recently, impaired autophagy has also been implicated as a factor contributing to tau oligomerization and accumulation [115].

Whether Aβ42 oligomers, and impaired functions of both the 26S proteasome and autophagy, both identified in s-IBM muscle fibers [11, 13, 28, 100], contribute to tau phosphorylation remains to be studied.

α-Syn and parkin

α-Syn, a 140 kDa protein of not-yet-well-understood normal cellular functions, is a major component of Lewy bodies in Parkinson disease brain (reviewed in [116, 117]) Abnormal expression of α-syn occurring spontaneously in brains of various neurodegenerative disorders has been associated with, and possibly causative of, oxidative stress, impaired proteasome function, and mitochondrial abnormalities [116, 117]. Oxidative stress can induce aggregation of α-syn into amyloid-like fibrils [117, 118].

Recently, α-syn has been shown associated with mitochondria (reviewed in [118]), and its overexpression induced mitochondria abnormalities. Previously, α-syn was demonstrated to be degraded by both the 26S proteasome and autophagy [119, 120], and the newest studies also indicate that impaired autophagy may contribute to decreased α-syn clearance and formation of α-syn aggregates within Parkinson disease Lewy bodies [121]. Lysosomal degradation of α-syn *in vivo* was also supported by detection of α-syn within the lysosomal lumen [119], and the clearance of α-syn by lysosomes was shown to be facilitated by chaperone-mediated autophagy [119]. Consequently, it has been proposed that abnormal accumulation of α-syn in various degenerative disorders is caused mainly by inhibition of autophagy, probably due to defective chaperone-mediated autophagy [122]. While abnormalities of α-syn were usually considered central to the Parkinson disease pathogenesis, and abnormalities of Aβ were considered specific to the Alzheimer disease pathogenesis, it has been recently proposed that α-syn and its oligomers might also play a role in Alzheimer disease pathogenesis [116]. This proposal was based on evidence that in experimental models (a) fragments of α-syn are found in amyloid plaques, (b) Aβ promotes α-syn aggregation; (c) α-syn is accumulated in Alzheimer disease and Down syndrome brains, and (d) α-syn was first isolated from Alzheimer disease brain (referenced in [116]).

The mechanisms involved in the induction of various pathologies by α-syn are not well understood, but α-syn oligomerization and its other postranslational modifications are suggested to play an important role.

In 2000, our studies were the first to demonstrate that abnormal accumulation of α-syn occurs in diseased human muscle and thus is not unique to brain disorders [30].

We demonstrated that α-syn is accumulated in the form of aggregates in s-IBM muscle fibers (Plate 7.2b), where it closely colocalized with Aβ [30]. By gold-immuno-electron microscopy, α-syn and Aβ were associated with the same subcellular components composed of 6–10 nm amyloid-like fibrils and amorphous and fibrillar material [30]). More recently, we have demonstrated a preferential presence of the 22 kDa *O*-glycosylated form of α-syn in s-IBM muscle fibers [31]. The 22 kDa form, but not the native 16 kDa form of α-syn, was shown by others to be a target of ubiquitination by parkin [123]. Currently unknown is whether the demonstrated inhibition of both the 26S proteasome and lysosomal degradation in s-IBM muscle fibers [11, 13] contributes to their preferential increase of the 22 kDa *O*-glycosylated form of α-syn. Recently, it was reported that lysosomal enzyme cathepsin D protects against α-syn toxicity [124]. Cathepsin D activity is decreased in s-IBM muscle fibers [13], but whether this mechanism contributes to a putative α-syn toxicity in s-IBM is not known.

Because oxidative- and nitric-oxide-induced stress, and mitochondrial abnormalities, are also aspects of the s-IBM muscle-fiber pathology (reviewed in [3, 4] and below), a putative toxicity of α-syn, in addition to the cytotoxicity of Aβ, may contribute to the muscle-fiber degeneration.

Parkin is an E3-ubiquitin ligase that ubiquitinates α-syn, and it has recently been demonstrated to promote "mitophagy' (degradation of mitochondria through the autophagosomal-lysosomal system) [125]. In s-IBM muscle fibers aggregates of parkin are accumulated, and parkin is increased by immunoblots [31]. In brains of sporadic Parkinson disease patients, parkin and α-syn accumulate in Lewy bodies [31]. Parkin, in addition to ubiquitinating several proteins, also protects cells against toxicity induced by α-syn, ER stress and other stresses, perhaps by helping to aggregate toxic α-syn oligomers and promote their degradation [126]. Accordingly, increase of parkin in s-IBM muscle fibers might be their attempt to protect themselves against toxicity induced by α-syn, ER and other stresses existing there. However, the 2.7-fold increase of parkin in s-IBM muscle fibers might not be sufficient to overcome a 6-fold increase of α-syn [31], or to protect against other continuing stresses. In addition, parkin has recently been reported to promote Aβ42 clearance in cultured neuroblastoma cells [127]. Whether this mechanism occurs in s-IBM muscle is not known.

Interestingly, in diseased human muscle, α-syn and parkin accumulate in ragged-red fibers [128]. This accumulation of α-syn and parkin is not related to their accumulation in s-IBM muscle fibers [129]. Ragged-red fibers, originally described in 1970 [129] using the Engel-modified trichrome staining [21], represent muscle fibers containing enlarged and otherwise abnormal mitochondria that are often accumulated at the periphery of the fibers [21]. Ragged-red fibers are abundantly present in muscle biopsies of patients with various mitochondriopathies, including ones with genetically determined mitochondrial DNA mutations. They are also present in muscle biopsies of some aging patients, and their number is significantly increased in s-IBM muscle biopsies [130].

Our recent studies have shown that ragged-red fibers in muscle biopsies in various neuromuscular disorders contain accumulated α-syn and parkin (Plate 7.5b–d) [128]. We propose that abnormal mitochondria within the ragged-red fibers are destined for autophagic degradation, and parkin is recruited to facilitate their clearance, as has been reported in other systems [125, 131].

Cellular prion protein

Normal *cellular prion protein (PrP^c)* is a mainly transmembrane protein present in virtually all tissues (recently reviewed in [132]). Initial interest in PrP^c was generated because the infectious scrapie prion is the product of postranslantionally modified PrP^c (reviewed in [133]). Interest in normal biological functions of PrP^c has been growing, and its binding properties to other proteins, including Aβ42 and its oligomers, have been subject of many studies (reviewed in [134]). Physiologically, PrP^c has been shown to have several functions, including cell-cycle regulation, differentiation, and intracellular signaling (recently reviewed in [132]). Experimental overexpression of PrP^c in transgenic mice resulted in neurodegeneration, which was not transmissible [135]. Several years ago we demonstrated that PrP^c and its mRNA are abnormally accumulated in

the form of inclusions in s-IBM abnormal muscle fibers [32, 136] (Plate 7.2c).

Still unknown is whether abnormally accumulated PrP^c in s-IBM muscle fibers results mainly from increased synthesis or defective clearance through the impaired proteasomal and autophagic degradations that are known to exist in s-IBM. Interestingly, in addition to s-IBM muscle, increased PrP^c and its mRNA have also been shown increased at the postsynaptic domain of normal neuromuscular junctions (NMJs) and in the regenerating muscle fibers in various diseases [136, 137]. Because both PrP^c and AβPP, including AβPP's proteolytic fragment Aβ, as well as the PrP^c and AβPP mRNAs, were increased at the postsynaptic domain of human NMJs [22, 73, 136, 137], it was proposed by ourselves and others [94, 136] that their colocalization at both sites might have a pathogenic role, possibly by influencing the properties and functions of each other. The correctness of these hypotheses is now being proven through the work by others, who have identified PrP^c as a binding receptor for Aβ42 and Aβ42 oligomers at central nervous system synapses (reviewed in [134]). Accordingly, the binding of PrP^c to Aβ42 oligomers is now proposed to play a role in Alzheimer disease pathogenesis, even though this influence is still mainly considered extraneuronal (review in [138]). However, in our view it seems likely that Aβ42-oligomer–PrP^c complexes can also occur intracellularly (both in muscle fibers and in neuron): such complexes might be cytotoxic, causing cell atrophy and eventual death.

Our previous observation of increased PrP^c and its mRNA in human regenerating muscle fibers [136] is now supported by a new study reporting that overexpression of PrP^c in adult mouse muscle promotes its regeneration [139].

Myostatin

Myostatin, a protein secreted from skeletal muscle, is considered a negative regulator of muscle growth during development and of muscle mass during adulthood [140]. In biopsied s-IBM muscle fibers, myostatin precursor protein (MSTNPP) and myostatin dimer were significantly increased on immunoblots, and MSTNPP immuno-colocalized with Aβ/

AβPP [33]. Interestingly, AβPP overexpression in cultured normal human muscle fibers increased MSTNPP expression, and subsequent experimental inhibition of proteasome caused accumulation and colocalization of both MSTNPP/myostatin and AβPP/Aβ, and their physical association [141]. The mechanism(s) by which overexpressed AβPP/Aβ increases MSTNPP is not known. Possibly, AβPP binding to MSTNPP causes its posttranslational modification that lessens its traffic and degradation, resulting in accumulation.

Recently, the importance of MSTNPP accumulation in s-IBM was emphasized by the studies of others [142] demonstrating that MSTNPP is capable of forming intracellular β-pleated-sheet amyloid. Since myostatin physically associates with AβPP/ Aβ [33, 141], it is possible, as we have previously proposed [33], that these two proteins might enhance each other's aggregation, oligomerization, and β-pleated-sheet formation.

Other proteins abnormally accumulated in s-IBM muscle fibers are described below in relation to other abnormalities, and are also referenced in Table 7.1.

Protein aggregation and misfolding, abnormalities of protein disposal, and accumulation of p62/SQSTM1

General considerations

All cells depend on intracellular mechanisms to maintain a proper quality and balance of their proteins and organelles. Quality-control mechanisms assure that any malfunctioning or damaged intracellular structures, including proteins and organelles, are identified and repaired or cleared (reviewed in [120, 122, 143–145]). This control or surveillance machinery is particularly important for the nondividing postmitotic cells because their abnormal proteins cannot be distributed during cell division [122]. The mechanisms for ensuring proper protein quality also influence protein transcription, thereby preventing proteins of being over- or underproduced. To eliminate misfolded proteins,

a cell recruits several mechanisms: (a) protein *refolding* through the *ER chaperones*; (b) protein *refolding* through *heat-shock proteins*; (c) protein *degradation* through the *26S UPS*; and (d) *protein degradation* through *autophagy*. The autophagic process involves formation of autophagosomes, their fusion with lysosomes, and degradation of proteins by lysosomal catabolic enzymes (reviewed in detail in [120, 122, 143, 146–149]). Under various pathological conditions, and in aging, protein quality control is disturbed (reviewed in [143, 150]). This results in accumulation and aggregation of pathologically modified proteins and damaged organelles.

Accumulation of misfolded multi-protein aggregates in s-IBM muscle fibers can result from increased production and/or inadequate clearance of accumulated proteins, or both. Protein aggregation is considered to be caused by binding of partly unfolded or misfolded polypeptides induced by interaction between their inappropriately exposed hydrophobic surfaces [17]. Normal cell proteins folded correctly are soluble, or associated with cellular membranes or other structures (reviewed in [17]). In s-IBM, insoluble aggregates of improperly folded proteins are usually cytoplasmic, infrequently nuclear. Although fully formed, insoluble amyloid fibrils may not be cytototoxic, their pre-amyloid oligomeric complexes or aggregates, either diffuse or in a protofibril stage, can be cytotoxic [151].

Unfolding or misfolding of proteins can occur *in vivo* and *in vitro* under several circumstances, including macromolecular crowding, defective protein disposal, oxidative stress, and "aging" [122].

Diseases characterized by protein misfolding and aggregation are termed "conformational diseases" (reviewed in [152]). Unfolding, misfolding, and aggregation might be attributed to increased transcription, impaired disposal (see below), and abnormal accumulation and crowding of proteins. Abnormal glycosylation and other deleterious chemical modifications can also lead to protein unfolding and misfolding, and cellular malfunction, with consequences for the proteins and cellular function.

Pathways leading to protein degradation and their abnormalities in s-IBM muscle fibers

In eukaryotic cells, two major pathways of cellular protein degradation relate to the 26S proteasome and the autophagic/lysosomal systems [146]. The 26S proteasome, also called the UPS, is a major degradation mechanism for (a) normal regulatory and other short-lived proteins, and (b) misfolded proteins exported from the ER through a ubiquitin-mediated ATP-independent process [16, 146]. In contrast, long-lived, structural proteins and/or variously damaged or misfolded proteins, and obsolescent cellular organelles, are degraded through "autophagy" [120, 145, 153]. Below we describe major characteristics of each system and their abnormalities in s-IBM muscle fibers.

UPS and its inhibition in s-IBM muscle fibers

The 26S proteasome is responsible for degradation of the majority of cellular proteins through a ubiquitin-mediated ATP-dependent pathway (reviewed in [143]). The proteasome is a large ($\approx$700 kDa) multi-subunit protease complex present in cytoplasm, endoplasmic reticulum, and nuclei of eukaryotic cells [143, 154–156]. 26S proteasomes are composed of a catalytic 20S core and a 19S regulatory complex. The 20S core is composed of 28 individual α and β subunits arranged in four stacked rings. Each ring contains either seven α or seven β subunits [143, 154, 155]. The two external rings, composed of α subunits, stabilize the complex, while the two inner rings, composed of β subunits, contain the protease-activity sites having trypsin-like (TL), chymotrypsin-like (CTL), and peptidyl glutamyl-peptide hydrolytic (PGPH) activities [154, 155].

19S, a distinct multimeric complex termed "PA700 proteasome activator," is thought to mediate the recognition of both polyubiquitinated moieties and unfolded proteins, thereby permitting their access into the interior of the 20S component to be catabolized [143, 154, 155]. Decreased proteasome function has been recently reported in several neurodegenerative diseases characterized by accumulation of multi-protein aggregates in the brain [16, 157, 158]. Aβ has been reported to inhibit proteasomal activity in cultured cells [158–160].

In s-IBM muscle fibers, our studies have demonstrated proteasomal abnormalities, as evidenced by: (a) abnormal accumulation of 26S proteasome subunits by immunocytochemistry and immuno-electron microscopy; (b) increased expression of 26S proteasome subunits by immunoblots; but, contrastingly (c) reduced activities of the three major proteasomal proteolytic enzymes [11]. This indicates accumulation of hypo-active/inactive proteasomal subunit proteins.

Our studies suggested that the AβPP/Aβ-proteasome interrelationship may be important in inducing proteasome abnormalities in s-IBM muscle fibers because: (a) Aβ and proteasome subunits colocalized by light microscopy and were associated electron microscopically with the same structures; (b) there was physical association of AβPP/Aβ and proteasome protein by immunoprecipitation studies; and (c) in cultured human muscle fibers overexpressing AβPP/Aβ proteasome activity was inhibited ([11], and also see our culture IBM model below). Other factors present in s-IBM muscle fibers that might contribute to inhibiting proteasome function include an aging muscle-fiber environment; protein overcrowding; oxidative stress [5, 6, 161]; and accumulated p-tau [5, 6, 161], α-syn [30], and UBB^{+1} [45]. All of these are capable of inhibiting proteasome activity in other systems [159, 160, 162–164].

In s-IBM muscle fibers, UBB^{+1}, a known inhibitor of proteasomal function, is accumulated in the form of aggregates. UBB^{+1} is a product of "molecular misreading," a phenomenon designating acquired, non-DNA-encoded dinucleotide deletions occurring within mRNAs, thus producing potentially toxic mutant proteins [164]. Our studies were the first to show accumulation of UBB^{+1} in muscle fibers in any muscle disease, demonstrating for the first time that molecular misreading can occur in diseased human muscle. We proposed that the aging cellular environment of s-IBM muscle fibers, combined with factors such as oxidative stress and perhaps other detrimental molecular events, leads to abnormal production and accumulation of UBB^{+1} [45].

A failure to degrade/remove surplus proteins, including abnormal damaged proteins, is presumably detrimental to muscle fibers as it is to other cells. Furthermore, accumulated ubiquitinated, misfolded, and oxidized protein aggregates by themselves can cause proteasome inhibition. Moreover, the still-soluble, early intermediates of protein aggregates, in the form of dimers and trimers can also induce proteasome inhibition [163], and they are highly toxic to cells [17, 97]. There are other diverse functions controlled by the UPS, including regulation of gene transcription through monoubiquitination and deubiquitination of histones, and major histocompatibility complex I (MHC-I) presentation (reviewed in [114]). Whether proteasomal abnormalities participate in antigen presentation and T-cell inflammation in s-IBM muscle fibers remains to be studied.

Autophagosomal-lysosomal pathway

In contrast to the UPS, which is a major degradation mechanism for (a) normal regulatory and other short-lived proteins, and (b) misfolded proteins exported from the ER through a ubiquitin-mediated ATP-independent process [16, 146], the autophagosomal-lysosomal pathway (ALP) is the major degrading mechanism for long-lived, structural proteins and/or damaged or misfolded proteins, and obsolescent cellular organelles [120, 145, 153]. ALP is composed of three main pathways: (a) macroautophagy, (b) chaperone-mediated-autophagy, and (c) microautophagy, all of which lead to lysosomes (reviewed in [120, 145, 146, 150]). Lysosomes are the main compartments in which degradation of a various proteins and molecules actually occurs, through the activity of various lysosomal proteolytic enzymes. The other components of the ALP serve mainly as crucial delivery pathways to the lysosomes of the molecules to be degraded. The term "autophagy" in reference to the lysosomal degradation, has been used for decades, but the molecular aspects of delivering the cargo destined for lysosomal degradation have been delineated only recently [120, 145, 150, 165]. In fact, the term "autophagy" should be reserved for lysosomal degradation, and it is misleading to refer

to "macroautophagy" as the autophagy (which often occurs in the literature).

Macroautophagy designates formation and maturation of "autophagosomes," which are structures carrying degradation-destined proteins and organelles to the lysosomes for their lysosomal degradation. After an autophagosome fuses with the lysosomal membrane, it disposes its cargo into the lysosome, where it is then degraded by the lysosomal enzymes [120, 145, 150, 166]. Autophagosomes proliferate and mature when the lysosomal function is inhibited, because the cargo that they are carrying cannot be received and cleared by the lysosomes. That situation is detrimental to the cell and can result in formation of autophagosomal vacuoles [166]. This occurs in s-IBM muscle fibers and in neurons of some of the neurodegenerative disorders (see below). In some situations, proliferation of autophagosomes in neurons has been associated with abnormal Aβ overproduction and vacuolization [153, 167]. Accordingly, before suggesting to s-IBM patients or to those with various neurodegenerative disorders the use of drugs to enhance macroautophagy, the function of the entire ALP must be evaluated. For example, inhibition, rather than stimulation of macroautophagy increased neuronal survival under some pathologic conditions (reviewed in [122]).

During *chaperone-mediated autophagy*, the cargo destined for lysosomal degradation is selectively recognized by a complex of chaperones that controls cargo delivery to the receptor on the lysosomal membrane (reviewed in [144, 168] and referenced therein). In this process, the protein cargo must be unfolded before being internalized into the lysosome (reviewed in [150]). Heat-shock cognate protein 70 (hsc70) and lysosomal-associated membrane protein (LAMP)-2 are two molecules indispensable for this process (reviewed in [168])

In the process of *microautophagy*, the entire lysosomal membrane protrudes to embrace the cytosolic component destined for degradation (reviewed in [122, 150]).

Although autophagic vacuoles associated with accumulated lysosomal-membranous structures in s-IBM muscle biopsies (Figure 7.2) have been known for many years ([169–171] and recently reviewed in [2, 7, 172]), the mechanism of

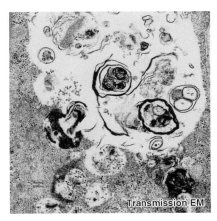

Figure 7.2 Transmission electron microscopy (EM) of an s-IBM vacuolated muscle fiber. Shown is a vacuole containing inclusions consisting of numerous various-sized membranous whorls of autophagosomal/lysosomal debris. Magnification: ×70,000.

their formation was not well understood. We have recently demonstrated [13] for the first time that in s-IBM muscle fibers there is increased formation and maturation of vacuolar autophagosomes, as indicated by: (a) the autophagosomal marker LC3-II [173], and (b) mammalian target of rapamycin (mTOR)-mediated phosphorylation of p70 S6 kinase [166, 173]. These observations suggest that activated macroautophagy is an important factor leading to formation of the vacuoles.

In contrast to several neurodegenerative diseases in which ALP functions have been extensively studied [120, 122, 145, 153], ALP functions in s-IBM muscle fibers have been virtually unexplored.

In addition to activated macroautophagy, our studies provided important evidence that autophagy related to lysosomal function is impaired in s-IBM muscle fibers. They showed a decrease of lysosomal cathepsin D and B enzymatic activities that appeared specific to s-IBM, because in polymyositis muscle fibers their activities were actually increased in our study [13] and in studies by others (referenced in [13]). In polymyositis macroautophagy was also increased but autophagic vacuoles and inclusions do not form, perhaps because the lysosomal system may be functioning adequately. Our results also suggest that lymphocytic inflammation, which is

present both in s-IBM and polymyositis, does not contribute to impairment of the autophagic/lysosomal degradation in s-IBM.

Impaired autophagy in s-IBM muscle fibers might be, at least partially, responsible for the abnormal accumulation of various proteins, including Aβ, α--syn, BACE1, and tau, all reported to be degraded through autophagy [120, 158, 174, 175]. Moreover, Aβ has been shown to be produced within the autophagosomes [153, 167, 176].

It is of interest that in adult rat skeletal muscle whose lysosomal enzyme activities were impaired by chloroquine treatment, Aβ was accumulated [177, 178]. Our newest studies demonstrated that inhibition of lysosomal activity in cultured human muscle fibers induces in them Aβ oligomerization ([100], and below).

p62/SQSTM1 is overexpressed and prominently accumulated in the form of inclusions

p62/SQSTM1 or "p62," is a shuttle protein transporting polyubiquitinated proteins to either proteasomal or lysosomal degradation [179, 180]. p62 is an integral component of inclusions in brains of various neurodegenerative disorders, for example in Alzheimer disease neurofibrillary tangles and Lewy bodies of Parkinson disease. In Alzheimer disease brain, the p62 localized in neurofibrillary tangles is associated with p-tau [181].

Our recent studies have demonstrated that in s-IBM muscle fibers p62 protein is increased at both the protein and mRNA levels, and it is strongly accumulated in aggregates within muscle fibers, where it closely colocalizes with p-tau by both the light- and electron-microscopic immunocytochemistry [48]. p62 immunocolocalized with p-tau by using two p-tau-recognizing antibodies, including AT100 (Plate 7.4a–c). By immuno-electron microscopy p62 associates with PHFs, and strongly embraces PHF clusters (Figure 7.3b).

Our p62 studies provided a new, reliable, and simple molecular marker of p-tau-containing PHF inclusions in s-IBM muscle fibers. The prominent p62 immunohistochemical positivity and pattern diagnostically distinguished s-IBM from polymyositis and dermatomyositis: we suggested using p62

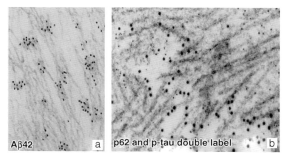

Figure 7.3 Single-label gold-immuno-electron microscopy of Aβ42, and double-label gold immuno-electron microscopy of p62 plus p-tau in s-IBM muscle fibers. (a) Aβ42 (5 nm gold particles) is immunolocalized to 6–10 nm amyloid-like fibrils, while in (b) p62 (10 nm gold particles) and p-tau (5 nm gold particles) intermingle on paired-helical filaments. Magnification: (a) ×80,000; (b) ×40,000.

immunoreactivity as an important diagnostic marker of s-IBM ([48], and see Chapter 10).

In normal cultured human muscle fibers, experimental inhibition of either proteasomal or lysosomal protein degradation caused substantial increase of p62 [48], suggesting that similar *in vivo* mechanisms known to be present in s-IBM muscle fibers might contribute to the p62 increase in them.

Transactive response DNA-binding protein 43

Transactive response DNA-binding protein 43 (TDP-43) is an RNA-/DNA-binding protein whose functions are not yet fully understood. It was reported to be involved in RNA processing, transcription, and exon skipping [182, 183]. Recent interest in TDP-43 was provoked by (a) discovering TDP-43-immunoreactive inclusions in the most common subtype of cerebral frontotemporal lobar degeneration (FTLD) associated with ubiquitin-positive inclusions, and in sporadic amyotrophic lateral sclerosis (ALS) [182, 183], and (b) identification of mainly missense mutations of TDP-43 in familial and sporadic ALS [182, 183]. TDP-43-immunoreactive cytoplasmic inclusions within s-IBM muscle fibers were reported by several investigators, including ourselves ([66] and referenced therein). Absence of the cytotoxic cleaved TDP-43 C-terminal fragment in s-IBM muscle fibers [68–70] might be against TDP-43 playing

an important pathogenic role. In s-IBM muscle, it is possible that TDP-43 could be considered a secondary pathology, as others have suggested for Alzheimer disease brains [182]. Experimentally, TDP-43 is increased when either autophagy or the 26S proteasome are inhibited [184, 185]. Because both protein-disposal systems are inhibited in s-IBM muscle fibers (reviewed above), their malfunctioning might contribute to the accumulation of TDP-43. However, our understanding of the consequences of TDP-43 accumulations in s-IBM muscle fibers awaits future studies.

Endoplasmic reticulum stress, decreased activity of SIRT1, oxidative stress, and putative role of αB-crystallin

ER stress and UPR

The ER is an organelle with an important role in the processing and folding of newly synthesized proteins, a function that is crucial for all cells. An efficient system of molecular chaperones in the ER is required to assure proper folding of misfolded native and abnormal proteins [148, 149, 186]. Upregulation of those ER chaperones, presumably reflecting the increased need for protein folding, occurs during the UPR [148, 149, 186]. The UPR involves the following: (a) transcriptional induction of ER chaperone proteins, whose function is to both increase the folding capacity of the ER and prevent protein aggregation; (b) translational attenuation to reduce protein overload and subsequent accumulation of unfolded proteins; and (c) removal of misfolded proteins for their degradation by 26S proteasome [148, 149, 186, 187]. The ER is also involved in "ER-associated degradation" [187]. Among various mechanisms associated with ER-associated degradation, HERP protein was proposed to play an important role functioning as an adapter protein connecting translocation of misfolded proteins from the ER with the ubiquitination process [187]. We have recently reported in s-IBM muscle fibers evidence of the UPR [14, 15]. We also demonstrated for the first time that the ER chaperones calnexin, calreticulin, GRP94, BiP/GRP78, and

ERp72 physically associate with AβPP in s-IBM muscle fibers, suggesting their playing role in AβPP folding and processing [15].

ER stress has been implicated in the pathogenesis of various neurodegenerative disorders, including Alzheimer and Parkinson diseases [20]. In Alzheimer disease brain, it has been postulated that prolonged ER stress leads to tau phosphorylation [188]. In Parkinson disease, ER stress and UPR activation have been suggested to contribute to neuronal cell death [189].

In mammals, there are three proximal sensors of ER stress that are localized to the ER membrane: (a) protein kinase RNA (PKR)-like ER protein kinase (PERK); (b) activating transcription factor 6 (ATF6); and (c) inositol-requiring enzyme 1 (IRE1) [149].

Our recent studies demonstrated that all three branches of the UPR are activated in s-IBM [190], which results in upregulation of major ER-resident chaperones, namely: GRP78, GRP94, calnexin, calreticulin, and ERp72 [15]. Also, HERP protein and mRNA are significantly increased in s-IBM muscle fibers [14].

ER stress most likely is induced in s-IBM muscle fibers by the accumulation of numerous misfolded proteins, as delineated above. In addition, oxidative and nitrosative stresses, and cholesterol accumulation, are known to occur in s-IBM muscle fibers [3, 55, 72], and in other systems they have been shown to lead to ER stress [191–193].

While UPR induction leading to upregulation of ER chaperones is supposed to decrease accumulation of abnormal proteins, this process does not seem effective in s-IBM muscle fibers, since abnormal proteins continue to accumulate leading us to propose that prolonged ER stress may aggravate muscle-fiber deterioration. Furthermore, in our experimental studies of cultured human muscle fibers (described below) experimentally induced ER stress leads to several detrimental mechanisms that we have also demonstrated in s-IBM muscle biopsies (details below).

In addition, ER stress may also be linked to the induction of inflammation in s-IBM muscle. For example, ER chaperones GRP78, calnexin, calreticulin, and PDI were shown to be involved in assembly and maturation of human MHC-I [194, 195], which is critical for muscle fibers to become antigen-presenting [1]. In various systems, the UPR has been shown to be involved in the induction of inflammatory cytokines such as tumor necrosis factor α, interleukins 2, 6, and 8 [186]. NFκB, which is a proinflammatory transcription factor known to be induced by ER stress and whose activation and acetylation are increased in s-IBM muscle fibers [75, 196, 197], may play a central role in this process. Therefore, we postulate that ER stress is an integral part of s-IBM pathogenesis.

Decreased deacetylase activity of SIRT1

SIRT1 belongs to the mammalian sirtuin family of NAD^+-dependent histone deacetylases (HDACs) [198, 199]. Targets known to be deacetylated by SIRT1 include histone 4 (H4), NFκB, and p53 [198, 199]. Through its deacetylase activity, SIRT1 is considered to control cellular metabolic homeostasis, and to play important roles in the regulation of gene expression, cell proliferation, differentiation, survival, and senescence [198, 199]. SIRT1 activation has been considered to play a crucial role in calorie-restriction-induced longevity in several species [200].

In addition, SIRT1 activation has been proposed to play a role in neuroprotection [198, 199]. For example, in an Alzheimer mouse model, increase of neuronal SIRT1 and its activation were reported to underlie the calorie-restriction prevention of Aβ-related Alzheimer disease-like neuropathology [198, 199]. In various cell lines, increase of SIRT1, or its activation, was reported to protect against Aβ toxicity by either decreasing the amount of Aβ through activation of α-secretase, or by inhibiting NFκB activation and its subsequent disturbance of signaling [198, 199].

Our most recent studies have shown that, in s-IBM muscle fibers as compared to age-matched controls, SIRT1 activity and deacetylation of its targets NFκB, H4, and p53 were significantly decreased [196]. Since increased acetylation, or decreased deacetylation, of NFκB leads to its increased activity [201], decreased SIRT1 deacetylase activity might be directly responsible for the presumably detrimental NFκB activation in s-IBM muscle fibers. Our study provides, to our knowledge, the first demonstration of decreased SIRT1 deacetylase activity in any human muscle disease, namely, s-IBM, a disease that is associated with aging. Abnormalities of SIRT1 in our ER-stress IBM human muscle culture model are described below.

Oxidative stress

Oxidative stress has been proposed for many years to play an important pathogenic role in neurodegenerative diseases [202, 203]. There is increasing evidence that free-radical toxicity may participate in the IBM pathogenesis as follows. Indicators of oxidative stress, as well as enzymes participating in the cellular defense against oxidative stress, are accumulated in s-IBM muscle fibers [55, 56, 60, 74]. Also, s-IBM muscle fibers contain increased and activated NFκB [59, 75].

In s-IBM muscle fibers we have recently reported abnormalities of the Parkinson disease-related DJ-1, a protein participating in amelioration of oxidative stress [12]. DJ-1 is a ubiquitously expressed protein of the ThiJ/PfpI/DJ-1 superfamily (reviewed in [204] and referenced in [12]). In s-IBM muscle fibers, DJ-1 is (a) highly oxidized and (b) abnormally accumulated in mitochondria [12]. Mutations in the *DJ-1* gene that prevent expression of DJ-1 protein are a cause of early-onset autosomal recessive Parkinson disease [204]. In sporadic Alzheimer and Parkinson disease brains, DJ-1 was reported to be increased and highly oxidized (referenced in [12]). Although its precise functions are not yet known, DJ-1 has been proposed to act as an antioxidant ([204] and referenced in [12]) and be an important mitochondrial protective agent (referenced in [12]). Increased oxidation of DJ-1 itself was proposed to decrease its antioxidant activity ([204] and referenced in [12]). We have proposed that in s-IBM muscle fibers the increased DJ-1 may be attempting to mitigate mitochondrial and oxidative damage, but being excessively oxidized may itself render it ineffective [1, 12]. Our studies indicated for the first time that DJ-1 might play a role in human muscle disease.

Abnormalities of αB-crystallin

αB-crystallin (αBC), a small heat-shock protein (sHSP) responding to stress, was shown immuno-

histochemically by others to be abnormally accumulated in muscle fibers of s-IBM and other myopathies [205]. It was reported that in s-IBM, but not in other myopathies, αBC was accumulated not only in the structurally abnormal, vacuolated, or otherwise obviously damaged muscle fibers, but also in many fibers termed by the authors "X-fibers," which did not display "significant" morphologic abnormality [205]. Therefore, it was proposed that increased αBC expression precedes other abnormalities in s-IBM muscle fibers [205]. The stressor(s) inducing αBC are not yet identified, and as such (a) might play a protective role [205], or (b) might, either by itself or bound to another protein, induce an inflammatory response [205, 206]. Since increased expression of αBC can occur under various stressful conditions (reviewed in [207]), we hypothesized that in morphologically "undamaged" s-IBM muscle fibers αBC might be induced in response to the early increase in them of "morphologically invisible" soluble Aβ oligomers (not in aggregates). Therefore, we studied αBC in cultured human muscle fibers shortly after overexpressing AβPP in them and before typical structural abnormalities characteristic to IBM had developed. We evaluated, both in cultured human muscle fibers and in s-IBM muscle fibers, whether αBC physically associates with AβPP/Aβ (details in [208]). Our studies showed that: (a) overexpression of AβPP into normal culture human muscle fibers significantly increased αBC; (b) additional inhibition of proteasome with epoxomicin further increased αBC; and (c) αBC physically associated with AβPP and Aβ oligomers [208]. Similarly, in biopsied s-IBM muscle fibers, αBC was significantly increased on the immunoblots and physically associated with AβPP and Aβ oligomers [208]. As an sHSP, αBC plays a role in the cellular defense against improperly degraded and accumulated toxic proteins by stabilizing the ones that have a propensity to aggregate and precipitate [207]. In Alzheimer brain, αBC binds to AβPP, and *in vitro*, αBC binds to Aβ and prevents Aβ fibrilization and aggregation [209, 210]. However, applied extracellularly together with Aβ to cultured rat neurons, αBC increases Aβ cytotoxicity, which is postulated to occur due to its influence in maintaining Aβ in the soluble oligomeric, highly cytotoxic form [211]. Even though the exact role of αBC in s-IBM muscle fibers awaits further elucidation, our studies clearly indicate that, in contrast to what was reported by others [212], αBC within the muscle fibers is increased by the increased intracellular AβPP/Aβ.

Mitochondrial abnormalities

Mitochondrial abnormalities in s-IBM muscle fibers include: (a) ragged-red fibers [129], (b) cytochrome c oxidase (COX)-negative muscle fibers, and (c) multiple mitochondrial DNA deletions (reviewed in [130]). These are more common in s-IBM muscle than expected for the patient's age (reviewed in [130]). Our newest studies confirmed that COX-negative muscle fibers were significantly increased in s-IBM muscle biopsies. While the COX-negative fibers were 90% type 2, there was a higher percent of type-1 COX-negative fibers than in controls [213]. We previously showed that excessive AβPP and Aβ contribute to the mitochondrial abnormalities in cultured human muscle fibers ([214] and below); this concept is now supported by studies in other systems, especially as putatively related to Alzheimer and Parkinson brain ([202, 215, 216] and referenced in [12]). Other as-yet-unknown mechanisms may also contribute to the prominent COX negativity in s-IBM muscle fibers, possibly including (a) toxic unaggregated oligomers of Aβ, α-syn, or other proteins; and (b) factors resulting from oxidative or ER stresses. Discovery of their cause could facilitate developing treatment strategies. The resultant mitochondrial abnormalities presumably contribute to the muscle-fiber malfunction and degeneration.

In seemingly otherwise-intact muscle fibers, the regions of COX negativity cannot produce ATP via oxidative phosphorylation; those presumably weakened regions must be surviving on ATP diffusing from adjacent COX-positive regions or produced locally by anaerobic glycolysis.

Another indication of mitochondrial abnormality was our demonstration that in s-IBM muscle fibers cytochrome c is aggregated within cytoplasm, where it is physically associated with AβPP and α-syn [217].

Cytochrome c is involved in electron transport within mitochondria, and its release from mitochondria is indicative of mitochondrial abnormality, which usually leads to apoptosis in mononucleated cells (reviewed in [218]). It is relevant that in s-IBM muscle fibers active/cleaved caspase-3 was not present [217], which is in agreement with our studies and others that apoptosis is not participating in the s-IBM pathogenic cascade (reviewed and referenced in [5]). However, in s-IBM muscle fibers the association of cytochrome c with AβPP and α-syn may enhance their oligomerization and fibrilization, thereby influencing their toxicity, as has been proposed for Alzheimer and Parkinson diseases [215].

Proteins accumulated in s-IBM muscle fibers are also increased at the postsynaptic domain of normal NMJs

Several years ago we emphasized that several proteins and their mRNAs accumulated within s-IBM muscle fibers are also present postsynaptically at the NMJs, and we termed this phenomenon "junctionalization of nonjunctional regions" [219]. During regeneration of normal muscle fibers, various proteins and their mRNAs are expressed within and along the length of the fiber. As a result of motor innervation, in normal mature fibers the same proteins, termed "junctional proteins," become increased at the *postsynaptic region* of the NMJ and suppressed everywhere in the fiber. This normal accumulation of proteins and their mRNAs postsynaptically we have termed "junctionalization" of the muscle fiber [5, 219]. Several of the "s-IBM proteins" and "s-IBM mRNAs" that are accumulated in nonjunctional regions of s-IBM muscle fibers are, in *normal innervated mature human muscle fibers*, also ones identified morphologically at the postsynaptic region of the NMJs [5, 219] (Table 7.2). p-Tau is the only "s-IBM protein" so far studied that was not found accumulated at normal NMJs [219]. In s-IBM muscle fibers we proposed that a possible pathogenic role of "extra-junctionalization" might be (a) partly related to normal attempts of the stricken fibers to regenerate, and (b) partly driven by ectopic

Table 7.2 Accumulation of the Same Proteins and Molecules within the aggregates of s-IBM muscle fibers and at the postsynaptic domain of human neuromuscular junctions (NMJs).

	s-IBM	NMJs
NMJ proteins		
nAchR protein/mRNA	+	+
43 kDa rapsyn	+	+
Aggregate-prone proteins		
AβPP/Aβ protein/mRNA	+	+
Prion protein, cellular protein/mRNA	+	+
α-synuclein	+	+
phosphorylated-tau	+	−
AβPP processing/Aβ deposition		
BACE1, BACE2	+	+
Cystatin C	+	+
Presenilin1	+	+
Markers of oxidative stress		
SOD1	+	+
nNOS, iNOS	+	+
α1-antichymotrypsin	+	+
Seleno-gluththione peroxidase-1	+	+
Catalase	+	+
Ref-1	+	+
NFκB	+	+
Malondialdehyde	+	+
Nitrotyrosine	+	−
Transcription/RNA metabolism		
RNA polymerase II	+	+
SMN	+	+
c-Jun, c-Fos	+	+
NFκB	+	+
Ref-1	+	+
Cholesterol metabolism		
ApoE	+	+
LDLR	+	+
VLDLR	+	+
Cytokines/growth factors		
FGF	+	+
TGF-1β	+	+
IL-1α	+	+
IL-1β	+	+
IL-6	+	+
Protein degradation		
Ubiquitin	+	+
Signal transduction components		
ERK	+	+
GSK-3β active	+	+
Other		
SIRT1	±	+

unrestrained extrajunctional expression of "junctional genes," possibly influenced by a pathologically unrestrained hypothetical normal "junctionalization master gene" [5, 7, 219]. A "master-gene product" might be serving, directly or indirectly, as a transcription factor activating genes for at least some of the "s-IBM-proteins," leading to a detrimental cascade. A normal junctionalization master gene, or possibly a specific "s-IBM master gene" might itself be activated by (a) an adjacently inserted viral gene (insertional mutagenesis), or (b) epigenetic influence. A pathologically deranged junctionalization master gene might also fail to properly form and maintain the junctional postsynaptic region. Some s-IBM fibers have abnormal NMJ structure [220]. Unlike cultured normal human muscle fibers, cultured muscle fibers overexpressing AβPP, either experimentally by AβPP gene transfer, or genetically in GNE-type h-IBM fibers, could not become innervated by co-cultured fetal rat spinal cord neurons [221]. We therefore postulated several years ago that AβPP overexpression in s-IBM patients' biopsied muscle fibers may cause the observed morphologic abnormalities, and an intracellular postsynaptic "myogenous dysinnervation" [5, 7, 221]. This proposal is gaining more interest now, because: (a) it was recently demonstrated that at some central nervous system synapses PrP^c is a "receptor" for Aβ42 and Aβ oligomers [134], and (b) we have shown that Aβ42 and its oligomers are accumulated in s-IBM fibers. The neuromuscular synapse pathology in s-IBM has a parallel in the occurrence of synapse pathology in Alzheimer disease [222], which, by analogy with s-IBM, we propose may, at least partly, reflect an *intracellular postsynaptic* mechanism.

Transthyretin gene mutation and s-IBM

We have described a 70-year-old African American man who had both s-IBM and *cardiac amyloidosis*, identified clinically by diphosphonate scan [7], and was homozygous for the transthyretin (TTR) Val122Ile mutation [223]. In addition to the skeletal muscle pathological features typical of s-IBM, there were unique aspects. They included: (a) congophilic deposits coimmunoreactive for both TTR and Aβ within vacuolated muscle fibers, where TTR is never present in ordinary s-IBM; and (b) prominent blood vessel congophilic amyloid, co-immunoreactive for both TTR and Aβ, neither occurring in blood vessels of ordinary s-IBM.

The TTR Val122Ile mutation is the most common cause of late-onset cardiac amyloidosis among African Americans [224]. Our patient's mutant TTR might be a *facilitating factor*, promoting the amyloid fibrillogenesis of Aβ within his muscle fibers and in muscle blood vessels. In other systems, non-mutant TTR can protectively sequester Aβ, prevent amyloid fibril formation *in vitro*, and mitigate Aβ cytotoxicity *in vivo* [225]. We have proposed that if our patient's cardiac amyloidosis, muscle blood vessel amyloidosis, and s-IBM all relate to his TTR mutation that would make it a *susceptibility-gene mutation* [223, 226]. By extension, perhaps other mutations or polymorphisms of TTR or other as-yet-unknown susceptibility genes – congenital or induced by viral, environmental, or aging factors – may be promoting s-IBM in many, if not all, other s-IBM patients. If the TTR Val122Ile mutation was a susceptibility factor in our patient, it probably had existed since conception, but his muscle weakness did not develop until after age 60. That would reemphasize the importance of an aging, or virally/environmentally modified cellular milieu for developing s-IBM.

Recently, a new mouse experimental model of s-IBM was described [227]. In it, two aspects are of particular interest to the possible pathogenesis of s-IBM: (a) overexpression of mutated gelsolin D187N within myofibers of aged mouse induced an intra-myofiber accumulation of misfolded and congophilic proteins, including Aβ and gelsolin; and (b) in addition to the intra-myofiber accumulation of gelsolin and the multi-protein aggregates it induced, these apparently being the primary events, there was also perivascular and endomysial lymphocytic cell infiltration, strongly suggesting – as we have previously proposed for s-IBM [1, 3] and reiterated in this chapter – that inflammation was secondary to protein abnormalities, rather than the reverse. This could explain why anti-inflammatory drugs do not produce enduring benefit in s-IBM [4]. This mutant gelsolin model is helpful because in patients' biopsies one cannot study the sequence of events.

Since overexpressed wild types of either gelsolin or TTR bind Aβ, prevent its aggregation, and protect from Aβ cytotoxicity [228, 229], we propose that their mutant forms lose these protective capabilities and allow intra-myofiber Aβ aggregation and amyloidosis. Accordingly, s-IBM patients should be studied for mutations or polymorphisms of gelsolin and TTR.

Experimental models designed to elucidate the IBM pathogenesis

One of our approaches to explore molecular mechanisms participating in the s-IBM pathogenesis involves utilizing well-differentiated cultured normal human muscle fibers, whose cellular microenvironment we experimentally modify to mimic various aspects of the s-IBM muscle-fiber milieu, thereby providing IBM human muscle culture models (IBM-HM-TC-Models). Others have utilized experimental transgenic mice models. These models will be summarized and referenced below.

Evidence suggesting pathogenic importance of experimental and genetically determined overexpression of AβPP in culture and *in vivo*

Overexpression of AβPP/Aβ in mature cultured normal human muscle fibers (AβPP$^{(+)}$-IBM-HM-TC-model)

Our AβPP$^{(+)}$-IBM-HM-TC-Model exhibits several aspects of the IBM pathologic phenotype including: (a) pronounced vacuolization of most of the muscle fibers; (b) congophilic inclusions in some of the muscle fibers; (c) aggresome formation; (d) nuclear PHFs; (e) mitochondria abnormalities including COX deficiency; (f) cholesterol accumulation; (g) increased αBC; (h) increased parkin; (i) increased myostatin; and (j) inability to become innervated [31, 141, 214, 221, 230, 231]. This cultured human muscle model clearly demonstrates that AβPP/Aβ overexpression can be central to the induction of IBM-characteristic phenotype.

Cultured muscle fibers from h-IBM due to GNE mutation

In our cultured muscle fibers of h-IBM due to a GNE mutation, the presumably genetically determined increase of AβPP/Aβ preceded other IBM-type abnormalities [221], including (a) their inability to become properly innervated by normal fetal spinal cord neurons, and (b) having morphologically abnormal NMJs [221]. We therefore postulated that spontaneous AβPP/Aβ overexpression in s-IBM patient muscle may be responsible for a "myogenous dysinnervation" [221] and for the observed NMJ structural abnormalities [220] (see above), and, by analogy, the same AβPP/Aβ-based mechanism may be occurring in h-IBM.

Experimental and genetically determined overexpression of AβPP/Aβ in transgenic mouse models

Support for our hypothesis that intracellular AβPP/Aβ cytotoxicity plays a detrimental role in the IBM pathogenesis has been provided by various transgenic mouse models. The first demonstration in transgenic mice of the importance of AβPP/Aβ in the induction of the IBM phenotype was provided in 1998 by Fukuchi et al. [232] and Jin et al. [233]. A newer mouse model in which experimental manipulation has led to the increased generation of Aβ42 had, in addition to some other aspects of IBM, (a) CD8 T-cell inflammation, (b) increased CD8 T-cell mRNA, (c) increased tau phosphorylation, and (d) increased expression of kinases GSK-3β and CDK5 [113], both of which participate in tau phosphorylation ([52, 53, 89], and see also above). Another aspect of those three AβPP transgenic mouse models was dependence on an aging milieu for the development of the IBM-like abnormalities [113, 232–234].

In another, recent, mouse model based on AβPP overexpression, abnormal calcium homeostasis due to increased Aβ was reported to be a very early abnormality [235]. Accordingly, the authors proposed that abnormal calcium homeostasis preceded by Aβ accumulation might be one of the earliest events in the s-IBM pathogenesis [235].

Interestingly, in a GNE-knockout mouse overexpressing the GNE V572L mutation, Aβ accumulation preceded by several weeks other identified muscle abnormalities, such as weakness, increased serum creatine kinase activity, muscle-fiber vacuolization, and general muscle atrophy ([236], and see Chapter 11). This model suggests that accumulation of Aβ, and perhaps its decreased sialylation, is an important upstream or midstream component of the h-IBM pathogenesis. In this model, as in other IBM animal models and s-IBM patients, aging also is a significant component contributing to both the weakness and abnormal pathological phenotype in those GNE mutant transgenic mice.

Evidence suggesting the importance of ER stress in the s-IBM pathogenic cascade

Experimental pharmacological induction of *ER stress* in well-differentiated cultured human muscle fibers created our ER$^{(+)}$-IBM-HM-TC-Model. This model exhibits several abnormalities that are present in s-IBM muscle biopsies, such as: (a) a strong induction of the UPR; (b) increased activation of NFκB; (c) increased myostatin mRNA and protein, as a response to abnormal NFκB activation; (d) decreased SIRT1 activity resulting in hyperacetylation and activation of NFκB; (e) increased BACE1 protein, its mRNA, and its noncoding regulatory transcript (BACE1 participates in abnormal processing of AβPP, which results in increased Aβ production; see above); (f) decreased NOGO-B, which might result in increased production of Aβ (NOGO-B prevents BACE1 binding to AβPP, and that subsequently decreases Aβ production); and (g) impaired autophagy as evidenced by (i) decreased activities of lysosomal proteolytic enzymes cathepsins D and B, (ii) increased LC3-II, and decreased phosphorylation of p70 S6 kinase; and (iii) decreased VMA21, a chaperone for assembly of lysosomal V-ATPase, which helps to maintain lysosomal acidic pH [13, 14, 40, 75, 76, 190, 196].

Consequence of 26S proteasome inhibition

Experimental inhibition of proteasome created our Prot$^{(-)}$-IBM-HM-TC-Model, which exhibits the following: (a) accumulation of ubiquitinated aggregates; (b) development of aggresomes; (c) αB-crystal-in increase and accumulation in aggregates; (d) parkin increase and aggregation; (e) myostatin aggregation; (f) GSK-3β activation; (g) induction of AβPP phosphorylation; and (h) increase of p62/SQSTM1 [11, 31, 34, 48, 141, 208].

Consequences of autophagy inhibition

Experimental inhibition of autophagy creates the Autoph$^{(-)}$-IBM-HM-TC-Model, which has been utilized only recently. However, it might be very important in the future, because inhibition of autophagy has been proposed to play an important role in the s-IBM pathogenesis [2, 13]. For example, we have recently reported that inhibition of autophagy leads to production of the putatively cytotoxic Aβ oligomers in normal, non-AβPP-overexpressing, cultured human muscle fibers [13]. Accordingly, our proposed detrimental intra-muscle-fiber toxicity and consequences of Aβ oligomers could be studied in this model. p62/SQSMT1 is also increased in this model [48], providing another similarity to the s-IBM phenotype [48, 66].

Below we describe how our results obtained in IBM-HM-TC-models might pertain to treatment of s-IBM patients.

Possible treatments of s-IBM

Current treatments are of only slight benefit for only some s-IBM patients, and do not stop the ongoing disease progression. A "right treatment" of s-IBM should produce actual increase of strength, because, ordinarily, injured muscle fibers, which are multi-nucleated cells, are able to repair and regenerate. However, s-IBM muscle fibers reportedly have impaired regeneration [237]. Therefore, a "right treatment" would need to: (a) stop degeneration: (b) stop inflammation (possibly by stopping the degeneration); and (c) allow, or promote repair and regeneration.

Until now, most treatment approaches have been directed toward stopping an inflammatory/dysimmune component of s-IBM, but they are considered largely ineffective, even though an occasional patient appeared to benefit [7, 238–240]. Attempted anti-dysimmune/anti-inflammatory treatments include: (a) corticosteroids; (b) methotrexate; (c) azathioprine; (d) mycophenolate; and (e) cyclosporine (reviewed in [7, 238–241]). In our unpublished experience, a few patients with s-IBM benefit to some degree from treatment with relatively modest single-dose (such as 15–45 mg) alternate-day (SDAD) prednisone. Endurance of limb strength in those responsive patients is clearly beneficial, repeatedly proven by worsening when the dose was lowered below a level critical for the given patient, e.g. 44, 38, 30, 18, or 14 mg SDAD prednisone. With muscle involvement, endurance for one's daily activities can be reduced before clinically tested "brute strength." (Endurance of larger muscles is typically not clinically tested, but should be, because even detailed quantitative strength testing can miss improvement in endurance.) Some patients have preferred continuing the slight prednisone benefit when their prednisone side effects were modest. Nevertheless, the underlying progressive muscle weakness is not stopped. In some patients, swallowing difficulty is slightly improved by prednisone (W. K. Engel, unpublished observations). But the overall failure of various forms of immunosuppression therapy to stop s-IBM progression [242] suggests that a dysimmune mechanism is neither paramount nor of major significance in causing the gradually increasing and disabling weakness.

Sometimes slight benefit can be achieved in some patients with intravenous IgG (IVIG). This may be related especially to a chronic immune dysschwannian polyneuropathy (CIDP) aspect demonstrable in some s-IBM patients. In some patients, swallowing difficulty can be improved by IVIG ([239] and references therein, and W.K. Engel, current observations). However, IVIG does not stop the underlying progression in the typical s-IBM patient.

Based on our own studies we propose that the most important general approach to developing treatment for s-IBM patients is to stop, and repair, deterioration and atrophy of the muscle fibers. The treatment approaches might need to be multifactorial, toward various intra-muscle-fiber detrimental aspects described above, including: (a) preventing abnormal accumulation and oligomerization of Aβ42, α-syn, and p-tau, and blocking their putative oligomeric toxicity on normal cellular components; and (b) decreasing adverse effects of ER stress by (i) improving protein degradation through the lysosomal and proteasomal pathways, and (ii) dispersing large protein aggregates; (iii) decreasing myostatin, a negative regulator of muscle mass; and, possibly, (iv) decreasing oxidative stress and improving mitochondrial function (however, the use of vitamin E, coenzyme Q, and L-carnitine have not been remarkably beneficial (unpublished results); (v) diminishing adverse effects of intra-muscle-fiber cholesterol (however, the use of statins is of uncertain benefit and potentially myotoxic for occasional patients); and (vi) greater understanding of molecular mechanisms to abrogate deleterious effects of "aging" of the human muscle-fiber milieu could provide new avenues toward s-IBM therapy.

Putative treatment approaches

Below we describe various putative treatment approaches. These are based on our IBM-culture models and various experimental Alzheimer disease models. However, for most of the compounds their possible toxicity and potential benefits in patients are not known.

Polyphenols

Various polyphenols recently have been reported to be beneficial in Alzheimer disease experimental mouse models and an IBM-culture model. They include the following.

Resveratrol (trans-3,4′,5-trihydroxystilbene) treatment of ER stress-induced cultured human muscle fibers (ERS$^{(+)}$-IBM-HM-TC-Model) significantly decreased in them myostatin mRNA and protein, which was associated with NFκB deacetylation (deactivation), and it increased muscle-fiber size [243]. Previously in Alzheimer mouse models, resveratrol was shown to decrease Aβ and diminish Alzheimer disease neuropathology [199, 244]. Resveratrol is an antioxidant polyphenol and potent activator of SIRT1 (reviewed in [244]). Accordingly, resveratrol, and/or other small molecules that activate SIRT1 (the activity of which is decreased in s-IBM muscle [196]), might be beneficial in treating s-IBM patients. Recently, SIRT1 activity was

reported to increase autophagy [245]. In s-IBM muscle fibers autophagy is impaired [13], and our studies suggest that resveratrol induces lysosomal cathepsin D activity [246] and decreases Aβ oligomers [247]. Accordingly, even though more studies are needed to fully support the use of resveratrol in s-IBM patients, including its optimal dose and potential side effects, there is a strong rationale that resveratrol might benefit s-IBM patients.

Other phenolic compounds, including curcumin and grape-seed-derived polyphenols, have been reported to decrease the amyloid burden and Aβ fibrilization in Alzheimer disease transgenic mice and *in vitro* [248–252].

Lithium

Lithium was reported to diminish tau and Aβ pathologies in various experimental models of Alzheimer disease (reviewed in [253]), but its clinical efficacy in treating Alzheimer disease patients is not established. In a transgenic mouse model whose skeletal muscle bears some aspects of IBM muscle fibers, lithium was reported to decrease tau phosphorylation through decreasing activity of GSK-3β [254].

Recently, we have shown that lithium treatment of cultured human muscle fibers in our AβPP$^{(+)}$-IBM-HM-TC-Model significantly decreased total AβPP, phosphorylated AβPP, and Aβ oligomers [34]. In addition, lithium significantly increased the inactive form of GSK-3β [34]. Accordingly, treating of s-IBM patients with lithium, which is widely used in treating bipolar disorder in humans, possibly would be beneficial.

Sodium phenylbutyrate

Phenylbutyrate is a chemical chaperone that has been reported to decrease α-syn toxicity in a Parkinson disease transgenic mice model and to reduce tau pathology in Alzheimer disease transgenic mice model, as well to reduce ER stress and decrease protein aggregation in cultured cell lines [255–257]. Sodium phenylbutyrate was tried in ALS patients, and doses up to 21 g/day were well tolerated [258]; however, no beneficial effect has yet been reported. In some patients with

Huntington disease, doses above 15 g/day were not well tolerated [259].

Improving lysosomal function

Improvement of lysosomal function might be useful in decreasing putatively toxic protein oligomers and their aggregation in s-IBM muscle. Recently attention has been given to small-molecule lysosomal modulators (review in [260]). Their effectiveness beyond experimental animal studies and culture systems is not known.

Decreasing myostatin

Myostatin is increased and aggregated in s-IBM muscle fibers (see above). Studies in our ERS$^{(+)}$-IBM-HM-TC-Model have shown that treatment with resveratrol (see above) decreases myostatin protein and mRNA, and increases the size of muscle fibers. Whether this effect will occur beneficially in patients is not known.

Role of physical therapy in helping s-IBM patients

1 Standard physical therapy, including active exercise, as tolerated, and maintaining range of motion.
2 Orthotics as needed, especially one self-locking knee brace on the weaker leg, and sometimes one or two simple lightweight drop-foot braces. Some patients have found that two self-locking knee braces are too awkward.
3 Mobility devices, as needed including a walker (with or without a seat, folding if necessary), electric seater, or motorized wheelchair.
4 Making the home environment safer and easier, including grab-bars and a raised toilet seat.
5 Assistive devices, such as to facilitate gripping utensils, and a simple seat-riser, consisting of a lightweight tote bag containing three to five 2.5 cm-thick pieces of styrofoam.

Acknowledgements

Research described in this chapter was supported over the years by grants from the National Institutes of Health, Muscular Dystrophy Association, Myositis Association, Myasthenia Gravis Foundation, and the Helen Lewis Research Fund. The authors are grateful to many research fellows in Dr Askanas' laboratory, whose work contributed to the results described herein. We are grateful to Dr P. Davies for his generous gift of the Alz-50 and PHF-1 antibodies.

References

1 Askanas V, Engel WK. (2008) Inclusion-body myositis: muscle-fiber molecular pathology and possible pathogenic significance of its similarity to Alzheimer's and Parkinson's disease brains. *Acta Neuropathol* **116**, 583–595.

2 Askanas V, Engel WK, Nogalska A. (2009) Inclusion body myositis: a degenerative muscle disease associated with intra-muscle fiber multi-protein aggregates, proteasome inhibition, endoplasmic reticulum stress and decreased lysosomal degradation. *Brain Pathol* **19**, 493–506.

3 Askanas V, Engel WK. (2007) Inclusion-body myositis, a multifactorial muscle disease associated with aging: current concepts of pathogenesis. *Curr Opin Rheumatol* **19**, 550–559.

4 Askanas V, Engel WK. (2006) Inclusion-body myositis: a myodegenerative conformational disorder associated with Abeta, protein misfolding, and proteasome inhibition. *Neurology* **66**, S39–S48.

5 Askanas V, Engel WK. (2001) Inclusion-body myositis: newest concepts of pathogenesis and relation to aging and Alzheimer disease. *J Neuropathol Exp Neurol* **60**, 1–14.

6 Askanas V, Engel WK. (2003) Proposed pathogenetic cascade of inclusion-body myositis: importance of amyloid-beta, misfolded proteins, predisposing genes, and aging. *Curr Opin Rheumatol* **15**, 737–744.

7 Engel WK, Askanas V. (2006) Inclusion-body myositis: clinical, diagnostic, and pathologic aspects. *Neurology* **66**, S20–S29.

8 Amouri R, Driss A, Murayama K et al. (2005) Allelic heterogeneity of GNE gene mutation in two Tunisian families with autosomal recessive inclusion body myopathy. *Neuromuscul Disord* **15**, 361–363.

9 Askanas V, Engel WK. (2008) Hereditary inclusion body myopathies. In: Rosenberg RN, Di Mauro S, Paulson HL et al. (eds), *The Molecular and Genetic Basis of Neurologic and Psychiatric Disease*, 4th edn. Wolters Kluwer, Lippincott Williams & Wilkins, Philadelphia, pp. 524–531.

10 Krause S, Schlotter-Weigel B, Walter MC et al. (2007) A novel homozygous missense mutation in the GNE gene of a patient with quadriceps-sparing hereditary inclusion body myopathy associated with muscle inflammation. *Neuromuscul Disord* **13**, 830–834.

11 Fratta P, Engel WK, McFerrin J et al. (2005) Proteasome inhibition and aggresome formation in sporadic inclusion-body myositis and in AbPP-overexpressing cultured human muscle fibers. *Am J Pathol* **167**, 517–526.

12 Terracciano C, Nogalska A, Engel WK et al. (2008) In inclusion-body myositis muscle fibers Parkinson-associated DJ-1 is increased and oxidized. *Free Radic Biol Med* **45**, 773–779.

13 Nogalska A, D'Agostino C, Terracciano C et al. (2010) Impaired autophagy in sporadic inclusion-body myositis and in endoplasmic reticulum stress-provoked cultured human muscle fibers. *Am J Pathol* **177**, 1377–1387.

14 Nogalska A, Engel WK, McFerrin J et al. (2006) Homocysteine-induced endoplasmic reticulum protein (Herp) is up-regulated in sporadic inclusion-body myositis and in endoplasmic reticulum stress-induced cultured human muscle fibers. *J Neurochem* **96**, 1491–1499.

15 Vattemi G, Engel WK, McFerrin J et al. (2004) Endoplasmic reticulum stress and unfolded protein response in inclusion body myositis muscle. *Am J Pathol* **164**, 1–7.

16 Keller JN, Hanni KB, Markesbery WR. (2000) Impaired proteasome function in Alzheimer's disease. *J Neurochem* **75**, 436–439.

17 Sherman MY, Goldberg AL. (2001) Cellular defenses against unfolded proteins: a cell biologist thinks about neurodegenerative diseases. *Neuron* **29**, 15–32.

18 Bossy-Wetzel E, Schwarzenbacher R, Lipton SA. (2004) Molecular pathways to neurodegeneration. *Nat Med* **10**(Suppl.) S2–S9.

19 Hindle JV. (2010) Ageing, neurodegeneration and Parkinson's disease. *Age Ageing* **39**, 156–161.

20 Lindholm D, Wootz H, Korhonen L. (2006) ER stress and neurodegenerative diseases. *Cell Death Differ* **13**, 385–392.

21 Engel WK, Cunningham GG. (1963) Rapid examination of muscle tissue and improved trichrome method for fresh-frozen biopsy sections. *Neurology* **13**, 919–923.

22 Askanas V, Alvarez RB, Engel WK. (1993) Beta-amyloid precursor epitopes in muscle fibers of inclusion body myositis. *Ann Neurol* **34**, 551–560.

23 Askanas V, Engel WK, Alvarez RB. (1992) Light and electron microscopic localization of beta-amyloid protein in muscle biopsies of patients with inclusion-body myositis. *Am J Pathol* **141**, 31–36.

24 Askanas V, Engel WK, Bilak M et al. (1994) Twisted tubulofilaments of inclusion body myositis muscle resemble paired helical filaments of Alzheimer brain and contain hyperphosphorylated tau. *Am J Pathol* **144**, 177–187.

25 Mirabella M, Alvarez RB, Bilak M et al. (1996) Difference in expression of phosphorylated tau epitopes between sporadic inclusion-body myositis and hereditary inclusion-body myopathies. *J Neuropathol Exp Neurol* **55**, 774–786.

26 Askanas V, Engel WK, Alvarez RB. (1993) Enhanced detection of congo-red-positive amyloid deposits in muscle fibers of inclusion body myositis and brain of Alzheimer's disease using fluorescence technique. *Neurology* **43**, 1265–1267.

27 Mendell JR, Sahenk Z, Gales T et al. (1991) Amyloid filaments in inclusion body myositis. Novel findings provide insight into nature of filaments. *Arch Neurol* **48**, 1229–1234.

28 Vattemi G, Nogalska A, King Engel W et al. (2009) Amyloid-beta42 is preferentially accumulated in muscle fibers of patients with sporadic inclusion-body myositis. *Acta Neuropathol* **117**, 569–574.

29 Askanas V, Engel WK, Alvarez RB et al. (1992) beta-Amyloid protein immunoreactivity in muscle of patients with inclusion-body myositis. *Lancet* **339**, 560–561.

30 Askanas V, Engel WK, Alvarez RB et al. (2000) Novel immunolocalization of alpha-synuclein in human muscle of inclusion-body myositis, regenerating and necrotic muscle fibers, and at neuromuscular junctions. *J Neuropathol Exp Neurol* **59**, 592–598.

31 Paciello O, Wojcik S, Engel WK et al. (2006) Parkin and its association with alpha-synuclein and AbetaPP in inclusion-body myositis and AbetaPP-overexpressing cultured human muscle fibers. *Acta Myol* **25**, 13–22.

32 Askanas V, Bilak M, Engel WK et al. (1993) Prion protein is abnormally accumulated in inclusion-body myositis. *Neuroreport* **5**, 25–28.

33 Wojcik S, Engel WK, McFerrin J et al. (2005) Myostatin is increased and complexes with amyloid-beta within sporadic inclusion-body myositis muscle fibers. *Acta Neuropathol* **110**, 173–177.

34 Terracciano C, Nogalska A, Engel WK et al. (2010) In AbetaPP-overexpressing cultured human muscle fibers proteasome inhibition enhances phosphoryla-

tion of AbetaPP751 and GSK3beta activation: effects mitigated by lithium and apparently relevant to sporadic inclusion-body myositis. *J Neurochem* **112**, 389–396.

35 Vattemi G, Engel WK, McFerrin J et al. (2001) Presence of BACE1 and BACE2 in muscle fibres of patients with sporadic inclusion-body myositis. *Lancet* **358**, 1962–1964.

36 Vattemi G, Engel WK, McFerrin J et al. (2003) BACE1 and BACE2 in pathologic and normal human muscle. *Exp Neurol* **179**, 150–158.

37 Vattemi G, Kefi M, Engel WK et al. (2003) Nicastrin, a novel protein participating in amyloid-beta production, is overexpressed in sporadic inclusion-body myositis muscle. *Neurology* **60**, A315.

38 Askanas V, Engel WK, Yang CC et al. (1998) Light and electron microscopic immunolocalization of presenilin 1 in abnormal muscle fibers of patients with sporadic inclusion-body myositis and autosomal-recessive inclusion-body myopathy. *Am J Pathol* **152**, 889–895.

39 Broccolini A, Gidaro T, Morosetti R et al. (2006) Neprilysin participates in skeletal muscle regeneration and is accumulated in abnormal muscle fibres of inclusion body myositis. *J Neurochem* **96**, 777–789.

40 Wojcik S, Engel WK, Yan R et al. (2007) NOGO is increased and binds to BACE1 in sporadic inclusion-body myositis and in A beta PP-overexpressing cultured human muscle fibers. *Acta Neuropathol* **114**, 517–526.

41 Vattemi G, Engel WK, McFerrin J et al. (2003) Cystatin C colocalizes with amyloid-beta and coimmunoprecipitates with amyloid-beta precursor protein in sporadic inclusion-body myositis muscles. *J Neurochem* **85**, 1539–1546.

42 Choi YC, Park GT, Kim TS et al. (2003) Sporadic inclusion body myositis correlates with increased expression and cross-linking by transglutaminases 1 and 2. *J Biol Chem* **275**, 8703–8710.

43 Askanas V, Serdaroglu P, Engel WK et al. (2003) Immunolocalization of ubiquitin in muscle biopsies of patients with inclusion body myositis and oculopharyngeal muscular dystrophy. *Neurosci Lett* **130**, 73–76.

44 Prayson RA, Cohen ML. (1997) Ubiquitin immunostaining and inclusion body myositis: study of 30 patients with inclusion body myositis. *Hum Pathol* **28**, 887–892.

45 Fratta P, Engel WK, Van Leeuwen FW et al. (2004) Mutant ubiquitin UBB + 1 is accumulated in sporadic inclusion-body myositis muscle fibers. *Neurology* **63**, 1114–1117.

46 Delaunay A, Bromberg KD, Hayashi Y et al. (2008) The ER-bound RING finger protein 5 (RNF5/RMA1) causes degenerative myopathy in transgenic mice and is deregulated in inclusion body myositis. *PLoS One* **3**, e1609.

47 Lunemann JD, Schmidt J, Schmid D et al. (2007) Beta-amyloid is a substrate of autophagy in sporadic inclusion body myositis. *Ann Neurol* **61**, 476–483.

48 Nogalska A, Terracciano C, D'Agostino C et al. (2009) p62/SQSTM1 is overexpressed and prominently accumulated in inclusions of sporadic inclusion-body myositis muscle fibers, and can help differentiating it from polymyositis and dermatomyositis. *Acta Neuropathol* **118**, 407–413.

49 Watts GD, Wymer J, Kovach MJ et al. (2004) Inclusion body myopathy associated with Paget disease of bone and frontotemporal dementia is caused by mutant valosin-containing protein. *Nat Genet* **36**, 377–381.

50 Ozturk A, McFerrin J, Engel W et al. (2004) HSP70 chaperone machinery in sporadic-inclusion-body myositis muscle fibers. *Neurology* **62**, A154.

51 Wilczynski GM, Engel WK, Askanas V. (2000) Association of active extracellular signal-regulated protein kinase with paired helical filaments of inclusion-body myositis muscle suggests its role in inclusion-body myositis tau phosphorylation. *Am J Pathol* **156**, 1835–1840.

52 Wilczynski GM, Engel WK, Askanas V. (2000) Cyclin-dependent kinase 5 colocalizes with phosphorylated tau in human inclusion-body myositis paired-helical filaments and may play a role in tau phosphorylation. *Neurosci Lett* **293**, 33–36.

53 Wilczynski GM, Broccolini A, Engel WK et al. (2001) Novel proposed role of glycogen synthase kinase 3beta in the pathogenesis of inclusion body myositis. *Neurology* **56** (Suppl. 3), A464.

54 Kannanayakal TJ, Mendell JR, Kuret J. (2008) Casein kinase 1 alpha associates with the tau-bearing lesions of inclusion body myositis. *Neurosci Lett* **431**, 141–145.

55 Yang CC, Alvarez RB, Engel WK et al. (1996) Increase of nitric oxide synthases and nitrotyrosine in inclusion-body myositis. *Neuroreport* **8**, 153–158.

56 Askanas V, Sarkozi E, Alvarez RB et al. (1996) Superoxide dismutase-1 gene and protein in vacuolated muscle fibers of sporadic inclusion-body myositis, hereditary inclusion-body myopathy, and cultured human muscle after beta-amyloid precursor protein gene transfer. *Neurology* **46**, A487.

57 Broccolini A, Engel WK, Alvarez RB et al. (1998) Possible pathogenic role of malondialdehyde, a toxic product of lipid peroxidation, in sporadic inclusion-body myositis. *Neurology* **50**, A367–A368.

58 Bilak M, Askanas V, Engel WK. (1994) Alpha 1-antichymotrypsin is strongly immunolocalized at normal human and rat neuromuscular junctions. *Synapse* **16**, 280–283.

59 Yang CC, Askanas V, Engel WK et al. (1998) Immunolocalization of transcription factor NF-kappaB in inclusion-body myositis muscle and at normal human neuromuscular junctions. *Neurosci Lett* **254**, 77–80.

60 Broccolini A, Mirault ME, Engel WK et al. (1999) Abnormal accumulation of seleno-glutathion peroxidase-1 and catalase and their mRNAs in sporadic inclusion-body myositis. *Neurology* **52** (Suppl. 2), A333.

61 Wilczynski GM, Engel WK, Askanas V. (2001) Novel cytoplasmic immunolocalization of RNA polymerase II in inclusion-body myositis muscle. *Neuroreport* **12**, 1809–1814.

62 Broccolini A, Engel WK, Alvarez RB et al. (2000) Paired helical filaments of inclusion-body myositis muscle contain RNA and survival motor neuron protein. *Am J Pathol* **156**, 1151–1155.

63 Nogalska A, Engel W, Askanas V. (2007) Abnormalities of peroxisome proliferator-activated receptor gamma in sporadic inclusion-body myositis muscle fibers. *Ann Neurol* **62**, S13.

64 Broccolini A, Engel WK, Alvarez RB et al. (2000) Redox factor-1 in muscle biopsies of patients with inclusion-body myositis. *Neurosci Lett* **287**, 1–4.

65 Broccolini A, Engel WK, Askanas V. (2000) Possible pathogenic role of redox factor 1 and Ap-1 transcription factor complex in sporadic inclusion-body myositis. *Neurology* **54** (Suppl. 3), A464.

66 D'Agostino C, Nogalska A, Engel WK et al. (2011) In sporadic inclusion-body myositis muscle fibres TDP-43-positive inclusions are less frequent and robust than p62-inclusions, and are not associated with paired helical filaments. *Neuropathol Appl Neurobiol* **37**, 315–320.

67 Küsters B, van Hoeve B, Schelhaas H et al. (2009) TDP-43 accumulation is common in myopathies with rimmed vacuoles. *Acta Neuropathol* **117**, 209–211.

68 Olive M, Janue A, Moreno D et al. (2009) TAR DNA-Binding protein 43 accumulation in protein aggregate myopathies. *J Neuropathol Exp Neurol* **68**, 262–273.

69 Salajegheh M, Pinkus JL, Taylor JP et al. (2009) Sarcoplasmic redistribution of nuclear TDP-43 in inclusion body myositis. *Muscle Nerve* **40**, 19–31.

70 Weihl CC, Temiz P, Miller SE et al. (2008) TDP-43 accumulation in inclusion body myopathy muscle suggests a common pathogenic mechanism with frontotemporal dementia. *J Neurol Neurosurg Psychiatry* **79**, 1186–1189.

71 Mirabella M, Alvarez RB, Engel WK et al. (1996) Apolipoprotein E and apolipoprotein E messenger RNA in muscle of inclusion body myositis and myopathies. *Ann Neurol* **40**, 864–872.

72 Jaworska-Wilczynska M, Wilczynski GM, Engel WK et al. (2002) Three lipoprotein receptors and cholesterol in inclusion-body myositis muscle. *Neurology* **58**, 438–445.

73 Sarkozi E, Askanas V, Johnson SA et al. (1993) beta-Amyloid precursor protein mRNA is increased in inclusion-body myositis muscle. *Neuroreport* **4**, 815–818.

74 Askanas V, Engel WK. (2005) Molecular pathology and pathogenesis of inclusion-body myositis. *Microsc Res Tech* **67**, 114–120.

75 Nogalska A, Wojcik S, Engel WK et al. (2007) Endoplasmic reticulum stress induces myostatin precursor protein and NF-kappaB in cultured human muscle fibers: relevance to inclusion body myositis. *Exp Neurol* **204**, 610–618.

76 Nogalska A, Engel WK, Askanas V. (2010) Increased BACE1 mRNA and noncoding BACE1-antisense transcript in sporadic inclusion-body myositis muscle fibers--Possibly caused by endoplasmic reticulum stress. *Neurosci Lett* **474**, 140–143.

77 Stockley JH, O'Neill C. (2008) Understanding BACE1: essential protease for amyloid-beta production in Alzheimer's disease. *Cell Mol Life Sci* **65**, 3265–3289.

78 De Strooper B. (2010) Proteases and proteolysis in Alzheimer disease: a multifactorial view on the disease process. *Physiol Rev* **90**, 465–494.

79 Li Y, Zhou W, Tong Y et al. (2006) Control of APP processing and Abeta generation level by BACE1 enzymatic activity and transcription. *FASEB J* **20**, 285–292.

80 Faghihi MA, Modarresi F, Khalil AM et al. (2008) Expression of a noncoding RNA is elevated in Alzheimer's disease and drives rapid feed-forward regulation of beta-secretase. *Nat Med* **14**, 723–730.

81 Vetrivel KS, Thinakaran G. (2006) Amyloidogenic processing of beta-amyloid precursor protein in

intracellular compartments. *Neurology* **66** (2 Suppl. 1), S69–S73.

82 Levy E, Sastre M, Kumar A et al. (2001) Codeposition of cystatin C with amyloid-beta protein in the brain of Alzheimer disease patients. *J Neuropathol Exp Neurol* **60**, 94–104.

83 Fielding CJ, Fielding PE. (2000) Cholesterol and caveolae: structural and functional relationships. *Biochim Biophys Acta Mol Cell Biol Lipids* **1529**, 210–222.

84 Kefi M, Vattemi G, Engel WK et al. (2002) Abnormal accumulation of caveolin-1 and its colocalization with cholesterol, amyloid-beta and phosphorylated tau in inclusion-body myositis (IBM) muscle. *Neurology* **58**, 391.

85 Broccolini A, Ricci E, Pescatori M et al. (2004) Insulin-like growth factor I in inclusion-body myositis and human muscle cultures. *J Neuropathol Exp Neurol* **63**, 650–659.

86 Shin RW, Ogino K, Shimabuku A et al. (2007) Amyloid precursor protein cytoplasmic domain with phospho-Thr668 accumulates in Alzheimer's disease and its transgenic models: a role to mediate interaction of Abeta and tau. *Acta Neuropathol* **113**, 627–636.

87 Lee MS, Kao SC, Lemere CA et al. (2003) APP processing is regulated by cytoplasmic phosphorylation. *J Cell Biol* **163**, 83–95.

88 Aplin AE, Gibb GM, Jacobsen JS et al. (1996) In vitro phosphorylation of the cytoplasmic domain of the amyloid precursor protein by glycogen synthase kinase-3beta. *J Neurochem* **67**, 699–707.

89 Hernández F, Gómez de Barreda E, Fuster-Matanzo A et al. (2010) GSK3: A possible link between beta amyloid peptide and tau protein. *Exp Neurol* **223**, 322–325.

90 Tanaka S, Shiojiri S, Takahashi Y et al. (1989) Tissue-specific expression of three types of beta-protein precursor mRNA: enhancement of protease inhibitor-harboring types in Alzheimer's disease brain. *Biochem Biophys Res Commun* **165**, 1406–1414.

91 Guerin C, Sinnreich M, Karpati G. (2008) Transcritional dysregulation in muscle fibers in sporadic inclusion body myositis (sIBM). *Neurology* **7** (Suppl. 3), A304.

92 Leroy K, Yilmaz Z, Brion JP. (2007) Increased level of active GSK-3beta in Alzheimer's disease and accumulation in argyrophilic grains and in neurones at different stages of neurofibrillary degeneration. *Neuropathol Appl Neurobiol* **33**, 43–55.

93 Jope RS. (2003) Lithium and GSK-3: one inhibitor, two inhibitory actions, multiple outcomes. *Trends Pharmacol Sci* **24**, 441–443.

94 Gambetti P, Perry G. (1994) Alzheimer's disease and prion proteins: a meeting made in muscle. *Am J Pathol* **145**, 1261–1264.

95 Askanas V, Engel WK. (1998) Does overexpression of betaAPP in aging muscle have a pathogenic role and a relevance to Alzheimer's disease? Clues from inclusion body myositis, cultured human muscle, and transgenic mice. *Am J Pathol* **153**, 1673–1677.

96 Selkoe DJ. (2003) Aging, amyloid, and Alzheimer's disease: a perspective in honor of Carl Cotman. *Neurochem Res* **28**, 1705–1713.

97 LaFerla FM, Green KN, Oddo S. (2007) Intracellular amyloid-beta in Alzheimer's disease. *Nat Rev Neurosci* **8**, 499–509.

98 El-Agnaf OM, Mahil DS, Patel BP et al. (2000) Oligomerization and toxicity of beta-amyloid-42 implicated in Alzheimer's disease. *Biochem Biophys Res Commun* **273**, 1003–1007.

99 Masuda Y, Uemura S, Ohashi R et al. (2009) Identification of physiological and toxic conformations in Abeta42 aggregates. *Chembiochem* **10**, 287–295.

100 Nogalska A, D'Agostino C, Engel WK et al. (2010) Novel demonstration of amyloid-beta oligomers in sporadic inclusion-body myositis muscle fibers. *Acta Neuropathol* **120**, 661–666.

101 Klein WL, Stine WB, Jr., Teplow DB. (2004) Small assemblies of unmodified amyloid beta-protein are the proximate neurotoxin in Alzheimer's disease. *Neurobiol Aging* **25**, 569–880.

102 Lambert MP, Barlow AK, Chromy BA et al. (1998) Diffusible, nonfibrillar ligands derived from Abeta1-42 are potent central nervous system neurotoxins. *Proc Natl Acad Sci USA* **95**, 6448–6453.

103 Honson NS, Kuret J. (2008) Tau aggregation and toxicity in tauopathic neurodegenerative diseases. *J Alzheimers Dis* **14**, 417–422.

104 Iqbal K, Liu F, Gong CX et al. (2009) Mechanisms of tau-induced neurodegeneration. *Acta Neuropathol* **118**, 53–69.

105 Ksiezak-Reding H, Dickson DW, Davies P et al. (1987) Recognition of tau epitopes by anti-neurofilament antibodies that bind to Alzheimer neurofibrillary tangles. *Proc Natl Acad Sci USA* **84**, 3410–3414.

106 Jicha GA, Lane E, Vincent I et al. (1997) A conformation- and phosphorylation-dependent antibody recognizing the paired helical filaments of Alzheimer's disease. *J Neurochem* **69**, 2087–2095.

107 Zheng-Fischhèofer Q, Biernat J, Mandelkow EM et al. (1998) Sequential phosphorylation of Tau by glycogen synthase kinase-3beta and protein kinase A at

Thr212 and Ser214 generates the Alzheimer-specific epitope of antibody AT100 and requires a paired-helical-filament-like conformation. *Eur J Biochem* **252**, 542–552.

108 Iqbal K, Wang X, Blanchard J et al. (2010) Alzheimer's disease neurofibrillary degeneration: pivotal and multifactorial. *Biochem Soc Trans* **38**, 962–966.

109 Spires-Jones TL, Stoothoff WH, de Calignon A et al. (2009) Tau pathophysiology in neurodegeneration: a tangled issue. *Trends Neurosci* **32**, 150–159.

110 Martinez A, Portero-Otin M, Pamplona R et al. (2009) Protein targets of oxidative damage in human neurodegenerative diseases with abnormal protein aggregates. *Brain Pathol* **20**, 281–297.

111 Reynolds MR, Berry RW, Binder LI. (2005) Site-specific nitration and oxidative dityrosine bridging of the tau protein by peroxynitrite: implications for Alzheimer's disease. *Biochemistry.* **44**, 1690–1700.

112 Zhang YJ, Xu YF, Chen XQ et al. (2005) Nitration and oligomerization of tau induced by peroxynitrite inhibit its microtubule-binding activity. *FEBS Lett* **579**, 2421–2427.

113 Kitazawa M, Green KN, Caccamo A et al. (2006) Genetically augmenting Abeta42 levels in skeletal muscle exacerbates inclusion body myositis-like pathology and motor deficits in transgenic mice. *Am J Pathol* **168**, 1986–1997.

114 Lehman NL. (2009) The ubiquitin proteasome system in neuropathology. *Acta Neuropathol* **118**, 329–347.

115 Wang Y, Martinez-Vicente M, Kruger U et al. (2009) Tau fragmentation, aggregation and clearance: the dual role of lysosomal processing. *Hum Mol Genet* **18**, 4153–4170.

116 Crews L, Tsigelny I, Hashimoto M et al. (2009) Role of synucleins in Alzheimer's disease. *Neurotox Res* **16**, 306–317.

117 Waxman EA, Giasson BI. (2009) Molecular mechanisms of [alpha]-synuclein neurodegeneration. *Biochim Biophys Acta Mol Basis Dis* **1792**, 616–624.

118 Devi L, Anandatheerthavarada HK. (2010) Mitochondrial trafficking of APP and alpha synuclein: Relevance to mitochondrial dysfunction in Alzheimer's and Parkinson's diseases. *Biochim Biophys Acta Mol Basis Dis* **1802**, 11–9.

119 Mak SK, McCormack AL, Manning-Bog AB et al. (2010) Lysosomal degradation of alpha-synuclein in vivo. *J Biol Chem* **285**, 13621–13629.

120 Martinez-Vicente M, Cuervo AM. (2007) Autophagy and neurodegeneration: when the cleaning crew goes on strike. *Lancet Neurol* **6**, 352–361.

121 Crews L, Spencer B, Desplats P et al. (2010) Selective molecular alterations in the autophagy pathway in patients with Lewy body disease and in models of alpha-synucleinopathy. *PLoS One* **5**, e9313.

122 Wong E, Cuervo AM. (2010) Autophagy gone awry in neurodegenerative diseases. *Nat Neurosci* **13**, 805–811.

123 Shimura H, Schlossmacher MG, Hattori N et al. (2001) Ubiquitination of a new form of alpha-synuclein by parkin from human brain: implications for Parkinson's disease. *Science* **293**, 263–269.

124 Qiao L, Hamamichi S, Caldwell K et al. (2008) Lysosomal enzyme cathepsin D protects against alpha-synuclein aggregation and toxicity. *Mol Brain* **1**, 17.

125 Narendra D, Tanaka A, Suen DF et al. (2008) Parkin is recruited selectively to impaired mitochondria and promotes their autophagy. *J Cell Biol* **183**, 795–803.

126 Tsai YC, Fishman PS, Thakor NV et al. (2003) Parkin facilitates the elimination of expanded polyglutamine proteins and leads to preservation of proteasome function. *J Biol Chem* **278**, 22044–22055.

127 Burns MP, Zhang L, Rebeck GW et al. (2009) Parkin promotes intracellular Abeta1-42 clearance. *Hum Mol Genet* **18**, 3206–3216.

128 Paciello O, Wojcik S, Engel WK et al. (2006) Alpha-synuclein and Parkin are novel proteins accumulated in ragged-red fibers. *Neuromuscul Disord* **16**, 657.

129 Engel WK. (1971) "Ragged-red fibers" in opthamoplegia syndromes and their differential diagnosis. *Excerpta Med Inter Cong Series* **237**, 28.

130 Oldfors A, Moslemi AR, Jonasson L et al. (2006) Mitochondrial abnormalities in inclusion-body myositis. *Neurology* **66**, S49–S55.

131 Wild P, Dikic I. (2010) Mitochondria get a Parkin' ticket. *Nat Cell Biol* **12**, 104–106.

132 Nicolas O, Gavin R, del Rio JA. (2009) New insights into cellular prion protein (PrPc) functions: the "ying and yang" of a relevant protein. *Brain Res Rev* **61**, 170–184.

133 Prusiner SB. (2001) Neurodegenerative Diseases and Prions. *N Engl J Med* **344**, 1516–1526.

134 Gunther EC, Strittmatter SM. Beta-amyloid oligomers and cellular prion protein in Alzheimer's disease. *J Mol Med* **88**, 331–338.

135 Chiesa R, Piccardo P, Biasini E et al. (2008) Aggregated, wild-type prion protein causes neurological dysfunction and synaptic abnormalities. *J Neurosci* **28**, 13258–13267.

136 Sarkozi E, Askanas V, Engel WK. (1994) Abnormal accumulation of prion protein mRNA in muscle fibers

of patients with sporadic inclusion-body myositis and hereditary inclusion-body myopathy. *Am J Pathol* **145**, 1280–1284.

137 Askanas V, Bilak M, Engel WK et al. (1993) Prion protein is strongly immunolocalized at the postsynaptic domain of human normal neuromuscular junctions. *Neurosci Lett* **159**, 111–114.

138 Nygaard HB, Strittmatter SM. (2009) Cellular prion protein mediates the toxicity of beta-amyloid oligomers: implications for Alzheimer disease. *Arch Neurol* **66**, 1325–1328.

139 Stella R, Massimino ML, Sandri M et al. (2010) Cellular prion protein promotes regeneration of adult muscle tissue. *Mol Cell Biol* **30**, 4864–4876.

140 Gonzalez-Cadavid NF, Bhasin S. (2004) Role of myostatin in metabolism. *Curr Opin Clin Nutr Metab Care* **7**, 451–457.

141 Wojcik S, Nogalska A, McFerrin J et al. (2007) Myostatin precursor protein is increased and associates with amyloid-beta precursor protein in inclusion-body myositis culture model. *Neuropathol Appl Neurobiol* **33**, 238–242.

142 Starck CS, Sutherland-Smith AJ. (2010) Cytotoxic aggregation and amyloid formation by the myostatin precursor protein. *PLoS One* **5**, e9170.

143 Ciechanover A. (2006) Intracellular protein degradation: from a vague idea thru the lysosome and the ubiquitin-proteasome system and onto human diseases and drug targeting. *Neurology* **66**, 7–19.

144 Cuervo AM, Wong ES, Martinez-Vicente M. (2010) Protein degradation, aggregation, and misfolding. *Mov Disord* **25**, S49–S54.

145 Shacka JJ, Roth KA, Zhang J. (2008) The autophagy-lysosomal degradation pathway: role in neurodegenerative disease and therapy. *Front Biosci* **13**, 718–736.

146 Ding WX, Yin XM. (2008) Sorting, recognition and activation of the misfolded protein degradation pathways through macroautophagy and the proteasome. *Autophagy*. **4**, 141–150.

147 Fink AL. (1999) Chaperone-mediated protein folding. *Physiol Rev* **79**, 425–449.

148 Yoshida H. (2007) ER stress and diseases. *FEBS J* **274**, 630–658.

149 Wu J, Kaufman RJ. (2006) From acute ER stress to physiological roles of the Unfolded Protein Response. *Cell Death Differ* **13**, 374–384.

150 Cuervo AM. (2008) Autophagy and aging: keeping that old broom working. *Trends Genet* **24**, 604–612.

151 Glabe CG, Kayed R. (2006) Common structure and toxic function of amyloid oligomers implies a common mechanism of pathogenesis. *Neurology* **66**, S74–S78.

152 Kopito RR, Ron D. (2000) Conformational disease. *Nat Cell Biol* **2**, E207–E209.

153 Nixon RA. (2007) Autophagy, amyloidogenesis and Alzheimer disease. *J Cell Sci* **120**, 4081–4091.

154 Bedford L, Paine S, Sheppard PW et al. (2010) Assembly, structure, and function of the 26S proteasome. *Trends in Cell Biol* **20**, 391–401.

155 Voges D, Zwickl P, Baumeister W. (1999) The 26S proteasome: a molecular machine designed for controlled proteolysis. *Annu Rev Biochem* **68**, 1015–1068.

156 Ciechanover A, Brundin P. (2003) The ubiquitin proteasome system in neurodegenerative diseases. Sometimes the chicken, sometimes the egg. *Neuron* **40**, 427–446.

157 McNaught KS, Belizaire R, Isacson O et al. (2003) Altered proteasomal function in sporadic Parkinson's disease. *Exp Neurol* **179**, 38–46.

158 Oddo S. (2008) The ubiquitin-proteasome system in Alzheimer's disease. *J Cell Mol Med* **12**, 363–373.

159 Cecarini V, Bonfili L, Amici M et al. (2008) Amyloid peptides in different assembly states and related effects on isolated and cellular proteasomes. *Brain Res* **1209**, 8–18.

160 Tseng BP, Green KN, Chan JL et al. (2008) A[beta] inhibits the proteasome and enhances amyloid and tau accumulation. *Neurobiol Aging* **29**, 1607–1618.

161 Askanas V, Engel WK. (2002) Inclusion-body myositis and myopathies: different etiologies, possibly similar pathogenic mechanisms. *Curr Opin Neurol* **15**, 525–531.

162 Keck S, Nitsch R, Grune T et al. (2003) Proteasome inhibition by paired helical filament-tau in brains of patients with Alzheimer's disease. *J Neurochem*. **85**, 115–122.

163 Lindersson E, Beedholm R, Hojrup P et al. (2004) Proteasomal inhibition by alpha-synuclein filaments and oligomers. *J Biol Chem* **279**, 12924–12934.

164 Dennissen FJA, Kholod N, Steinbusch HWM et al. (2010) Misframed proteins and neurodegeneration: a novel view on Alzheimer's and Parkinson's diseases. *Neurodegenerative Dis* **7**, 76–79.

165 He C, Klionsky DJ. (2009) Regulation mechanisms and signaling pathways of autophagy. *Annu Rev Genet* **43**, 67–93.

166 Nixon RA. (2006) Autophagy in neurodegenerative disease: friend, foe or turncoat? *Trends Neurosci* **29**, 528–535.

167 Nixon RA, Wegiel J, Kumar A et al. (2005) Extensive involvement of autophagy in Alzheimer disease: an

immuno-electron microscopy study. *J Neuropathol Exp Neurol* **64**, 113–122.

168 Cuervo AM. (2010) Chaperone-mediated autophagy: selectivity pays off. *Trends Endocrinol Metab* **21**, 142–150.

169 Carpenter S, Karpati G, Heller I et al. (1978) Inclusion body myositis: a distinct variety of idiopathic inflammatory myopathy. *Neurology* **28**, 8–17.

170 Kumamoto T, Ueyama H, Tsumura H et al. (2004) Expression of lysosome-related proteins and genes in the skeletal muscles of inclusion body myositis. *Acta Neuropathol* **107**, 59–65.

171 Tsuruta Y, Furuta A, Furuta K et al. (2001) Expression of the lysosome-associated membrane proteins in myopathies with rimmed vacuoles. *Acta Neuropathol* **101**, 579–584.

172 Mikol J, Engel AG. (2004) Inclusion body myositis. In: Engel AG (ed.) *Myology*. 3rd edn. McGraw-Hill Book Co., New York, pp. 1367–1388.

173 Klionsky DJ, Abeliovich H, Agostinis P et al. (2008) Guidelines for the use and interpretation of assays for monitoring autophagy in higher eukaryotes. *Autophagy* **4**, 151–175.

174 Hamano T, Gendron TF, Causevic E et al. (2008) Autophagic-lysosomal perturbation enhances tau aggregation in transfectants with induced wild-type tau expression. *Eur J Neurosci* **27**, 1119–1130.

175 Koh YH, von Arnim CA, Hyman BT et al. (2005) BACE is degraded via the lysosomal pathway. *J Biol Chem* **280**, 32499–32504.

176 Yu WH, Cuervo AM, Kumar A et al. (2005) Macroautophagy–a novel beta-amyloid peptide-generating pathway activated in Alzheimer's disease. *J Cell Biol* **171**, 87–98.

177 Ikezoe K, Furuya H, Arahata H et al. (2009) Amyloid-beta accumulation caused by chloroquine injections precedes ER stress and autophagosome formation in rat skeletal muscle. *Acta Neuropathol* **117**, 575–582.

178 Tsuzuki K, Fukatsu R, Takamaru Y et al. (1995) Amyloid beta protein in rat soleus muscle in chloroquine-induced myopathy using end-specific antibodies for Abeta40 and Abeta42: immunohistochemical evidence for amyloid beta protein. *Neurosci Lett* **202**, 77–80.

179 Bjorkoy G, Lamark T, Johansen T. (2006) p62/SQSTM1: a missing link between protein aggregates and the autophagy machinery. *Autophagy* **2**, 138–139.

180 Seibenhener ML, Babu JR, Geetha T et al. (2004) Sequestosome 1/p62 is a polyubiquitin chain binding protein involved in ubiquitin proteasome degradation. *Mol Cell Biol* **24**, 8055–8068.

181 Kuusisto E, Salminen A, Alafuzoff I. (2002) Early accumulation of p62 in neurofibrillary tangles in Alzheimer's disease: possible role in tangle formation. *Neuropathol App Neurobiol* **28**, 228–237.

182 Chen-Plotkin AS, Lee VM, Trojanowski JQ. (2010) TAR DNA-binding protein 43 in neurodegenerative disease. *Nat Rev Neurol* **6**, 211–220.

183 Gendron TF, Josephs KA, Petrucelli L. (2010) Review: transactive response DNA-binding protein 43 (TDP-43): mechanisms of neurodegeneration. *Neuropathol Appl Neurobiol* **36**, 97–112.

184 Moscat J, Diaz-Meco MT, Wooten MW. (2007) Signal integration and diversification through the p62 scaffold protein. *Trends Biochem Sci* **32**, 95–100.

185 Wang X, Fan H, Ying Z et al. (2010) Degradation of TDP-43 and its pathogenic form by autophagy and the ubiquitin-proteasome system. *Neurosci Lett* **469**, 112–116.

186 Schroder M. (2008) Endoplasmic reticulum stress responses. *Cell Mol Life Sci* **65**, 862–894.

187 Vembar SS, Brodsky JL. (2008) One step at a time: endoplasmic reticulum-associated degradation. *Nat Rev Mol Cell Biol* **9**, 944–957.

188 Hoozemans JJ, van Haastert ES, Nijholt DA et al. (2009) The unfolded protein response is activated in pretangle neurons in Alzheimer's disease hippocampus. *Am J Pathol* **174**, 1241–1251.

189 Hoozemans JJ, van Haastert ES, Eikelenboom P et al. (2007) Activation of the unfolded protein response in Parkinson's disease. *Biochem Biophys Res Commun* **354**, 707–711.

190 Nogalska A, Engel WK, Askanas V. (2010) Putative pathogenic role of the endoplasmic reticulum stress in sporadic inclusion-body myositis. *Acta Myol* **29**, 143–144.

191 Hanada S, Harada M, Kumemura H et al. (2007) Oxidative stress induces the endoplasmic reticulum stress and facilitates inclusion formation in cultured cells. *J Hepatol* **47**, 93–102.

192 Li Y, Ge M, Ciani L et al. (2004) Enrichment of endoplasmic reticulum with cholesterol inhibits sarcoplasmic-endoplasmic reticulum calcium ATPase-2b activity in parallel with increased order of membrane lipids: implications for depletion of endoplasmic reticulum calcium stores and apoptosis in cholesterol-loaded macrophages. *J Biol Chem* **279**, 37030–37039.

193 Uehara T, Nakamura T, Yao D et al. (2006) S-Nitrosylated protein-disulphide isomerase links protein misfolding to neurodegeneration. *Nature* **441**, 513–517.

194 Kang K, Park B, Oh C et al. (2009) A role for protein disulfide isomerase in the early folding and assembly of MHC class I molecules. *Antioxid Redox Signal* **11**, 2553–2561.

195 Paulsson K, Wang P. (2003) Chaperones and folding] of MHC class I molecules in the endoplasmic reticulum. *Biochim Biophys Acta* **1641**, 1–12.

196 Nogalska A, D'Agostino C, Engel WK et al. (2010) Decreased SIRT1 deacetylase activity in sporadic inclusion-body myositis muscle fibers. *Neurobiol Aging* **31**, 1637–1648.

197 Pahl HL, Baeuerle PA. (1997) The ER-overload response: activation of NF-kappa B. *Trends Biochem Sci* **22**, 63–67.

198 Albani D, Polito L, Forloni G. (2010) Sirtuins as novel targets for Alzheimer's disease and other neurodegenerative disorders: experimental and genetic evidence. *J Alzheimers Dis* **19**, 11–26.

199 Tang BL. (2009) Sirt1's complex roles in neuroprotection. *Cell Mol Neurobiol* **29**, 1093–1103.

200 Michan S, Sinclair D. (2007) Sirtuins in mammals: insights into their biological function. *Biochem J* **404**, 1–13.

201 Yeung F, Hoberg JE, Ramsey CS et al. (2004) Modulation of NF-kappaB-dependent transcription and cell survival by the SIRT1 deacetylase. *EMBO J* **23**, 2369–2380.

202 Abou-Sleiman PM, Muqit MM, Wood NW. (2006) Expanding insights of mitochondrial dysfunction in Parkinson's disease. *Nat Rev Neurosci* **7**, 207–219.

203 Reddy VP, Zhu X, Perry G et al. (2009) Oxidative Stress in Diabetes and Alzheimer's Disease. *J Alzheimers Dis* **16**, 763–774.

204 Choi J, Sullards MC, Olzmann JA et al. (2006) Oxidative damage of DJ-1 is linked to sporadic Parkinson and Alzheimer diseases. *J Biol Chem* **281**, 10816–10824.

205 Banwell BL, Engel AG. (2000) AlphaB-crystallin immunolocalization yields new insights into inclusion body myositis. *Neurology* **54**, 1033–1041.

206 Karpati G, Hohlfeld R. (2000) Biologically stressed muscle fibers in sporadic IBM: a clue for the enigmatic etiology? *Neurology* **54**, 1020–1021.

207 Sun Y, MacRae TH. (2005) The small heat shock proteins and their role in human disease. *FEBS J* **272**, 2613–2627.

208 Wojcik S, Engel WK, McFerrin J et al. (2006) AbetaPP-overexpression and proteasome inhibition increase alphaB-crystallin in cultured human muscle: relevance to inclusion-body myositis. *Neuromuscul Disord* **16**, 839–844.

209 Raman B, Ban T, Sakai M et al. (2005) AlphaB-crystallin, a small heat-shock protein, prevents the amyloid fibril growth of an amyloid beta-peptide and beta2-microglobulin. *Biochem J* **392**, 573–581.

210 Stege GJ, Renkawek K, Overkamp PS et al. (1999) The molecular chaperone alphaB-crystallin enhances amyloid beta neurotoxicity. *Biochem Biophys Res Commun* **262**, 152–156.

211 Vicart P, Caron A, Guicheney P et al. (1998) A missense mutation in the alphaB-crystallin chaperone gene causes a desmin-related myopathy. *Nat Genet* **20**, 92–95.

212 Muth IE, Barthel K, Bähr M et al. (2009) Proinflammatory cell stress in sporadic inclusion body myositis muscle: overexpression of αB-crystallin is associated with amyloid precursor protein and accumulation of β-amyloid. *J Neurol Neurosurg Psychiatry* **80**, 1344–1349.

213 Terracciano C, Engel W, Askanas V. (2008) In sporadic inclusion-body myositis muscle biopsies, cytochrome oxidase (COX) negative muscle fibers do not correlate with either inflammation or with aggregates containing amyloid-beta or phosphorylated tau. *Neurology* **70**, A304.

214 Askanas V, McFerrin J, Baque S et al. (1996) Transfer of beta-amyloid precursor protein gene using adenovirus vector causes mitochondrial abnormalities in cultured normal human muscle. *Proc Natl Acad Sci USA* **93**, 1314–1319.

215 Hashimoto M, Rockenstein E, Crews L et al. (2003) Role of protein aggregation in mitochondrial dysfunction and neurodegeneration in Alzheimer's and Parkinson's diseases. *Neuromolecular Med* **4**, 21–36.

216 Hong WK, Han EH, Kim DG et al. (2007) Amyloid-beta-peptide reduces the expression level of mitochondrial cytochrome oxidase subunits. *Neurochem Res* **32**, 1483–1488.

217 Wojcik S, Paciello O, Engel WK et al. (2007) In sporadic inclusion-body myositis muscle fiber cytoplasm, cytochrome c aggregates with a-synuclein and amyloid-beta precursor protein, but does not activate caspase-3. *Neuromuscul Disord* **17**, 853.

218 Borutaite V. (2010) Mitochondria as decision-makers in cell death. *Environ Mol Mutagen* **51**, 406–416.

219 Askanas V, Engel WK, Alvarez RB. (1998) Fourteen newly recognized proteins at the human neuromuscular junctions--and their nonjunctional accumulation in inclusion-body myositis. *Ann NY Acad Sci* **841**, 28–56.

220 Alvarez RB, Engel W, Askanas V. (2000) Ultrastructural abnormalities of neuromuscular juunctions in

sporadic inclusion-body myositis. *Neurology* **54**, A240–A241.

221 McFerrin J, Engel WK, Askanas V. (1998) Impaired innervation of cultured human muscle overexpressing betaAPP experimentally and genetically: relevance to inclusion-body myopathies. *Neuroreport* **9**, 3201–3205.

222 Terry RD. (1996) The pathogenesis of Alzheimer disease: an alternative to the amyloid hypothesis. *J Neuropathol Exp Neurol* **55**, 1023–1025.

223 Askanas V, Engel WK, Alvarez RB et al. (2000) Inclusion 'body myositis, muscle blood vessel and cardiac amyloidosis, and transthyretin Val122Ile allele. *Ann Neurol* **47**, 544–549.

224 Jacobson DR, Pastore RD, Yaghoubian R et al. (1997) Variant-sequence transthyretin (isoleucine 122) in late-onset cardiac amyloidosis in black Americans. *N Engl J Med* **336**, 466–473.

225 Stein TD, Johnson JA. (2002) Lack of neurodegeneration in transgenic mice overexpressing mutant amyloid precursor protein is associated with increased levels of transthyretin and the activation of cell survival pathways. *J Neurosci* **22**, 7380–7388.

226 Askanas V, Engel WK, McFerrin J et al. (2003) Transthyretin Val122Ile, accumulated Abeta, and inclusion-body myositis aspects in cultured muscle. *Neurology* **61**, 257–260.

227 Page LJ, Suk JY, Bazhenova L et al. (2009) Secretion of amyloidogenic gelsolin progressively compromises protein homeostasis leading to the intracellular aggregation of proteins. *Proc Natl Acad Sci USA* **106**, 11125–11130.

228 Chauhan V, Ji L, Chauhan A. (2008) Anti-amyloidogenic, anti-oxidant and anti-apoptotic role of gelsolin in Alzheimer's disease. *Biogerontology* **9**, 381–389.

229 Buxbaum JN, Ye Z, Reixach N et al. (2008) Transthyretin protects Alzheimer's mice from the behavioral and biochemical effects of Abeta toxicity. *Proc Natl Acad Sci USA* **105**, 2681–2686.

230 Askanas V, McFerrin J, Alvarez RB et al. (2010) Beta APP gene transfer into cultured human muscle induces inclusion-body myositis aspects. *Neuroreport* **8**, 2155–2158.

231 McFerrin J, Engel WK, Leclerc N et al. (2002) Combined influence of amyloid-beta precursor protein (AbPP) gene transfer and cholesterol excess on cultured humen muscle fibers. *Neurology* **58**, 489.

232 Fukuchi K, Pham D, Hart M et al. (1998) Amyloid-beta deposition in skeletal muscle of transgenic mice: possible model of inclusion body myopathy. *Am J Pathol* **153**, 1687–1693.

233 Jin LW, Hearn MG, Ogburn CE et al. (1998) Transgenic mice over-expressing the C-99 fragment of betaPP with an alpha-secretase site mutation develop a myopathy similar to human inclusion body myositis. *Am J Pathol* **153**, 1679–1686.

234 Sugarman MC, Yamasaki TR, Oddo S et al. (2002) Inclusion body myositis-like phenotype induced by transgenic overexpression of beta APP in skeletal muscle. *Proc Natl Acad Sci USA* **99**, 6334–6339.

235 Lopez JR, Shtifman A. (2010) Intracellular β-amyloid accumulation leads to age-dependent progression of $Ca2+$ dysregulation in skeletal muscle. *Muscle Nerve* **42**, 731–738.

236 Malicdan MC, Noguchi S, Nonaka I et al. (2007) A Gne knockout mouse expressing human V572L mutation develops features similar to distal myopathy with rimmed vacuoles or hereditary inclusion body myopathy. *Hum Mol Genet* **16**, 115–128.

237 Morosetti R, Mirabella M, Gliubizzi C et al. (2006) MyoD expression restores defective myogenic differentiation of human mesoangioblasts from inclusion-body myositis muscle. *Proc Natl Acad Sci USA* **103**, 16995–17000.

238 Griggs RC. (2006) The current status of treatment for inclusion-body myositis. *Neurology* **66**, S30–S32.

239 Dalakas MC. (2010) Immunotherapy of myositis: issues, concerns and future prospects. *Nat Rev zRheumatol* **6**, 129–137.

240 Needham M, Mastaglia FL. (2007) Inclusion body myositis: current pathogenetic concepts and diagnostic and therapeutic approaches. *Lancet Neurol* **6**, 620–631.

241 Barohn RJ, Herbelin L, Kissel JT et al. (2006) Pilot trial of etanercept in the treatment of inclusion-body myositis. *Neurology* **66**, S123–S124.

242 Benveniste O, Guiguet M, Freebody J et al. (2010) Immunosuppresive-treatment does not alter natural history of sporadic-inclusion body myositis (sIBM): the Pitie-Salpetriere/Oxford study. *Acta Myol* **29**, 144–145.

243 Nogalska A, D'Agostino C, Engel WK et al. (2008) Resveratrol, a polyphenol found in red wine, reduces NF-kB activation and myostatin in endoplasmic reticulum stress (ERS)-provoked cultured human muscle fibers:relevance to treatment of sporadic inclusion-body myositis. *Ann Neurol* **64**, S9.

244 Cucciolla V, Borriello A, Oliva A et al. (2007) Resveratrol: from basic science to the clinic. *Cell Cycle* **6**, 2495–2510.

245 Lee IH, Cao L, Mostoslavsky R et al. (2008) A role for the NAD-dependent deacetylase Sirt1 in the

regulation of autophagy. *Proc Natl Acad Sci USA* **105**, 3374–3379.

246 Nogalska A, D'Agostino C, Engel WK et al. (2010) Resveratrol, naturally occuring polyphenol found in red wine, increases cathepsin D activity in edoplasmic reticulul stres (ERS)-provoked cultured human muscle fibers: relevance to treatment of sporadic inclusion-body myositis. *Acta Myol* **29**, 111.

247 Nogalska A, D'Agostino C, Engel W et al. (2009) Treatment with resveratrol, trans-3,4',5-trihydroxystilbene polyphenol decreases amyloid beta precursor protein, amyloid beta oligomerization and myostatin in AβPP overexpressing cultured human muscle fibers (AβPP$^+$-CHMF IBM Model): relevance to treatment of sporadic-IBM patients. *Neurology* **72**, A104.

248 Hamaguchi T, Ono K, Murase A et al. (2009) Phenolic compounds prevent Alzheimer's pathology through different effects on the amyloid-beta aggregation pathway. *Am J Pathol* **175**, 2557–2565.

249 Hamaguchi T, Ono K, Yamada M. (2010) Curcumin and Alzheimer's Disease. *CNS Neurosci Ther* **16**, 285–297.

250 Kim J, Lee HJ, Lee KW. (2010) Naturally occurring phytochemicals for the prevention of Alzheimer's disease. *J Neurochem* **112**, 1415–1430.

251 Ono K, Condron MM, Ho L et al. (2008) Effects of grape seed-derived polyphenols on amyloid beta-protein self-assembly and cytotoxicity. *J Biol Chem* **283**, 32176–32187.

252 Wang J, Ho L, Zhao W et al. (2008) Grape-derived polyphenolics prevent Abeta oligomerization and attenuate cognitive deterioration in a mouse model of Alzheimer's disease. *J Neurosci* **28**, 6388–6392.

253 Engel T, Goni-Oliver P, Gomez de Barreda E et al. (2008) Lithium, a potential protective drug in Alzheimer's disease. *Neurodegener Dis* **5**, 247–249.

254 Kitazawa M, Trinh DN, LaFerla FM. (2008) Inflammation induces tau pathology in inclusion body myositis model via glycogen synthase kinase-3beta. *Ann Neurol* **64**, 15–24.

255 Ono K, Ikemoto M, Kawarabayashi T et al. (2009) A chemical chaperone, sodium 4-phenylbutyric acid, attenuates the pathogenic potency in human alpha-synuclein A30P + A53T transgenic mice. *Parkinsonism Relat Disord* **15**, 649–654.

256 de Almeida SF, Picarote G, Fleming JV et al. (2007) Chemical chaperones reduce endoplasmic reticulum stress and prevent mutant HFE aggregate formation. *J Biol Chem* **282**, 27905–27912.

257 Ricobaraza A, Cuadrado-Tejedor M, Perez-Mediavilla A et al. (2009) Phenylbutyrate ameliorates cognitive deficit and reduces tau pathology in an Alzheimer's disease mouse model. *Neuropsychopharmacology* **34**, 1721–1732.

258 Cudkowicz ME, Andres PL, Macdonald SA et al. (2009) Phase 2 study of sodium phenylbutyrate in ALS. *Amyotroph Lateral Scler* **10**, 99–106.

259 Hogarth P, Lovrecic L, Krainc D. (2007) Sodium phenylbutyrate in Huntington's disease: a dose-finding study. *Mov Disord* **22**, 1962–1964.

260 Bahr BA. (2009) Lysosomal modulatory drugs for a broad strategy against protein accumulation disorders. *Curr Alzheimer Res* **6**, 438–445.

CHAPTER 8

Inflammatory and autoimmune features of inclusion-body myositis

Marinos C. Dalakas

Chair, Clinical Neurosciences, Neuromuscular Diseases, Imperial College London, London, UK

Introduction

Sporadic inclusion-body myositis (s-IBM), polymyositis (PM), necrotizing autoimmune myositis, and dermatomyositis (DM) comprise the four main subsets of acquired inflammatory myopathies [1–6]. Among them, IBM is most common in people above the age of 50, with the majority of patients manifesting their first symptoms between 50 and 65 years of age. Because s-IBM has a very slow and insidious onset, it is likely that the disease has started decades before patients seek medical attention, as supported by finding advanced signs of myopathology even in muscles that appear clinically healthy (Dalakas, unpublished observations). Consequently, s-IBM may not necessarily be a disease of old age but rather of middle age. s-IBM remains the most enigmatic disorder because it is characterized by inflammatory and degenerative features that are prominent from the early stages of the disease and persist even in the most advanced phase. This is puzzling, especially for the inflammation that in most of patients remains intense throughout the course of the disease. Further, IBM although immunopathologically similar to PM, follows a slow, indolent, and protracted course, and does not readily respond to immunotherapies.

Our observations with hundreds of s-IBM muscle specimens, including sequential biopsies from Chief, Neuroimmunology Unit, Department of Pathophysiology, University of Athens Medical School, Athens Greece the same patients over time, have consistently revealed that in IBM the inflammatory cells invade healthy-looking, nonvacuolated fibers, whereas the vacuolated fibers are rarely invaded by T-cells, suggesting that the autoimmune inflammatory features coexist with degeneration and the two processes may progress either in parallel or independently [5–7]. This observation has led us to investigate the interrelationship between molecules involved in inflammation and degeneration in an effort to explore therapies that may have an impact on both processes.

This review is focused on the pertinent immunopathologic features of s-IBM, the specificity of the inflammatory response, the association with viral infections, the interrelationship between inflammatory and degenerative molecules, and the responses to various immunotherapies. It does not address the degenerative component because it is extensively discussed in other chapters. A hypothesis on how a primary inflammatory process can lead to a self-sustaining degenerative disease resistant to immunotherapies will be also presented.

Immunopathogenesis of s-IBM

A series of clinical observations, disease associations, and immunopathological studies indicate that immune mechanisms play a fundamental role in the pathogenesis of s-IBM, even from the outset of the disease, as detailed below and summarized in Box 8.1.

Muscle Aging, Inclusion-Body Myositis and Myopathies, First Edition. Edited by Valerie Askanas and W. King Engel.

Box 8.1 Factors supporting the immuno-pathogenesis of s-IBM

1 Immunogenetic association with DR$\beta_1$0301 and DQ$\beta_1$0201 alleles and the B$_8$-DR$_3$-DR$_{52}$-DQ2 haplotype; the human leukocyte antigen A (HLA-A) haplotype is associated with earlier disease onset.

2 s-IBM can occur in family members of the same generation (familial inflammatory IBM), as seen with other autoimmune disorders.

3 Association with other autoimmune disorders and autoantibodies in frequencies analogous to the one seen in other autoimmune disorders (i.e. Myasthenia gravis, Lampert-Eaton myasthenic syndrome MG, LEMS).

4 Increased association with paraproteinemia (22.8%) in frequencies significantly higher than age-matched controls (2%).

5 Association with common variable immunodeficiency and natural killer cells.

6 Association with HIV and human T-cell lymphotropic virus type 1 (HTLV-1) infection, with increasingly recognized frequency (more than 40 cases reported).

7 The CD8$^+$ autoinvasive T-cells: (a) surround major histocompatibility complex (MHC)-I-expressing fibers (MHC-I/CD8$^+$ lesion); (b) express perforin and activation markers of cytotoxicity; (c) are clonally expanded with restricted amino acid sequences in the CDR3 region of the T-cell receptor (TCR); and (d) TCR families persist over time even in different muscles.

8 There is ubiquitous upregulation of MHC-I antigen and the costimulatory molecules BB1, ICOS-L, and CD40 on muscle fibers, even on those not invaded by T-cells, while the counterreceptors CD28, CTLA-4, ICOS, and CD40L are overexpressed on the autoinvasive T-cells.

9 There is strong upregulation of cytokines, chemokines, and their receptors at the protein, mRNA, and gene levels.

10 Some patients may transiently respond to immunotherapies to some degree but they soon become resistant.

Association with other autoimmune disorders and autoantibodies

Based on a series of 99 consecutive patients with s-IBM, it was found that in at least 20% of them the disease is associated with systemic autoimmune or connective tissue disorders or with various autoantibodies directed against nuclear or cytoplasmic antigens [1, 8]. Although antibodies against various synthetases, translation factors, and proteins of the signal-recognition particles were less commonly found in IBM compared to PM and DM, they were still noted in at least 5% of the patients [8]. As with other inflammatory myopathies, the significance of these antibodies remains unclear, but they support an ongoing autoimmune process and abnormal immunoregulation. In another series of 52 IBM patients, 33% of them had other autoimmune disorders, such as multiple sclerosis, autoimmune thyroid disease, rheumatoid arthritis, or Sjögren syndrome [9]. Interestingly, the frequency of the associated autoimmune disorders in this series was the same as the one noted for Lambert–Eaton myasthenic syndrome [9], a classic autoimmune disorder. The frequency of IBM in patients with chronic dermatomyositis is also of interest and not fortuitous. It has been observed in at least five cases of others and ours who had classic DM under treatment, but developed many years later the typical clinicohistological features of IBM, including unresponsiveness to immunotherapies [3, 10].

Immunogenetic associations

An increased frequency of DR$\beta_1$0301 and DQ$\beta_1$0201 alleles associated with DR and DQ haplotypes has been observed [2, 4] and documented in up to 75% of our patients [11]. Further, the B$_8$-DR$_3$-DR$_{52}$-DQ2 haplotype is found in 67% of patients, regardless of whether they have another autoimmune disease, in frequencies identical to that seen in other autoimmune disorders such as myasthenia gravis or myasthenic syndrome [9]. The human leukocyte antigen A (HLA-A) haplotype appears to be associated with earlier disease onset [9], suggesting that immunoregulatory genes are inherently connected with the manifestation of symptoms.

The classic clinical and histological phenotype of s-IBM, with prominent endomysial inflammation, has been seen in other family members of the same generation [12]. This association, which we have called "familial inflammatory IBM," is analogous to the familiar occurrence of other autoimmune disorders, such as myasthenia gravis, rheumatoid arthritis, or lupus, in several family members of the same generation [12].

Association with dysproteinemia, paraproteinemia, and immunodeficiency

A benign IgG, IgM, or IgA monoclonal gammopathy has been observed in 16 of 70 (22.8%) IBM patients, mean age 60.6 years (range 35–77 years), compared to 2% in age-matched controls (mean age 66.1 years; range 42–80 years) [13]. The monoclonal IgG extracted from the serum of IBM patients, more often than the controls, recognized various muscle proteins of 35–145 kDa, indicating disturbed immunoregulation or continuous B-cell activation [13]. The latter is consistent with clonal expansion of B-cells noted in the muscles of patients with s-IBM. [14]. In addition, IBM has been seen in patients with agammaglobulinemia and common variable immunodeficiency [15, 16]. The patients with IBM and immunodeficiency have been younger by a mean period of 15 years and have responded to intravenous immunoglobulin (IVIG) or steroids for a period of time [15, 16]. In our two reported cases, we have found, in addition to CD8$^+$ cells invading major histocompatibility complex I (MHC-I)-expressing muscle fibers, a high number of endomysial natural killer cells (NK cells) invading intercellular cell adhesion molecule 1 (ICAM-1)-positive muscle fibers [15]. Based on these findings, we have proposed that in patients with immunodeficiency/IBM the lymphocyte-induced cytotoxicity is of two types, one mediated by CD8$^+$ cytotoxic T-cells invading MHC-I-expressing muscle fibers and the other mediated by NK cells invading MHC-I-negative but ICAM-positive fibers [15].

The autoinvasive CD8$^+$ T-Cells are Activated, Appear Early, and are Cytotoxic

In IBM there is evidence of an antigen-directed cytotoxicity mediated by the autoinvasive CD8$^+$ T-cells in a pattern identical to the one observed in PM [1, 17–19]. The fundamental role of T-cell-mediated myocytotoxicity in s-IBM is supported by the following.

• T-cell invasion of nonnecrotic fibers is found early and in higher frequency than the Congo-red-positive fibers [20] suggesting that inflammation precedes the accumulation of amyloid and related stressor molecules.

• The autoinvasive T-cells are activated, as evidenced by their expression of ICAM-I, MHC-I, CD45RO, and inducible costimulator (ICOS) on their surface [19–22], suggesting an active participation, rather than a bystander effect, in muscle-fiber injury.

• The CD8$^+$ cells surround healthy, but MHC-I-class-expressing, nonnecrotic muscle fibers that eventually invade [22–24]. The CD8/MHC-I lesion is characteristic of IBM and PM [22–24] because it does not occur in inflammatory dystrophies or non-immune myopathies.

• By immuno-electron microscopy, CD8$^+$ cells and macrophages send spike-like processes into nonnecrotic muscle fibers, which traverse the basal lamina and focally displace or compress the muscle fibers [18].

• The endomysial CD8$^+$ T-cells, contain perforin and granzyme granules, as demonstrated with double immunocytochemistry and confirmed by finding increased mRNA expression of perforin [19]. In IBM, the perforin granules are prominent among the autoinvasive CD8$^+$ T-cells, especially those that are activated and express costimulatory molecules [19]. Perforin granules are vectorially directed towards the surface of the muscle fiber, inducing necrosis upon release, as demonstrated for PM [25]. These cells are also cytotoxic *in vitro* when exposed to autologous myotubes [26, 27]. Consequently, as in PM, the perforin pathway seems to be the major cytotoxic effector mechanism in IBM. In contrast, the Fas-/Fas-L-dependent apoptotic process is not functionally involved, despite expression of the Fas antigen on muscle fibers and of Fas-L on autoinvasive CD8$^+$ cells [28–31]. Whether the coexpression of the antiapoptotic molecules Bcl2, FLICE (Fas-associated death domain-like IL-1-converting enzyme)-inhibitory protein (FLIP), and human IAP-like protein (h1LP) confers resistance of muscle to Fas-mediated apoptosis remains unclear [30, 31].

Formation of immunological synapses between the autoinvasive cytotoxic CD8⁺ T-Cells with the MHC-I-Expressing Muscle Fibers

Muscle fibers normally do not express detectable amounts of MHC class I or II antigens. In IBM, however, widespread overexpression of MHC is an early event that can be seen even in areas remote from the inflammation [22, 32]. Based on *in vitro* studies, MHC-I is induced by cytokines and chemokines such as interferon γ (IFN-γ) or tumor necrosis factor α (TNFα) [33–36]. Because several of these cytokines are detected at a given time in increased levels in the muscle tissue of s-IBM patients [21, 37–41], the upregulation of MHC class I on the sarcolemma is probably related to continuous overexpression of cytokines. In transgenic mice, the MHC class I may act as an inciting event triggering an atypical, noninflammatory myopathy with "myositis-specific" antibodies, presumably via the MHC-I-induced cell stress [42]. In other chronic myopathies including the inflammatory dystrophies, and in contrast to s-IBM, the muscle fibers do not express the MHC-I antigen or the costimulatory molecules described below in a ubiquitous and consistent pattern [32], while the few T-cells in the proximity to the muscle fibers are clonally diverse and do not break the sarcolemma to release cytotoxic granules, as seen in IBM.

A fundamental observation in the immunopathology of s-IBM is the formation of immunological synapses between the MHC-I-expressing muscle fibers, which serve as antigen-presenting cells, and the activated CD8⁺ T-cells that invade the fibers [21, 24], as supported by the following.

Rearrangement of the *TCR* gene of the endomysial T-cells

The T-cells recognize an antigen via the T-cell receptor (TCR), a heterodimer of two α and β chains, encoded by multiple gene families in the V (variable), D (diversity), J (joining), and C (constant) regions of the TCR. The part of the TCR that recognizes an antigen is the CDR3 region, which is encoded by genes in the V-J and V-D-J segments of the *TCR* gene. If the endomysial T-cells are selectively recruited by a specific autoantigen, the use of the *V* and *J* genes of the TCR should be restricted and the amino acid sequence in their CDR3 region should be conserved. In patients with IBM, but not in those with DM or dystrophies, only certain T-cells of specific TCRα and TCRβ families are recruited to the muscle from the circulation [43–46]. Cloning and sequencing of the amplified endomysial or autoinvasive *TCR* gene families has demonstrated a restricted use of the *J*β gene with conserved amino acid sequence in the CDR3 region, indicating that these cells are specifically selected by antigens and clonally expanded *in situ* [43–46]. Immunocytochemistry combined with polymerase chain reaction and sequencing of the most prominent TCR families has shown that it is the autoinvasive, but not the perivascular, CD8⁺ cell population that clonally expands [43–46]. Sequential muscle biopsy specimens obtained during a 19–22 month period from three of our IBM patients, demonstrated that the clonal restriction of the same Vβ families not only persists among the autoinvasive CD8⁺ cells but these cells also exhibit conserved amino acid sequence homology in the complementary CDR3-determining region, indicating specific recruitment within the muscle to recognize heretofore unknown antigens [45]. That identical T-cell clones with restricted amino acid sequence persist in different muscles of IBM patients has now been confirmed in several studies [44, 46], suggesting that the same antigens in a given patient drive the T-cell-activation process. Examination with spectratyping of the CDR3 region of the TCR Vβ chains of lymphocytes concurrently obtained from the peripheral blood and muscles has confirmed in a large number of patients the clonality of the autoinvasive T-cells compared to those in the peripheral blood [47]. With this study we have concluded that in IBM the T-cell clones expand *in situ* within the muscle microenvironment after recognizing local antigens [47].

Presence of costimulatory molecules for synapse formation

The clonally expanded CD8⁺ cells are primed to receive antigenic peptides presented by the MHC-I molecule of the antigen-presenting cells, in conjunction with costimulatory molecules to form immunological synapses. The muscle fibers could serve as antigen-presenting cells provided they possess the B7 family of costimulatory molecules (B7-1, B7-2, BB1, or inducible costimulator ligand (ICOS-L)) and bind to their respective counterreceptors CD28, CTLA-4, or ICOS on the autoinvasive CD8 + T-cells. Indeed, several studies have demonstrated that in s-IBM muscles the BB1 (CD80) as well as ICOS-L are expressed on MHC-I-positive muscle fibers which make cell-to-cell contact with the CD28/CTLA-4 or

ICOS ligands on the autoinvasive CD8 + T-cells [19, 48–51] (Figure 8.1). Of importance, the ICOS-positive T-cells are cytotoxic, expressing perforin granules [19]. Because both BB1 and ICOS-L are functional molecules induced by IFN-γ or TNFα on human myoblasts, in s-IBM the BB1/CD28 and the ICOS–ICOS-L interactions would participate in antigen presentation, clonal expansion, and costimulation of memory T-cells [50].

The upregulation of these molecules offers the potential for therapeutic manipulations because of the availability of humanized monoclonal antibodies

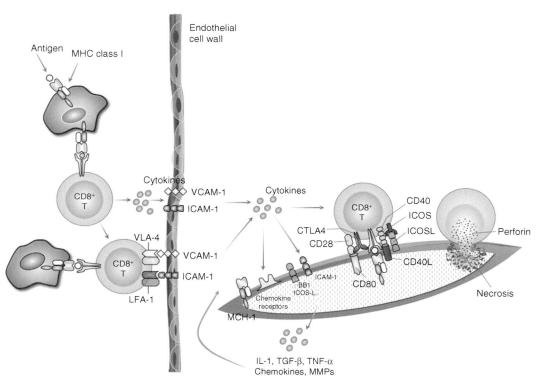

Figure 8.1 Molecules, receptors, and their ligands involved in the transgression of T-cells through the endothelial cell wall and recognition of antigens on muscle fibers of patients with s-IBM. LFA-1/ICAM-1 binding and TCR scanning for antigen initiates the formation of an immunological synapse between MHC-I and TCR. Stimulation is supported and enhanced by the engagement of costimulatory molecules BB1, ICOS, and CD40 on the muscle fibers and their ligands CD28, CTLA-4, ICOS-L, and CD40L on the autoinvasive T-cells. Metalloproteinases facilitate the migration of T-cells and their attachment to the muscle surface. Muscle-fiber necrosis occurs via the perforin granules released by the autoaggressive T-cells. A direct myocytotoxic effect exerted by the released IFN-γ, interleukin 1 (IL-1), or TNFα may also play a role. Death of the muscle fiber is mediated by a form of necrosis rather than apoptosis. (Reproduced from Dalakas [21].)

against CD28, CTLA4, or CD40L. These agents are strong inhibitors of T-cell activation and may be considered for experimental trials in patients with s-IBM.

Upregulation of cytokines, cytokine signaling, chemokines, and metalloproteinases

Cytokines and chemokines are essential in enhancing the activation of T-cells and the induction of costimulatory molecules for formation of the synapses, as discussed above. Various cytokines, including interleukins (IL-1, IL-2, IL-6, and IL-10), TNFα, IFN-γ, signal transducer and activation of transcription (STAT), and transforming growth factor β (TGF-β), are variably overexpressed in the muscle of patients with IBM [33–41]. Using gene array studies, the upregulated chemokine and cytokine genes were much higher in the muscles of patients with IBM compared to those with DM [53].

Chemokines, a class of small cytokines, are important molecules in leukocyte recruitment and activation at the sites of inflammation. Among them, MCP-1 and MIP-1a are strongly upregulated in IBM muscles at the protein and mRNA levels [38, 40, 41, 52]. The IFN-γ-inducible chemokines Mig and IP-10, and the Mig's receptor CXCR3, are also strongly expressed on the muscle fibers and on a subset of autoinvasive CD8$^+$ cells [39]. Because Mig and IP-10 are produced by myotubes upon IFN-γ stimulation, they could facilitate the recruitment of activated T-cells to the muscle and contribute to the self-sustaining nature of endomysial inflammation [21, 24]. Furthermore, MCP-1 and MIP-1a have a fibrogenic effect and their presence in the extracellular matrix along with their *in situ* synthesis may have an effect in promoting tissue fibrosis in the late stages of IBM. Various adhesion and extracellular matrix molecules such as vascular cell adhesion molecule (VCAM), ICAM, and thrombospondins are also upregulated in the tissues of patients with IBM [54, 55] and may enhance the inflammatory response or promote tissue fibrosis in the late stages of the disease.

Another important group of molecules facilitating the adhesion and transmigration of lymphocytes is the metalloproteinases (MMPs), a family of calcium-dependent zinc endopeptidases involved in the remodeling of the extracellular matrix. Pathologically, MMPs propagate the inflammatory response by facilitating T-cell adhesion to matrices and endothelial cells and the exit of lymphoid cells from the circulation to targeted tissues. Among MMPs, the MMP-9 and MMP-2 are upregulated on the nonnecrotic and MHC-I-class-expressing muscle fibers of patients with PM and IBM [54]. Further, MMP-2 immunostains the autoinvasive CD8$^+$ T-cells, which make cell-to-cell contact with muscle fibers. Because collagen IV is prominent on the muscle membrane, the overexpression of MMPs in IBM may facilitate T-cell adhesion and enhance T-cell-mediated cytotoxicity by degrading extracellular matrix proteins [54]. Targeting MMPs with pharmacologic agents may offer therapeutic options in the management of patients with IBM.

What has been a critical observation for the pathogenesis of IBM and the chronicity of the disease is that the muscle, *in vivo* and *in vitro*, can secrete proinflammatory cytokines upon cytokine stimulation in an autoamplificatory mechanism that facilitates the recruitment of activated T-cells to the muscle and contributes to the self-sustaining nature of endomysial inflammation [19, 21, 24]

Other immune cells support the autoimmune process in s-IBM but lack specificity

Myeloid dendritic cells, potent cells in antigen presentation, are abundantly found in the endomysial infiltrates of all inflammatory myopathies including PM, DM, and IBM [56]. These cells may present local antigens to T-cells and B-cells and contribute to muscle-fiber injury. A large number of plasma cells and clonally expanded B-cells are also found in IBM, PM, and DM muscles [14, 56], suggesting an antigen-specific humoral immune response. These cells, however, lack specificity for IBM, as they are frequently noted in the targeted tissues in several autoimmune disorders. Their presence simply denotes that different effector mechanisms of T-cells and B-cells concurrently play an active role in the autoimmune process. The suggestion that in PM and

IBM there is a humoral response associated with *in situ* production of autoantibodies [14, 56] remains unproven and highly speculative.

Association with retroviral infections (HIV, HTLV-1)

Although several viruses, including coxsackie-viruses, influenza, paramyxoviruses, cytomegalovirus, and Epstein–Barr virus have been indirectly associated with IBM, sensitive methodologies have not proven any connection with these viruses [57]. The exception has been with HIV and human T-cell lymphotropic virus type 1 (HTLV-1) infection where s-IBM has been seen with rather unusual frequency [57–62]. More than 40 cases of HIV-/ HTLV-1-positive patients with IBM have been reported or are known to us, indicating that this association is not fortuitous. It appears that in HIV-positive patients who live longer and harbor the virus for several years the disease is more frequently recognized. The clinical phenotype and muscle histology of HIV/IBM patients are identical to retroviral-negative IBM except that the disease starts before the age of 50 but several years after the first manifestations of the retroviral infection. The predominant endomysial cells are CD8$^+$ cytotoxic T-cells, which, along with macrophages, invade or surround MHC-class-I-antigen-expressing nonnecrotic muscle fibers [57–60]. Using *in situ* hybridization, polymerase chain reaction, immunocytochemistry, and electron microscopy, viral antigens could not be detected within the muscle fibers but only in occasional endomysial macrophages [57, 58]. Molecular immunological studies using tetramers have shown that retrovirally specific cytotoxic T-cells, whose TCR contains amino acid residues for specific HLA/viral peptides, are recruited within the clonally expanded T-cells and invade muscle fibers [60–62]. We have interpreted these observations to suggest that in HIV/HTLV-1-IBM there is no evidence of persistent infection of the muscle fibers with the virus or viral replication within the muscle, but rather that the chronic retroviral infection, in genetically susceptible individuals, triggers a persistent inflammatory process that leads to s-IBM [62]. The retrovirally infected endomysial macrophages may facilitate the *in situ* autoimmune process by secreting cytokines, chemokines, or NO, thereby upregulating MHC-I or costimulatory molecules and perpetuating the disease.

The development of IBM in HIV-positive patients should be distinguished from a toxic myopathy related to long-term therapy with zidovudine, which is characterized by fatigue, myalgia, mild muscle weakness, and mild elevation of serum creatine kinase activity [63]. Zidovudine-induced myopathy, which generally improves when the drug is discontinued, is a mitochondrial disorder characterized histologically by the presence of "ragged-red/-blue" fibers. Abnormal muscle mitochondria and depletion of the muscle mitochondrial DNA by zidovudine result from inhibition of γ-DNA polymerase, an enzyme found solely in the mitochondrial matrix [57, 63].

Amyloid and degeneration-related molecules in s-IBM: an interrelationship with inflammation

IBM is a complex disorder because in addition to the clear immunopathogenic events described above, there is an equally strong degenerative process as evidenced by the presence of rimmed vacuoles (almost always in fibers not invaded by T-cells), intracellular deposition of Congo-red-positive amyloid, and the presence of cytoplasmic filaments with accumulation of β-amyloid-related molecules including APP, phosphorylated tau, apolipoprotein E, γ-tubulin, clusterin, gelsolin, and a number of molecules indicative of cell stress, as reviewed in Chapter 7 in this volume. These accumulations, although extensively studied in s-IBM, do not seem to be unique to this disease, because they have been also observed in myofibrillar and other vacuolar myopathies [64–68]. Inhibition of the 26S proteasome and impaired autophagy appear to occur in s-IBM [69, 70], as discussed elsewhere in this volume by Askanas et al. What appears a unique association in IBM, however, compared to other chronic vacuolar myopathies, is the concomitant accumulation of the aforementioned molecules with a strong primary inflammatory response and the overexpression of pro-inflammatory mediators and MHC class I on all the fibers, vacuolated or not. Regardless of whether the primary event is an inflammatory or protein dysregulation process, the unique coexistence of the two processes has led our laboratory to explore whether there is an interrelationship between inflammation and degeneration in an effort to understand what drives each process and to design targeted therapeutic strategies.

Inflammation may trigger or enhance accumulation of β-amyloid

The main inflammatory molecules CCL-3, CCL-4, CXCL-9, IFN-γ, and IL-1β are expressed to a higher degree in s-IBM muscle compared to PM or DM [53]. Most importantly, in s-IBM these molecules appear to be produced by the muscle fibers themselves, whereas in PM and DM the majority of the signal is localized to immune cells, the connective tissue,

and the capillaries [71]. In s-IBM, but not in PM or DM, there is also a significant correlation between the mRNA expression of APP, as a key relevant degenerative marker, with the inflammatory mediators IFN-γ and CXCL-9 which also colocalize with APP/β-amyloid proteins. Further, exposure of muscle cells to pro-inflammatory cytokines IL-1β and IFN-γ induces an overexpression of APP with subsequent accumulation of protein aggregates. On this basis, we have proposed that in s-IBM a continuous stimulation of inflammatory factors may, after a long period, induce a higher basal expression of APP and an increased sensitivity to *de novo* pro-inflammatory cytokines that triggers a self-perpetuating cycle [2, 24, 72] (Figure 8.2). The association between inflammation and accumulation of β-amyloid in skeletal muscle has recently been shown in a mouse model of s-IBM, where lipopolysaccharide-induced inflammation enhanced the accumulation of proteins such as tau and β-amyloid [73].

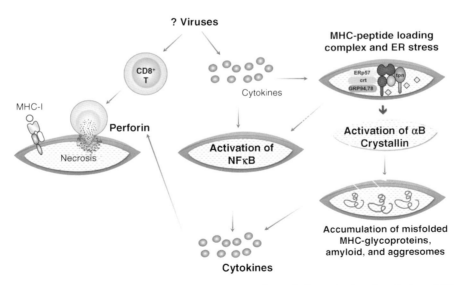

Figure 8.2 Proposed mechanism of the interplay between inflammation and degeneration in IBM. Viral or inflammatory triggers lead to clonal expansion of CD8 T-cells and T-cell-mediated cytotoxicity in the perforin pathway. The released cytokines upregulate MHC class I molecules and increase levels of the MHC-peptide loading complex, because the abundance of generated peptides cannot be conformationally assembled with the MHC to exit the endoplasmic reticulum (ER). As a result, there is an endoplasmic reticulum stress response, which leads to activation of the transcription factor nuclear factor κB (NFκB) and further cytokine release with subsequent accumulation of misfolded MHC glycoproteins, including phosphorylated tau and amyloid-related proteins. (Reproduced from Dalakas [72].)

αB-crystallin and APP as cell stress markers

Almost 10 years ago, αB-crystallin has been demonstrated in healthy-looking muscle fibers (termed "X-fibers") in IBM muscle [74]. αB-crystallin is a heat-shock protein which can chaperone proteins in skeletal muscle, and is associated with cell stress or β-amyloid clearance. In a quantitative assessment of multilabeling and serial immunohistochemistry, a positive correlation between αB-crystallin and β-amyloid-associated markers was found in s-IBM muscles [75]. The normal-appearing muscle fibers that were positive for αB-crystallin were often double-positive for APP while the degenerating/vacuolated fibers displaying β-amyloid accumulations, colabeled with αB-crystallin, APP, and markers of degeneration/regeneration. A significant colocalization between APP/β-amyloid and markers of cell stress and regeneration/degeneration, such as NCAM and desmin, was also noted. On this basis, it appears that in the muscle fibers of s-IBM, αB-crystallin is an early event associated with a stress response that precedes accumulation of β-amyloid. These observations were strengthened by *in vitro* studies which demonstrated that accumulation of β-amyloid, upon pro-inflammatory cell stress, was preceded by upregulation of APP and αB-crystallin [75]. Interestingly, in cultured human muscle fibers genetic overexpression of AβPP induces αB-crystallin [76].

Reconciling the immunopathogenesis of IBM with the relative resistance of the disease to conventional immunotherapies

In spite of the above-described primary immune factors, s-IBM remains resistant to most immunotherapies, justifying the contention that it could be more of a degenerative disease rather than an autoimmune disease. The general connotation, however, that IBM is totally resistant to immunotherapy is not entirely correct. In many clinics that use immunotherapies, including our own, a small number of patients may transiently respond to common immunotherapeutic agents such as corticosteroids, azathioprine, methotrexate, or mycophenolate early in the disease. Up to 25% of patients in a controlled study have also responded transiently to IVIG [77]. IVIG has also improved the dysphagia of IBM in both a controlled study and in uncontrolled series [77–80]. The benefits from these immunotherapies are limited and short-lived, however; IBM remains a steadily progressive disease with overall relative resistance to therapies. This pattern of transient therapeutic response resembles the one seen in various other autoimmune diseases where immune and degenerative features coexist from the outset. Primary progressive multiple sclerosis is a classic example as many of these patients partially respond for a period of time but afterwards they become resistant to all therapies.

The following reasons may explain the lack of treatment efficacy in s-IBM [5, 6].

• s-IBM is a chronic disease and therapy is always initiated late, when the degenerative cascade has already begun, due to insidious onset and very slow disease progression. After having seen hundreds of IBM patients, we have come to recognize that the disease starts long before the patients develop clinical symptoms, as there is a critical threshold above which weakness is clinically manifested. It is striking that even patients with minimal clinical weakness already exhibit muscle atrophy and extensive pathology in certain muscle groups (revealed by histology or muscle imaging).

• The observations discussed above show that αB-crystallin is, along with pro-inflammatory markers, an early event associated with cell stress response that seems to precede the accumulation of β-amyloid. Since chronic inflammation can enhance the degenerative features and accumulation of misfolded proteins [24, 72], early initiation of anti-inflammatory therapy may arrest progression to clinical IBM. The following two recent cases support this concept and emphasize that even the typical IBM histology can be reversed with early treatment. One was a rapidly progressive patient with DM who had the typical pathological features consistent with IBM, but sustained complete remission with immunotherapy [81]; the second was a patient of ours who presented with rapidly progressive proximal myopathy –

clinically suspected to be PM – whose biopsy was consistent with IBM; she too, had complete remission with prednisone and mycophenolate. Such cases – albeit anecdotal – are not rare; they have been seen before by others and us and highlight the concept that early treatment in patients with histological IBM who have not yet developed the clinical IBM phenotype may lead to complete remission.

• The production of pro-inflammatory mediators by the muscle fibers themselves may pose a problem in arresting the process because the standard immunosuppressants may not be able to suppress the factors that trigger the continuous production of cytokines by the muscle fibers themselves [6].

• The immunopathology is secondary, so that even a maximal immunosuppression would have a limited effect on the continuing degenerative process. This is unlikely because, as outlined above, the immune response in IBM is primary and antigen-driven and may even precede degeneration. Regardless, however, of whether the inflammation or the degeneration is the dominant factor, it is likely that in IBM two processes coexist from the outset and progress in parallel. Consequently, we believe that an effective treatment may need to concurrently suppress both the degenerative and the inflammatory component from the outset. The noted interaction of the two processes suggests that application of agents with double effect may be therapeutically rewarding. Such agents include rapamycin and the Interleukin-1β (IL-1β) antagonists, because they concurrently suppress inflammation and stressor molecules; both of these agents are currently being considered for experimental studies by our group.

• The correct anti-dysimmune/inflammatory agent has not yet been found as targeted immunotherapy. Conducting small but intense bench-to-bedside studies like the one performed with Alemtuzumab [82] possibly is the way to proceed. The latter study has suggested that suppression of endomysial inflammation might have an effect on some degeneration- or regeneration-associated molecules such as αB-crystallin and desmin with resulting short-term clinical stability. This study seems to suggest that new anti-lymphocyte therapies, if proven safe for long-term therapy, might have an effect not only on inflammatory mediators but also in halting some

elements of degeneration and cell stress if therapy is applied for long periods. It is a new way of thinking with implications beyond inflammatory myopathies [72]. As the industry is generating new such agents, we should take advantage if there are no long-term safety concerns. The same applies to agents suppressing the "degenerative" molecules. In Alzheimer disease, where these very same molecules are abundant in the patients' brains, no therapy has been effective. Possibly in support of the neuroinflammatory effect, IVIG, a drug that has anti-inflammatory properties, currently shows some promise in Alzheimer disease [83–86].

References

1 Dalakas MC. (1991) Polymyositis, dermatomyositis and inclusion-body myositis. *N Engl J Med* **325**, 1487–1498.

2 Mastaglia FL, Garlepp MJ, Phillips BA, Zilko PJ. (2003) Inflammatory myopathies: clinical, diagnostic and therapeutic aspects. *Muscle Nerve* **27**, 407–425.

3 Lotz BP, Engel AG, Nishino H et al. (1989) Inclusion body myositis. *Observations in 40 patients. Brain* **112**, 727–747.

4 Needham M, Mastaglia FL. (2007) Inclusion body myositis: current pathogenetic concepts and diagnostic and therapeutic approaches. *Lancet Neurol* **6**(7), 620–631.

5 Dalakas MC. (2010) Inflammatory muscle diseases: a critical review on pathogenesis and therapies. *Curr Opin Pharmacol* **10**(3), 346–352.

6 Schmidt J, Dalakas MC. (2010) Pathomechanisms of inflammatory myopathies: recent advances and implications for diagnosis and therapies. *Exp Opin* **4**, 241–250.

7 Dalakas MC. (2006) Inflammatory, immune, and viral aspects of inclusion-body myositis. *Neurology* **66** (2 Suppl. 1), S33–S38.

8 Koffman BM, Rugiero M, Dalakas MC. (1998) Autoimmune diseases and autoantibodies associated with sporadic inclusion body myositis. *Muscle Nerve* **21**, 115–117.

9 Bandrising UA, Schrender GMTH, Giphart MJ et al. (2004) Associations with autoimmune disorders and HLA Class I, and II antigens in inclusion body myositis. *Neurology* **63**, 2396–2398.

10 McCoy AL, Bubb MR, Plotz PH, Davis JC. (1999) Inclusion body myositis long after dermatomyositis: a report of two cases. *Clin Exp Rheumatol* **141**, 926–930.

11 Koffman BM, Sivakumar K, Simonis T et al. (1998) HLA allele distribution distinguishes sporadic inclusion body myositis from hereditary inclusion body myopathies. *J Neuroimmunol* **84**, 139–142.

12 Sivakumar K, Semino-Mora, Dalakas MC. (1997) An inflammatory, familial, inclusion body myositis with autoimmune features and a phenotype identical to sporadic inclusion body myositis: studies in 3 families. *Brain* **120**, 653–661.

13 Dalakas MC, Illa I, Gallardo E, Juarez C. (1997) Inclusion body myositis and paraproteinemia: incidence and immunopathologic correlations. *Ann Neurol* **41**, 100–104.

14 Bradshaw EM, Orihuela A, McArdel SL et al. (2007) A local antigen-driven humoral response is present in the inflammatory myopathies. *J Immunol* **178**(1), 547–556.

15 Dalakas MC, Illa I. (1995) Common variable immunodeficiency and inclusion body myositis: a distinct myopathy mediated by natural killer cells. *Ann Neurol* **37**, 806–810.

16 Lindberg C, Persson LI, Bjorkander J, Oldfors A. (1994) Inclusion body myositis: clinical, morphological, physiological and laboratory findings in 18 cases. *Acta Neurol Scand* **89**, 123–131.

17 Arahata, K, Engel AG. (1984) Monoclonal antibody analysis of mononuclear cells in myopathies. I: Quantitation of subsets according to diagnosis and sites of accumulation and demonstration and counts of muscle fibres invaded by T cells. *Ann Neurol* **16**, 193–208.

18 Arahata K, Engel AG. (1986) Monoclonal antibody analysis of mononuclear cells in myopathies III. Immunoelectron microscopy aspects of cell-mediated muscle fiber injury. *Ann Neurol* **19**, 112–125.

19 Schmidt J, Rakocevic G, Raju R, Dalakas MC. (2004) Upregulated inducible costimulator and ICOS-ligand in inclusion body myositis muscle: significance for CD8+ T cell cytotoxicity. *Brain* **127**, 1182–1190.

20 Pruitt 2nd JN, Showalter CJ, Engel AG. (1996) Sporadic inclusion body myositis: counts of different types of abnormal fibers. *Ann Neurol* **39**(1), 139–143.

21 Dalakas MC. (2006) Mechanisms of disease: signaling pathways and immunobiology of inflammatory myopathies. *Nat Clin Pract Rheumatol* **2**(4), 219–227.

22 Emslie-Smith AM, Arahata K, Engel AG. (1989). Major histocompatibility complex class I antigen expression, immunologicalization of interferon subtypes, and T cell-mediated cytotoxicity in myopathies. *Hum Pathol* **20**, 224–231.

23 Dalakas MC. (2004) Inflammatory disorders of muscle: progress in polymyositis, dermatomyositis and inclusion body myositis. *Curr Opin Neurol* **17**, 561–567.

24 Dalakas MC. (2006) Sporadic inclusion body myositis: diagnosis, pathogenesis and therapeutic strategies. *Nat Clin Prac Neurol* **2**, 437–447.

25 Goebels N, Michaelis D, Engelhardt M et al. (1996) Differential expression of perforin in muscle-infiltrating T cell in polymyositis and dermatomyositis. *J Clin Invest* **97**, 2905–2910.

26 Wiendl H, Hohlfeld R, Kieseier BC. (2005) Immunobiology of muscle: advances in understanding an immunological microenvironment. *Trends Immunol* **26**, 373–380.

27 Hohlfeld R, Engel AG. (1991) Coculture with autologous myotubes of cytotoxic T cells isolated from muscle in inflammatory myopathies. *Ann Neurol* **29**, 498–507.

28 Behrens L, Bender A, Johnson MA, Hohlfeld R. (1997) Cytotoxic mechanisms in inflammatory myopathies: co-expression of Fas and protective Bcl-2 in muscle fibres and inflammatory cells. *Brain* **120**, 929.

29 Schneider C, Gold R, Dalakas MC et al. (1996) MHC class I mediated cytotoxicity does not induce apoptosis in muscle fibers nor in inflammatory T cells: studies in patients with polymyositis, dermatomyositis, and inclusion body myositis. *J Neuropath Exp Neurol* **55**, 1205–1209.

30 Nagaraju K, Casciola-Rosen L, Rosen A et al. (2000) The inhibition of apoptosis in myositis and in normal muscle cells. *J Immunol* **164**, 5459–5465.

31 Li M, Dalakas MC. (2000) Expression of human IAP-like protein in skeletal muscle: An explanation for the rare incidence of muscle fiber apoptosis in T-cell mediated inflammatory myopathies. *J Neuroimmunol* **106**, 1–5.

32 Karpati G, Pouliot Y, Carpenter S. (1988). Expression of immunoreactive major histocompatability complex products in human skeletal muscles. *Ann Neurol* **23**, 64–72.

33 Mantegazza R, Hughes SM, Mitchell D et al. (1991) Modulation of MHC class II antigen expression in human myoblasts after treatment with IFN-gamma. *Neurology* **41**, 1128.

34 Bao SS, King NJ, dos Remedios CG. (1990) Elevated MHC class I and II antigens in cultured human embryonic myoblasts following stimulation with gamma-interferon. *Immunol Cell Biol* **68**, 235–241.

35 Hohlfeld R, Engel AG. (1990) Induction of HLA-DR expression on human myoblasts with interferon-gamma. *Am J Pathol* **136**, 503.

36 Roy R, Danserau G, Tremblay JP et al. (1991) Expression of major histocompatibility complex antigens on human myoblasts. *Transplant Proc* **23**, 799.

37 Lundberg I, Brengman JM, Engel AG. (1995) Analysis of cytokine expression in muscle in inflammatory myopathies, Duchenne's dystrophy and non-weak controls. *J Neuroimmunol* **63**, 9–16.

38 Tews DS, Goebel HH. (1996) Cytokine expression profiles in idiopathic inflammatory myopathies. *J Neuropathol Exp Neurol* **55**, 342–347.

39 De Bleecker JL, Meire VI, Declercq W, Van Aken HE. (1999) Immunolocalization of tumor necrosis factor-alpha and its receptors in inflammatory myopathies. *Neuromusc Disord* **9**, 239.

40 Figarella-Branger D, Civate M, Bartoli C, Pellissier JF. Cytokines, chemokines, and cell adhesion molecules in inflammatory myopathies. *Muscle and Nerve* 2003) **28**(6), 659–682.

41 Raju R, Vasconcelos OM, Semino-Mora C et al. (2003) Expression of interferon-gamma inducible chemokines in the muscles of patients with inclusion body myositis. *J Neuroimmunol* **141**, 125–131.

42 Nagaraju K, Raben N, Loeffler L et al. (2000) Conditional up-regulation of MHC class I in skeletal muscle leads to self-sustaining autoimmune myositis and myositis-specific autoantibodies. *Proc Natl Acad Sci USA* **97**, 9209–9214.

43 Bender A, Behrens L, Engel AG, Hohlfeld R. (1998) T-cell heterogeneity in muscle lesions of inclusion body myositis. *J Neuroimmunol* **84**, 86–91.

44 Fyhr IM, Moslemi AR, Mosavi AA et al. (1997) Oligoclonal expansion of muscle infiltrating T cells in inclusion body myositis. *J Neuroimmunol* **79**, 185–189.

45 Amemiya K, Granger RP, Dalakas MC. (2000) Clonal restriction of T-cell receptor expression by infiltrating lymphocytes in inclusion body myositis persists over time:studies in repeated muscle biopsies. *Brain* **123**, 2030–2039.

46 Muntzing K, Lindberg C, Moslemi AR, Oldfors A. (2003) Inclusion body myositis: clonal expansions of muscle-infiltrating T cells persist over time. *Scand J Immunol* **58**, 195–200.

47 Salajegheh M, Rakocevic G, Raju R et al. (2007) T cell receptor profiling in muscle and blood lymphocytes in sporadic inclusion body myositis. *Neurology* **69**, 1672–1679.

48 Behrens L, Kerschensteiner M, Misgeld T et al. (1998) Human muscle cells express a functional costimulatory molecule distinct from B7.1 (CD80) and B7.2 (CD86) in vitro and in inflammatory lesions. *J Immunol* **161**, 5943–5951.

49 Murata K, Dalakas MC. (1999) Expression of the costimulatory molecule BB-1, the ligands CTLA-4 and CD28 and their mRNA in inflammatory myopathies. *Am J Pathol* **155**, 453–460.

50 Wiendel H, Mitsdoerffer M, Schneider D et al. (2003) Muscle fibers and cultured muscle or cells express the B7.1/2 related costimulatory molecule ICOSL: implications for the pathogenesis of inflammatory myopathies. *Brain* **126**, 1026–1035.

51 Dalakas MC. (2001) The molecular and cellular pathology of inflammatory muscle diseases. *Curr Opin Pharmacol* **1**, 300–306.

52 De Bleecker JL, De Paepe B, Vanwalleghem IE, Schroder JM. (2002) Differential expression of chemokines in inflammatory myopathies. *Neurology* **58**, 1779–1785.

53 Raju R, Dalakas MC. (2005) Gene expression profile in the muscles of patients with inflammatory myopathies: effect of therapy with IVIg and biological validation of clinically relevant genes. *Brain* **128**(Pt 8) 1887–1896.

54 Choi YC, Dalakas MC. (2000) Expression of matrix metalloproteinases in the muscle of patients with inflammatory myopathies. *Neurology* **54**, 65–71.

55 Salajegheh M, Raju R, Schmidt J et al. (2007) Upregulation of thrombospondin-1(TSP-1) and its binding partners, CD36 and CD47 in sporadic inclusion body myositis. *J Neuroimmunol* **187**, 166–174.

56 Greenberg SA, Pinkus GS, Amato AA et al. (2007) Myeloid dendritic cells in inclusion-body myositis and polymyositis. *Muscle Nerve* **35**, 17–23.

57 Dalakas MC. (2004) Viral related muscle disease. In: Engel AG (ed.), *Myology* (3rd edn). McGraw Hill, New York, pp. 1389–1417.

58 Cupler EJ, Leon-Monzon M, Miller J et al. (1996) Inclusion body myositis in HIV-I and HTLV-I infected patients. *Brain* **119**, 1887–1893.

59 Ozden S, Gessain A, Gout O, Mikol J. (2001) Sporadic inclusion body myositis in a patient with human T cell leukemia virus type 1-associated myelopathy. *Clin Infect Dis* **32**, 510–514.

60 Ozden S, Cochet M, Mikol J et al. (2004) Direct evidence for a chronic CD8 + -T-cell-mediated immune reaction to tax within the muscle of a human T-cell leukemia/lymphoma virus type 1-infected patient with sporadic inclusion body myositis. *J Virol* **78**, 10320–10327.

61 Saito M, Higuchi I, Saito A et al. (2002) Molecular analysis of T cell clonotypes in muscle-infiltrating lymphocytes from patients with human T lymphotropic virus type 1 polymyositis. *J Infect Dis* **186**, 1231–1241.

62 Dalakas MC, Rakocevic G, Shatunov A et al. (2007) IBM with HIV infection: 4 new cases with clonal expansion of viral-specific T cells. *Ann Neurol* **61**, 466–475.

63 Dalakas MC, Illa I, Pezeshkpour GH et al. (1990) Mitochondrial myopathy caused by long-term zidovudine therapy. *N Engl J Med* **332**, 1098–1105.

64 Fidzianska A, Rowinska-Marcinska K, Hausmanowa-Petrusewicz I. (2004) Coexistence of X-linked recessive Emery-Dreifuss muscular dystrophy with inclusion body myositis-like morphology. *Acta Neuropathol* **104**, 197–203.

65 Semino-Mora C, Dalakas MC. (1988) Rimmed vacuoles with B-Amyloid and ubiquitinated filamentous deposits in the muscles of patients with long-standing denervation (post-poliomyelitis muscular atrophy): similarities with inclusion body myositis. *Hum Pathol* **29**, 1128–1133.

66 Selcen D, Ohno K, Engel AG. (2004) Myofibrillar myopathy: clinical, morphological and genetic studies in 63 patients. *Brain* **127**, 439–451.

67 Ferrer I, Martin B, Castano JG et al. (2004) Proteasomal expression, induction of immunoproteasome subunits, and local MHC class I presentation in myofibrillar myopathy and inclusion body myositis. *J Neuropathol Exp Neurol* **63**, 484–498.

68 Ferrer I, Carmona M, Blanco R et al. (2005) Involvement of clusterin and the aggresome in abnormal protein deposits in myofibrillar myopathies and inclusion body myositis. *Brain Pathol* **15**, 101–108.

69 Fratta P, Engel WK, McFerrin J et al. (2005) Proteasome inhibition and aggresome formation in sporadic inclusion-body myositis and in AbPP-overexpressing cultured human muscle fibers. *Am J Pathol* **167**, 517–526.

70 Nogalska A, D'Agostino C, Terracioano C et al. (2010) Impaired autophagy in sporadic inclusion-body myositis and in endoplasmic reticulum stress-provoked cultured human muscle fibers. *Am J Pathol* **177**(3), 1377–1387.

71 Schmidt J, Barthel K, Wrede A, Salajegheh M, Bähr M, Dalakas MC. (2008) Interrelation of inflammation and APP in sIBM: IL-1 beta induces accumulation of beta-amyloid in skeletal muscle. *Brain* **131**, 1228–1240.

72 Dalakas MC. (2008) Molecular links between inflamation and degeneration: Lessons on "Neuroinflammation" using IBM as a model. *Ann Neurol* **64**, 1–3.

73 Kitazawa M, Trinh DN, LaFerla FM. (2008) Inflammation induces tau pathology in inclusion body myositis model via glycogen synthase kinase-3beta. *Ann Neurol* **64**(1), 15–24.

74 Banwell BL, Engel AG. (2000). AlphaB-crystallin immunolocalization yields new insights into inclusion body myositis. *Neurology* **54**(5), 1020–1021.

75 Muth IE, Barthel K, Bähr M et al. (2009) Proinflammatory cell stress in sporadic inclusion body myositis muscle: overexpression of alphaB-crystallin is associated with amyloid precursor protein and accumulation of beta-amyloid. *J Neurol Neurosurg Psychiatry* **80**(12), 1344–1349.

76 Wojcik S, Engel WK, McFerrin J et al. (2006) AbPP overexpression & proteasome inhibition increase αB-crystallin in cultured human muscle: relevance to inclusion-body myositis. *Neuromusc Disord* **16**, 839–844.

77 Dalakas MC. (2003) Therapeutic strategies in inflammatory myopathies. *Semin Neurol* **23**, 199–206.

78 Dalakas MC, Sekul EA, Cupler EJ, Sivakumar K. (1997) The efficacy of high dose intravenous immunoglobulin (IVIg) in patients with inclusion-body myositis (IBM). *Neurology* **48**, 712–716.

79 Dalakas MC. (2010) Advances in the treatment of myositis. *Nat Rev Rheumatol* **6**, 129–137.

80 Cherin P, Pelletier S, Teixeira A et al. (2002) Intravenous immunoglobulin for dysphagia of inclusion body myositis. *Neurology* **58**, 326.

81 Layzer R, Lee HS, Iverson D, Margeta M. (2009) Dermatomyositis with inclusion body myositis pathology. *Muscle Nerve* **40**(3), 469–471.

82 Dalakas MC, Rakocevic G, Schmidt J et al. (2009) Effect of Alemtuzumab (CAMPATH 1-H) in patients with inclusion-body myositis. *Brain* **132**(Pt 6) 1536–1544.

83 Hughes RA, Dalakas MC, Cornblath DR et al. (2009) Clinical applications of intravenous immunoglobulins in neurology. *Clin Exp Immunol* **158** (Suppl. 1), 34–42.

84 Relkin NR, Szabo P, Adamiak B et al. (2009) 18-month study of intravenous immunoglobulin for treatment of mild Alzheimer disease *Neurobiol Aging* **30**(11), 1728–1736.

85 Fillit H, Hess G Hill J et al. (2009) IV immunoglobulin is associated with reduced risk of Alzheimer disease and related disorders *Neurology* **73**, 180–185.

86 Dalakas MC. (2008) IVIG in other autoimmune neurological disorders: current status and future prospects. *J Neurol* **255** (Suppl. 3), 12–16.

CHAPTER 9

Sporadic inclusion-body myositis: clinical symptoms, physical findings, and diagnostic investigations

Frank L. Mastaglia

Centre for Neuromuscular and Neurological Disorders, University of Western Australia, Queen Elizabeth II Medical Centre, Perth, WA, Australia

Introduction

Sporadic inclusion-body myositis (s-IBM) is a chronic progressive and disabling condition which affects males more often than females. The age of onset of symptoms is variable but is usually after the age of 40 years (Figure 9.1) and the condition eventually leads to loss of manual control, impaired mobility, and increasing dependency over 15–25 years [1, 2]. The clinical phenotype is also quite variable in terms of the presenting symptoms and severity of muscle weakness when the patient first presents depending on the stage of the disease and its duration. As the tempo of the condition is very insidious, and as the initial symptoms are relatively nonspecific, many patients do not present to their medical practitioner until the disease is quite advanced and there is often a further delay before appropriate investigations are carried out and the diagnosis of s-IBM is confirmed [3]. Moreover, it is not uncommon for the condition to be misdiagnosed on initial presentation.

Presenting symptoms

The earliest and most common complaints are usually related to weakness or fatigue of the lower limbs and include difficulty rising from the squatting position or from low chairs, and walking up and down stairs. Less frequently foot-drop is the presenting symptom while in some cases falls are the initial presenting complaint. Exercise-related myalgia of the thighs and knee pain are not uncommon, particularly if there is some pre-existing osteoarthritis of the knees. Some patients present because of noticeable wasting of the thighs. Less common presenting complaints are difficulty with activities involving gripping, such as holding hand tools or golf clubs, or using keys, spray cans, or perfume sprays due to weakness of the long flexors of the thumb and fingers. Dysphagia is common once the disease is established and in some patients it may be the presenting symptom and reason for referral. The diagnosis of s-IBM may be made at an earlier stage in such cases when the involvement of the limb muscles is still relatively mild.

Clinical course

The natural history of s-IBM is for the weakness to be progressive but the rate of deterioration in strength varies in different patients. The rate of progression appears to be more rapid in patients with disease onset after the age of 60 years [4]. A quantitative

Muscle Aging, Inclusion-Body Myositis and Myopathies, First Edition. Edited by Valerie Askanas and W. King Engel.
© 2012 Blackwell Publishing Ltd. Published 2012 by Blackwell Publishing Ltd.

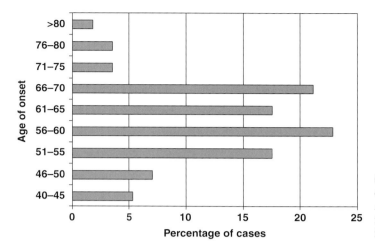

Figure 9.1 Distribution of age at onset of first symptoms in a series of 56 Australian cases of s-IBM. (Reproduced from Needham et al. [3], with permission from the BMJ Publishing Group.)

myographic study of 11 patients showed a 4% mean rate of decline in strength over a 6 month period, but in a third of cases there was no change in strength over this period, or even a slight improvement in some cases [5]. As the condition continues to progress patients have increasing difficulty with a variety of everyday activities such as handwriting, cutting up food, using other utensils, dressing, personal hygiene, and mobility and they become increasingly dependent on their partners or carers. Most patients need a walking aid (cane or walker) after 5–10 years and a minority of patients become wheelchair-bound after 10–15 years [3, 6]. A 10-point IBM-functional rating scale (IBM-FRS) has been developed to quantify and monitor the severity of such disabilities over time (Table 9.1) [7].

Most s-IBM patients experience falls at some stage of the disease which may result in fractures, severe soft tissue injuries, or other more serious injuries. Falls can occur both in the early stages and late stages, and tend to be less frequent during the intermediate stages of the disease, presumably because of the use of compensatory strategies and a reduction in mobility.

The majority of s-IBM patients develop dysphagia at some stage of the disease, the frequency varying from 40–80% in different series [6, 8, 9]. While in many cases this is relatively mild and may not even be mentioned by the patients, in some it may lead to recurrent episodes of choking and aspiration pneumonia, and may interfere with adequate nutrition. Videofluoroscopy during swallowing shows abnormal function of the cricopharyngeal sphincter in many patients [9]. In some the dysphagia responds to treatment with intravenous immunoglobulin [10], but others require dilatation or botulinum toxin injection of the sphincter, or a cricopharyngeal myotomy [11].

Patterns of muscle involvement

The pattern of muscle weakness and atrophy in s-IBM is characteristically selective and differs from that in other inflammatory myopathies such as polymyositis and dermatomyositis. In the upper limbs the muscles first affected are the long flexors of the fingers and thumb, with particular involvement of the flexor digitorum profundus and flexor pollicis longus. As the disease progresses, weakness of the superficial finger and wrist flexors and of the finger extensors also develops and there is progressive wasting of the forearm muscles, particularly of the flexor compartment. In longstanding cases there is progressive loss of the ability to grip, to close the hand and to oppose the fingers and thumb, and contractures of the interphalageal joints frequently develop [3, 6]. The weakness of the forearm muscles is often asymmetric and in most cases is more severe on the nondominant side [12] (Figure 9.2). As the disease progresses there is also increasing weakness of more proximal muscle groups such as the elbow flexors and extensors and the deltoids.

Table 9.1 IBM functional rating scale (IBM-FRS) (Reproduced from Jackson et al. [7]).

1. Swallowing
   – 4 Normal
   – 3 Early eating problems—occasional choking
   – 2 Dietary consistency changes
   – 1 Frequent choking
   – 0 Needs tube feeding
2. Handwriting (with dominant hand prior to IBM onset)
   – 4 Normal
   – 3 Slow or sloppy; all words are legible
   – 2 Not all words are legible
   – 1 Able to grip pen but unable to write
   – 0 Unable to grip pen
3. Cutting food and handling utensils
   – 4 Normal
   – 3 Somewhat slow and clumsy, but no help needed
   – 2 Can cut most foods, although clumsy and slow; some help needed
   – 1 Food must be cut by someone, but can still feed slowly
   – 0 Needs to be fed
4. Fine motor tasks (opening doors, using keys, picking up small objects)
   – 4 Independent
   – 3 Slow or clumsy in completing task
   – 2 Independent but requires modified techniques or assistive devices
   – 1 Frequently requires assistance from caregiver
   – 0 Unable
5. Dressing
   – 4 Normal
   – 3 Independent but with increased effort or decreased efficiency
   – 2 Independent but requires assistive devices
   – 1 Requires assistance from caregiver for some clothing items
   – 0 Total dependence
6. Hygiene (bathing and toileting)
   – 4 Normal
   – 3 Independent but with increased effort or decreased activity
   – 2 Independent but requires use of assistive devices (shower chair, raised toilet seat, etc.)
   – 1 Requires occasional assistance from caregiver
   – 0 Completely dependent
7. Turning in bed and adjusting covers
   – 4 Normal
   – 3 Somewhat slow and clumsy but no help needed
   – 2 Can turn alone or adjust sheets, but with great difficulty
   – 1 Can initiate, but not turn or adjust sheets alone
   – 0 Unable or requires total assistance

8. Sit to stand
   – 4 Independent (without use of arms)
   – 3 Performs with substitute motions (leaning forward, rocking) but without use of arms
   – 2 Requires use of arms
   – 1 Requires assistance from a device or person
   – 0 Unable to stand
9. Walking
   – 4 Normal
   – 3 Slow or mild unsteadiness
   – 2 Intermittent use of an assistive device (ankle–foot orthosis, cane, walker)
   – 1 Dependent on assistive device
   – 0 Wheelchair-dependent
10. Climbing stairs
    – 4 Normal
    – 3 Slow with hesitation or increased effort; uses hand rail intermittently
    – 2 Dependent on hand rail
    – 1 Dependent on hand rail and additional support (cane or person)
    – 0 Cannot climb stairs

In the lower limbs the quadriceps femoris muscles are most severely affected and undergo progressive atrophy, particularly of the vastus medialis and lateralis, with relative sparing of the rectus femoris (Figure 9.2). As in the upper limbs the weakness is often more severe on the nondominant side. Weakness of the ankle dorsiflexors is also common but severe foot-drop occurs infrequently. Other muscle groups such as the hip extensors and abductors and ankle plantar flexors are usually only mildly affected.

The neck flexors are often weak, while the extensors are usually spared. However, in some cases there is more severe weakness of the neck extensor and paraspinal muscles resulting in a "dropped-head" or "bent-spine" syndrome [13]. The cranial muscles are usually spared apart from mild, or rarely more severe, weakness of the facial muscles.

Other clinical findings

Some patients with s-IBM have features of a mild peripheral neuropathy with depressed lower limb

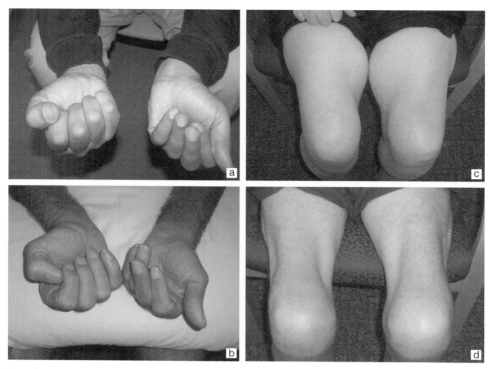

Figure 9.2 (a,b) Asymmetric weakness of the finger flexors, more severe in the left hand, in two s-IBM patients. (c,d) Quadriceps wasting in s-IBM patients.

reflexes and distal sensory impairment [14, 15]. Evidence of a subclinical neuropathy on nerve conduction studies has been reported in 1.5–33% of cases in different studies [15, 16].

Associated conditions

Unlike dermatomyositis and polymyositis, s-IBM is not usually associated with other systemic features such as interstitial lung disease or myocardial involvement. However, some s-IBM patients have another associated autoimmune disease such as Sjögren syndrome, systemic lupus erythematosus, scleroderma, rheumatoid arthritis, or thrombocytopenic purpura [17], and there are also rare reports of s-IBM developing in patients who have previously had dermatomyositis [18]. s-IBM has also been reported to be associated with HIV or human T-cell

lymphotropic virus type 1 (HTLV-1) infection [19], and with common variable immunoglobulin deficiency in some cases [20]. There are rare reports of the association of s-IBM with macrophagic myofasciitis [21], sarcoidosis [22], Creutzfeldt–Jakob disease [23], and cardiac amyloidosis [24].

Few studies have investigated the association with malignant disease but it is usually held that the frequency is not increased in s-IBM [2]. However, a population-controlled Australian study in Victoria found that there was a 2.4-fold increase in the risk of concurrent or subsequent malignancy in patients with s-IBM [25]. The frequency of malignant disease in this study was similar to that reported by Lotz et al. [8], who found that 15% of their series of 40 s-IBM cases had an associated malignancy. These observations therefore suggest that s-IBM patients should undergo thorough screening for malignancy.

Diagnosis and differential diagnosis

The diagnosis of s-IBM can usually be made on clinical grounds based upon the characteristic pattern of muscle weakness and atrophy and insidiously progressive clinical course. Muscle magnetic resonance imaging (MRI) scans may be helpful by confirming the pattern of muscle involvement in the upper and lower limbs. However, definitive confirmation of the diagnosis requires a muscle biopsy. Proposed criteria for the diagnosis of s-IBM are listed in Table 9.2, and the muscle-biopsy criteria are described in Chapter 10 in this volume.

The differential diagnosis of s-IBM is broad and includes amyotrophic lateral sclerosis (ALS), particularly in patients with asymmetric distal upper-limb weakness and atrophy and when there is associated dysphagia; and late-onset forms of distal myopathy and muscular dystrophy. Differentiation from other forms of inflammatory myopathy such as polymyositis and dermatomyositis can usually be made on the basis of the proximal pattern of upper- and lower-limb weakness and lack of finger weakness in these conditions. Common misdiagnoses in patients with s-IBM include ALS, polymyositis, arthritis, and old age [3]. In patients with a previous history of poliomyelitis earlier in life the onset of s-IBM may be misinterpreted as the postpoliomyelitis syndrome [26].

Laboratory investigations

Biochemical studies

The serum creatine kinase (CK) level is usually mildly elevated and there is rarely more than a 10-fold elevation, but the level may be normal in some cases [8, 27]. It is therefore not helpful diagnostically apart from being an indicator of a myopathic process if it is found to be elevated.

The cardiac troponin T (cTnT) level has been reported to be elevated in the majority of patients with s-IBM and to remain stable over time. In a study of 42 s-IBM cases Lindberg et al. [28] found that 62% of cases had cTnT levels of over 0.05 μg/L which is the usual cut-off level for the diagnosis of myocardial infarction. The finding of an elevated cTnT level in a patient with s-IBM is not therefore necessarily indicative of myocardial ischemia unless the level is known to have previously been within the normal range.

The possible diagnostic value of plasma amyloid-β (Aβ) levels was investigated in a group of 31 s-IBM patients. The levels of Aβ42 were found to be significantly elevated in s-IBM patients when compared to controls and patients with polymyositis but there was a considerable overlap between the groups and Aβ42 levels were also found to be elevated in patients with dermatomyositis [29].

Serum autoantibodies

No specific autoantibody has been associated with s-IBM. However, patients with s-IBM may have various other autoantibodies such as antinuclear antibody and anti-SSA/-SSB antibodies. Such autoantibodies were found in 20% of s-IBM cases in one large series [17]. A monoclonal gammopathy may also occur and was found in 22% of cases in one series [30].

Human leukocyte antigen studies

In white populations around 75% of s-IBM patients carry the major histocompatibility complex (MHC)

Table 9.2 Proposed diagnostic criteria for s-IBM (Modified with permission from Phillips BA, Mastaglia FL. [42]).

Characteristic features

A. Clinical features
- Duration of illness more than 6 months
- Age at onset is older than 30 years (but rare under 50 years)
- Slowly progressive muscle weakness and atrophy; selective pattern with quadriceps femoris and finger flexors affected first, followed by other muscle groups; frequently asymmetric and more severe on nondominant side
- Dysphagia occurs in the majority of cases

B. Laboratory features
- Serum creatine kinase (CK) levels variable elevated (less than 10 times normal), but may be normal; cardiac troponin (cTn) is often elevated
- Electromyogram: mixed pattern with short- and long-duration motor-unit potentials; fibrillations and positive waves may be present
- Muscle-biopsy diagnostic criteria (see Chapter 10)

---

class II allele human leukocyte antigen (HLA)-DRB1*0301 (serological specificity DR3) and other allelic components of the 8.1 MHC ancestral haplotype (HLA-A1, B8) [31]. It has been estimated that carriers of HLA-DRB1*0301 have a 10-fold-higher risk of developing s-IBM [32]. However, the sensitivity and specificity of this association is not sufficiently high to be of diagnostic value. HLA alleles have also been reported to have modifying effects on the clinical phenotype of the disease [3, 32]. The HLA-DR3 allele has been associated with more severe disease, while HLA-DR1/DR3 heterozygotes were found to have an earlier age of disease onset and more rapidly progressive weakness in an Australian s-IBM cohort (Figure 9.3).

Electrophysiological studies

Concentric needle electromyography demonstrates a pattern of early-recruiting, short-duration, low-amplitude polyphasic motor-unit action potentials (MUAPs) in affected muscles. In addition, larger long-duration MUAPs are often also present, as well as fibrillation potentials, positive waves, and in-creased insertion activity [8, 33]. In some patients these findings may lead to a mistaken diagnosis of a neurogenic disorder such as amyotrophic lateral sclerosis [34]. While large polyphasic MUAPs can also be seen in other chronic myopathies, this "mixed" electromyogram (EMG) pattern with both myopathic- and neuropathic-appearing MUAPs is very characteristic of s-IBM and should alert the electromyographer to the diagnosis. Quantitative EMG, macro-EMG, and single-fiber EMG studies have failed to show any evidence of a neurogenic component in s-IBM [33, 35–37]. Nerve-conduction studies may show reduced amplitude sensory nerve action potentials as well as reduced motor nerve conduction velocities and delayed F-wave latencies in some patients, but evidence of a diffuse peripheral neuropathy is uncommon [16].

Muscle imaging

Muscle MRI scanning is a useful investigation in patients with suspected s-IBM, particularly when the muscle biopsy findings are inconclusive or if a biopsy is not possible, and allows recognition of the

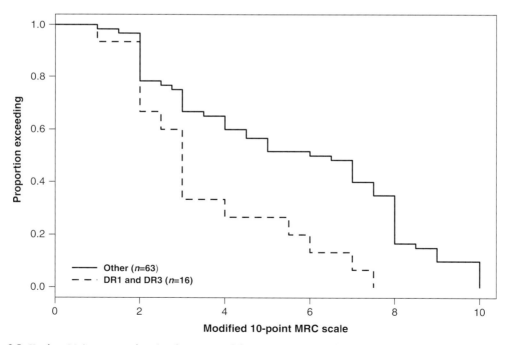

Figure 9.3 Kaplan–Meier curves showing faster rate of deterioration in quadriceps muscle strength in s-IBM patients carrying the HLA-DR1/DR3 genotype compared with other HLA-DRB1 genotypes.

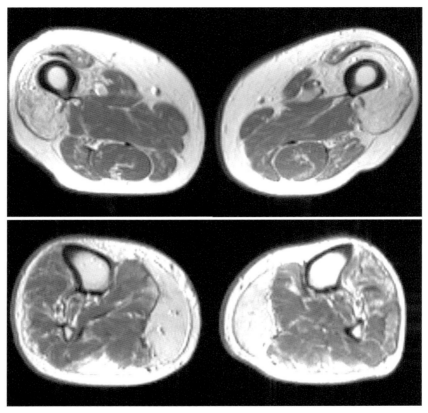

Figure 9.4 Proton-density-weighted MRI scans of the thighs (upper panels) and calves (lower panels) in a 78-year-old man with longstanding s-IBM showing signal change in the quadriceps and medial gastrocnemius muscles.

selective pattern of muscle involvement which is characteristic of s-IBM [38, 39]. Atrophy and changes in signal properties are typically found in the quadriceps femoris and medial gastrocnemius

muscles in the lower limbs and in the forearm flexor muscles on proton-density-weighted images (Figures 9.4 and 9.5)[38], and also on T1- and T2-weighted images and with a fat-suppressive short

Figure 9.5 MRI scan at mid-forearm level showing selective signal change in the flexor digitorum profundus (FDP; arrow) and not in the flexor digitorum sublimis (FDS; arrowhead). FPL, flexor pollicis longus; R, radius; U, ulna; II and V refer to the portions of those muscles – i.e., FDP and FDS – that flex the second (II) and fifth (V) digits of the hand. (Reproduced from Takamure et al. [39], with permission of the author and publisher.)

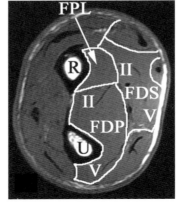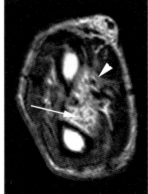

tau inversion recovery (STIR) sequence [40, 41]. MRI demonstrates the preferential involvement of the vasti with relative sparing of the rectus femoris in the quadriceps muscle complex, of the medial head of gastrocnemius with sparing of the lateral head, and of the flexor digitorum profundus within the forearm flexor muscle complex [38].

References

1 Needham M, Mastaglia FL. (2007) Inclusion body myositis: current pathogenetic concepts and diagnostic and therapeutic approaches. *Lancet Neurol* **6**(7), 620–631.

2 Amato AA, Barohn RJ. (2009) Inclusion body myositis: old and new concepts. *J Neurol Neurosurg Psychiatry* **80**(11), 1186–1193.

3 Needham M, James I, Corbett A et al. (2008) Sporadic inclusion body myositis: phenotypic variability and influence of HLA-DR3 in a cohort of 57 Australian cases. *J Neurol Neurosurg Psychiatry* **79**(9), 1056–1060.

4 Peng A, Koffman BM, Malley JD, Dalakas MC. (2000) Disease progression in sporadic inclusion body myositis: observations in 78 patients. *Neurology* **55**(2), 296–298.

5 Rose MR, McDermott MP, Thornton CA et al. (2001) A prospective natural history study of inclusion body myositis: implications for clinical trials. *Neurology* **57**(3), 548–550.

6 Badrising UA, Maat-Schieman ML, van Houwelingen JC et al. (2005) Inclusion body myositis. Clinical features and clinical course of the disease in 64 patients. *J Neurol* **252**(12), 1448–1454.

7 Jackson CE, Barohn RJ, Gronseth G et al. (2008) Inclusion body myositis functional rating scale: a reliable and valid measure of disease severity. *Muscle Nerve* **37**(4), 473–476.

8 Lotz BP, Engel AG, Nishino H et al. (1989) Inclusion body myositis. Observations in 40 patients. *Brain* **112**(3), 727–747.

9 Cox FM, Verschuuren JJ, Verbist BM et al. (2009) Detecting dysphagia in inclusion body myositis. *J Neurol* **256**(12), 2009–2013.

10 Cherin P, Pelletier S, Teixeira A et al. (2002) Intravenous immunoglobulin for dysphagia of inclusion body myositis. *Neurology* **58**(2), 326.

11 Oh TH, Brumfield KA, Hoskin TL et al. (2007) Dysphagia in inflammatory myopathy: clinical characteristics, treatment strategies, and outcome in 62 patients. *Mayo Clin Proc* **82**(4), 441–447.

12 Felice KJ, Relva GM, Conway Sr., (1998) Further observations on forearm flexor weakness in inclusion body myositis. *Muscle Nerve* **21**(5), 659–661.

13 Hund E, Heckl R, Goebel HH, Meinck HM. (1995) Inclusion body myositis presenting with isolated erector spinae paresis. *Neurology* **45**(5), 993–994.

14 Lindberg C, Oldfors A, Hedstrom A. (1990) Inclusion body myositis: peripheral nerve involvement. Combined morphological and electrophysiological studies on peripheral nerves. *J Neurol Sci* **99**(2–3) 327–338.

15 Amato AA, Gronseth GS, Jackson CE et al. (1996) Inclusion body myositis: clinical and pathological boundaries. *Ann Neurol* **40**(4), 581–586.

16 Khurana H, Luciano CA. (1996) Nerve conduction studies in inclusion body myositis: Observations in 63 patients. *Muscle Nerve* **19**(9), 1192.

17 Koffman BM, Rugiero M, Dalakas MC. (1998) Immune-mediated conditions and antibodies associated with sporadic inclusion body myositis. *Muscle Nerve* **21**(1), 115–117.

18 McCoy AL, Bubb MR, Plotz PH, Davis JC. (1999) Inclusion body myositis long after dermatomyositis: a report of two cases. *Clin Exp Rheumatol* **17**(2), 235–239.

19 Cupler EJ, Leon-Monzon M, Miller J et al. (1996) Inclusion body myositis in HIV-1 and HTLV-1 infected patients. *Brain* **119** (Pt 6) 1887–1893.

20 Dalakas MC, Illa I. (1995) Common variable immunodeficiency and inclusion body myositis: a distinct myopathy mediated by natural killer cells. *Ann Neurol* **37**(6), 806–810.

21 Cherin P, Menard D, Mouton P et al. (2001) Macrophagic myofasciitis associated with inclusion body myositis: a report of three cases. *Neuromuscul Disord* **11**(5), 452–457.

22 Danon MJ, Perurena OH, Ronan S, Manaligod Jr., (1986) Inclusion body myositis associated with systemic sarcoidosis. *Can J Neurol Sci* **13**(4), 334–336.

23 Kovacs GG, Lindeck-Pozza E, Chimelli L et al. (2004) Creutzfeldt-Jakob disease and inclusion body myositis: abundant disease-associated prion protein in muscle. *Ann Neurol* **55**(1), 121–125.

24 Askanas V, Engel WK, Alvarez RB et al. (2000) Inclusion body myositis, muscle blood vessel and cardiac amyloidosis, and transthyretin Val122Ile allele. *Ann Neurol* **47**(4), 544–549.

25 Buchbinder R, Forbes A, Hall S et al. (2001) Incidence of malignant disease in biopsy-proven inflammatory myopathy. A population-based cohort study. *Ann Intern Med* **134**(12), 1087–1095.

26 Parissis D, Karkavelas G, Taskos N, Milonas I. (2003) Inclusion body myositis in a patient with a presumed diagnosis of post-polio syndrome. *J Neurol* **250**(5), 619–621.

27 Griggs RC, Askanas V, DiMauro S et al. (1995) Inclusion body myositis and myopathies. *Ann Neurol* **38**(5), 705–713.

28 Lindberg C, Klintberg L, Oldfors A. (2006) Raised troponin T in inclusion body myositis is common and serum levels are persistent over time. *Neuromuscul Disord* **16**(8), 495–497.

29 Abdo WF, van Mierlo T, Hengstman GJ et al. (2009) Increased plasma amyloid-beta42 protein in sporadic inclusion body myositis. *Acta Neuropathol* **118**(3), 429–431.

30 Dalakas MC, Illa I, Gallardo E, Juarez C. (1997) Inclusion body myositis and paraproteinemia: incidence and immunopathologic correlations. *Ann Neurol* **41**(1), 100–104.

31 Needham M, Mastaglia FL, Garlepp MJ. (2007) Genetics of inclusion-body myositis. *Muscle Nerve* **35**(5), 549–561.

32 Mastaglia FL, Needham M, Scott A et al. (2009) Sporadic inclusion body myositis: HLA-DRB1 allele interactions influence disease risk and clinical phenotype. *Neuromuscul Disord* **19**(11), 763–765.

33 Oh SJ, Claussen GC. (1995) Single-fiber EMG findings in inclusion body myopathy. *Muscle Nerve* **18**, 1050.

34 Dabby R, Lange DJ, Trojaborg W et al. (2001) Inclusion body myositis mimicking motor neuron disease. *Arch Neurol* **58**(8), 1253–1256.

35 Luciano CA, Dalakas MC. (1997) Inclusion body myositis: no evidence for a neurogenic component. *Neurology* **48**(1), 29–33.

36 Brannagan TH, Hays AP, Lange DJ, Trojaborg W. (1997) The role of quantitative electromyography in inclusion body myositis. *J Neurol Neurosurg Psychiatry* **63**(6), 776–779.

37 Barkhaus PE, Periquet MI, Nandedkar SD. (1999) Quantitative electrophysiologic studies in sporadic inclusion body myositis. *Muscle Nerve* **22**(4), 480–487.

38 Phillips BA, Cala LA, Thickbroom G.W et al. (2001) Patterns of muscle involvement in inclusion body myositis: clinical and magnetic resonance imaging study. *Muscle Nerve* **24**(11), 1526–1534.

39 Takamure M, Murata KY, Kawahara M, Ueno S. (2005) Finger flexor weakness in inclusion body myositis. *Neurology* **64**(2), 389.

40 Fraser DD, Frank JA, Dalakas M et al. (1991) Magnetic resonance imaging in the idiopathic inflammatory myopathies. *J Rheumatol* **18**(11), 1693–1700.

41 Sekul EA, Chow C, Dalakas MC. (1997) Magnetic resonance imaging of the forearm as a diagnostic aid in patients with sporadic inclusion body myositis. *Neurology* **48**(4), 863–866.

42 Phillips BA, Mastaglia FL. (2002) Idiopathic inflammatory myopathies: epidemiology, classification and diagnostic criteria. *Rheum Dis Clin N Am* **28**, 723–741.

CHAPTER 10

Pathologic diagnostic criteria of sporadic inclusion-body myositis and hereditary inclusion-body myopathy muscle biopsies

Valerie Askanas and W. King Engel

Departments of Neurology and Pathology, University of Southern California Neuromuscular Center, University of Southern California Keck School of Medicine, Good Samaritan Hospital, Los Angeles, CA, USA

Introduction

The sporadic inclusion-body myositis (s-IBM) muscle biopsy has very characteristic pathologic abnormalities. Proper evaluation of the muscle biopsy, consisting of the reactions below, is the most important aspect of the s-IBM diagnosis, including its distinction from polymyositis and hereditary inclusion-body myopathies (h-IBMs). Even though clinical features of s-IBM are quite typical (see Chapter 9 in this volume), s-IBM patients are often misdiagnosed as having polymyositis, especially at earlier stages of the disease. However, s-IBM patients do not satisfactorily respond to anti-dysimmune treatment, in contrast to polymyositis, which is usually responsive to this treatment ([1, 2] and see Chapters 3, 7, and 8). The correct diagnosis of s-IBM would prevent s-IBM patients from prolonged unsuccessful anti-dysimmune treatment with drugs that can induce undesirable side effects.

s-IBM patients can be mistakenly diagnosed as polymyositis because of (a) the various degrees of lymphocytic inflammation (with some macrophages), and (b) the expression on muscle fibers of major histocompatibility complex I (MHC-I) and their associated molecules: these are both present in polymyositis and s-IBM muscle biopsies. Accordingly, we do not consider expression of MHC-I to be a diagnostic criterion of s-IBM muscle biopsies. We prefer to utilize specific light-microscopic and electron-microscopic pathologic diagnostic criteria, described below, as the essential tools for distinguishing s-IBM from polymyositis.

Light-microscopic diagnostic abnormalities of the s-IBM muscle biopsy

Vacuolated muscle fibers

All our stainings are routinely performed on 10 μm sections of fresh-frozen muscle biopsies. The characteristic features of s-IBM that are evident on the Engel trichrome staining [3] (the standard general stain used for fresh-frozen sections of muscle biopsies) are muscle fibers containing one or a few vacuoles, in a given transverse section. Many of the vacuoles appear to be autophagic, containing poorly differentiated pinkish material within the vacuoles or at the periphery. Reddish-pinkish material on trichrome staining indicates lipoprotein membranous material [3, 4]. Occasional vacuoles have such

Muscle Aging, Inclusion-Body Myositis and Myopathies, First Edition. Edited by Valerie Askanas and W. King Engel.
© 2012 Blackwell Publishing Ltd. Published 2012 by Blackwell Publishing Ltd.

reddish material accumulated mainly on the periphery, and those vacuoles are sometimes referred to as "red-rimmed." However, "rimmed" vacuoles are rare: most s-IBM vacuoles do not have a distinctive reddish rim, and many appear somewhat empty. However, under higher-power magnification those vacuoles, in contrast to freezing artifact holes, often contain a greenish-gray or reddish material characteristic of proteinaceous or membranous material (see Plate 10.6a–c). We therefore routinely use the simpler term "vacuolated muscle fibers," instead of "muscle fibers with rimmed vacuoles." In general, the number of vacuolated muscle fibers in a given section of an s-IBM muscle biopsy is between three and 40, or sometimes more, depending on the size of the biopsy. On a given section of a biopsy, we consider three or four vacuolated muscle fibers diagnostic, if they are accompanied by other characteristic s-IBM criteria as described below.

Occasionally vacuolated muscle fibers can be invaded by mononucleated cells (Plate 10.6c). The number of muscle fibers containing vacuoles differs not only among various s-IBM patients, but also on different transverse sections of the same muscle biopsy. Moreover, two adjacent pieces of the same muscle biopsy obtained at the same time often have different numbers of vacuoles, as well as different other features, such as various degrees of inflammation. Therefore, we consider unreliable and sometimes misleading evaluation of muscle biopsies before and after a specific treatment, as is done in some therapeutic trials as a supposed criterion of treatment efficacy.

Intracellular amyloid deposits

Congo red staining fluorescence

Intra-muscle-fiber β-pleated-sheet amyloid was first discovered in s-IBM muscle fibers by Mendell et al. using Congo red staining under polarized light [5]. We have described a more reliable fluorescence-enhanced Congo red technique [6] that we routinely use to identify amyloid in s-IBM muscle fibers (Plate 10.6d,e). Accordingly, multiple or single foci of amyloid as identified by the Congo red fluorescence visualized through Texas red filters are evident within about 40–70% of the s-IBM vacuolated muscle fibers in a given transverse section, mostly occurring in the nonvacuolated regions of those

fibers, and only very rarely actually within the vacuoles. However, the seemingly "amyloid-negative" fibers can have amyloid foci at other levels of those same fibers (which are a few centimeters long and multinucleated). In addition, a number of seemingly nonvacuolated, normal-appearing muscle fibers also contain amyloid deposits. This fluorescence-enhanced Congo red technique is the best and most sensitive method for highlighting amyloid inclusions, which sometimes can be very small or few. Our double-staining results indicate that in s-IBM intra-muscle-fiber amyloid deposits, as evidenced by their fluorescence-enhanced Congo red staining, contain either amyloid β (Aβ)42 or paired helical filament (PHF) tau ([7, 8] and illustrated in Chapter 7), each of which is known to self-aggregate to form β-pleated-sheet congophilic amyloid in Alzheimer brain (referenced in Chapter 7). In s-IBM, intracellular Aβ42-containing amyloid deposits appear under the light microscope in the form of small round plaques, or "plaquettes," while amyloid deposits containing PHF tau appear mainly as squiggly inclusions [7] (see also Chapter 7). A number of other proteins accumulated in s-IBM muscle fibers, including prion, α-synuclein, and others, also have the propensity to self-aggregate into β-pleated-sheet amyloid (reviewed in Chapter 7).

Congo red visualized in polarized light is a widely used amyloid-seeking method; however, it is the least precise and most difficult to interpret, and should not be used for s-IBM diagnosis.

Crystal violet

Crystal violet metachromasia staining can also show the intra-myofiber amyloid deposits in s-IBM muscle fibers (Plate 10.6f). This method is more convenient because it does not require fluorescence microscopy, but is less precise because small amyloid deposits are difficult to identify.

Among several of our patients with other non-IBM vacuolar myopathies, including acid-maltase deficiency, hypokalemic periodic paralysis, myofibrillar myopathy, and undefined types, none had true amyloid deposits as identified by crystal violet staining. Abnormal muscle fibers in myofibrillar myopathy (as originally reported by De Bleecker et al. [9]) indeed have fluorescence-enhanced congophilic accumulations, but we doubt that in those patients congophilia represents true amyloid deposits because in none of our four myofibrillar myopathy patients was the congophilic material positive with crystal violet, and it did not produce an orange fluorescence with thioflavin-T, as it is typical for "real" amyloid (Askanas, unpublished observations). The only muscle disease, in addition to s- IBM, in which we have found definite and prominent amyloid deposits is h-IBMs due to valo-sin-containing-peptide (VCP) mutation (see below).

Identification of intra-muscle-fiber bundles of phosphorylated-tau-containing PHFs

p62/SQTSM1

p62/SQSTM1 or simply "p62," is a shuttle protein transporting polyubiquitinated proteins to both pro-teasomal and lysosomal degradation (referenced in Chapter 7). In s-IBM muscle fibers p62 is an integral component of PHFs containing tau ([10], and also referenced and illustrated in Chapter 7). Because, in s-IBM, light-microscopic staining of p62 is very abundant and distinctive (Plate 10.7a,b), we strong-ly recommend it to be included in pathologic in-vestigations of s-IBM muscle biopsies [10]. Advan-tages of p62 immunoreactivity are: (a) it is not immunoreactive in muscle-fiber nuclei nor in nuclei of inflammatory or connective tissue cells; and (b) at the ultrastructural level p62 embraces clusters of PHFs in the form of a thick shell, which enhances its light-microscopic detectability [10].

For diagnostic purposes, we recommend light-microscopic HRP-immunohistochemical staining of p62, which appears in the form of strongly immu-noreactive, various-sized, mainly squiggly, linear, or small rounded aggregates (Plate 10.7a,b). These are in the nonvacuolated cytoplasm of approximately 80% of the vacuolated muscle fibers, and in about 20–25% of the muscle fibers that are nonvacuolated on a given 10 µm transverse section.

SMI-31 monoclonal antibody

Immunostaining with SMI-31 antibody, which was originally made against the phosphorylated neuro-filament heavy-chain protein, recognizes the phos-phorylated tau (p-tau) of PHFs in s-IBM muscle and in Alzheimer brain on immunoblots [11, 12], and it

identifies squiggly inclusions containing p-tau in s-IBM muscle fibers [12]. Previously, we have recom-mended SMI-31 immunostaining as diagnostic [13], but currently we favor p62 immunoreactivity, be-cause its staining is stronger and more specific, and it does not stain muscle-fiber nuclei.

Ubiquitin immunoreactivity

If neither p62 nor SMI-31 antibodies are available, ubiquitin immunoreactivity within muscle fibers can be used to differentiate s-IBM from polymyosi-tis [14]. Ubiquitin-positive inclusions were also identifiable in formalin-fixed paraffin-embedded muscle biopsies of s-IBM patients, but not in any other inflammatory myopathies [15]. This is impor-tant for some laboratories when freshly frozen mus-cle biopsy specimens are not available (we do not know whether p62 antibodies detect PHFs in paraf-fin-embedded s-IBM sections).

Alkaline phosphatase staining

In s-IBM, absent or only very faint alkaline phos-phatase staining of perimysial connective tissue is characteristic; even in regions of active disease peri-mysial connective tissue lacks the typically strong alkaline-phosphatase-positivity seen in similarly ac-tive regions of polymyositis and dermatomyositis, which is attributable to active fibroblasts [16, 17] (Plate 10.7c,d). Regenerating/degenerating (regen-degen) muscle fibers (containing regenerating fea-tures and increased acid phosphatase), which are very strongly positive with alkaline phosphatase staining, are typically moderate to abundant in polymyositis and dermatomyositis, and a number of other myopathies. However, those fibers are rare-ly detectable in s-IBM biopsies, which corresponds to the recently demonstrated decreased regenerative capability of s-IBM muscle fibers [18].

Ultrastructural diagnostic abnormalities within s-IBM muscle fibers

Clusters of PHFs, which individually are 15–21 nm-diameter twisted filaments containing p-tau, are characteristic of s-IBM (illustrated and referenced in Chapter 7). They are most commonly located in nonvacuolated areas of vacuolated muscle fibers, and they are also present in nonvacuolated muscle fibers. They are essentially identical to PHFs of Alzheimer disease brain, and are immunopositive with several antibodies reacting with various epitopes of p-tau, including the ones that specifically recognize conformationally modified p-tau of Alzheimer brain [12] (Nogalska et al, unpublished work, and illustrated in Figure 7.1a–d in this volume).

The s-IBM muscle-fiber cytoplasm also contains (a) collections of 6–10 nm amyloid-like fibrils; (b) fine flocculo-membranous material; and (c) amorphous material: these three contain Aβ immunoreactivity [19]. We recently demonstrated that 6–10 nm amyloid-like fibrils preferentially contain Aβ42 immunoreactivity [8] (see Figure 7.3a in this volume). The combination of tau-positive PHFs plus Aβ42-positive collections of 6–10 nm amyloid-like fibrils within muscle fibers is currently considered diagnostic of s-IBM.

s-IBM intranuclear clusters (inclusions) of 15–21 nm-diameter "tubulofilaments," which on favorable sections sometimes appear as PHFs like those in the cytoplasm, are often immunopositive with p-tau (Figure 7.1e,f in this volume). These nuclear PHFs are sparse, present in only 2–4% of s-IBM muscle nuclei, and comprise less than 1% of all the p-tau-positive structures within s-IBM muscle fibers (reviewed in [7, 20, 21]). (In some h-IBM patients with mutant VCP, intranuclear p-tau-positive PHFs can be frequent [38, 39].)

Light-microscopic aspects that are important but not diagnostic

MHC-I immunoreactivity

This was proposed by some as diagnostic for s-IBM muscle biopsies [22–24]; however, the same degree of, or even more intense, MHC-I immunoreactivity of muscle fibers is present in polymyositis biopsies. In our opinion, MHC-I immunostaining should not be used as a diagnostic criterion of s-IBM.

TDP-43 immunoreactivity

Transactive response DNA-binding protein 43 (TDP-43) is a predominantly RNA-/DNA-binding protein, whose functions are not yet fully understood. It was reported to be involved in RNA processing, transcription, and exon skipping (reviewed in [25, 26]). TDP-43-immunoreactive cytoplasmic inclusions within s-IBM muscle fibers were reported by several investigators [27–30], and confirmed by us [31]. However, quantitative comparison of TDP-43-immunoreactive inclusions to those of p62 inclusions in 15,600 muscle fibers on adjacent serial sections of 10 s-IBM biopsies revealed that fibers positive for p62 inclusions were three times more frequent than those containing TDP-43 inclusions [31]. Moreover, p62 inclusions were larger and more distinctive, and two biopsies containing a number of p62 inclusions did not contain any TDP-43 inclusions. Therefore, we do not recommend TDP-43 for diagnostic evaluation of s-IBM biopsies. (Interestingly, TDP-43 cytoplasmic inclusions are prominent in the VCP-mutant h-IBM; see below.)

Small angular muscle fibers, presumably denervated

These are: (a) histochemically dark with the pan-esterase and NADH-tetrazolium reductase reactions, (b) indistinguishable from those in ordinary denervation diseases, and (c) generally considered indicative of "recent denervation" (our preferred term) [4] (reviewed in [1]). They are a characteristic feature of s-IBM muscle biopsies and probably contribute significantly to the clinical weakness (reviewed in [1, 21]), but are not diagnostic.

Mitochondrial abnormalities

These include (a) cytochrome *c* oxidase (COX)-negative muscle fibers [32] and (b) ragged-red fibers [33]. They can be more evident in s-IBM muscle biopsies than in age-matched controls [32], but are not diagnostic.

Ultrastructurally characteristic, but nondiagnostic abnormalities

These include: (a) numerous, various-sized membranous whorls such as myelin-like whorls, multilaminar bodies, osmophilically dark amorphous material, and other types of lysosomal debris (illustrated in Figure 7.2 in in this volume); and (b) abnormal mitochondria, some containing paracrystalline inclusions.

Pathologic characteristics of h-IBM muscle biopsies

h-IBM due to *GNE* gene mutation (GNE-h-IBM)

Clinical aspects of this h-IBM are described in Chapter 12. We introduced the term "hereditary inclusion-body myopathy" (h-IBM) in 1993 [34] to specify hereditary muscle diseases with pathologic features like those of s-IBM except for a lack of lymphocytic inflammation; hence the term "myopathy" instead of "myositis." However, older h-IBM patients may have slight inflammation in their muscle biopsies [35–37].

• On Engel trichrome staining there are various-sized vacuoles in abnormal muscle fibers, which are generally similar to those in s-IBM (Plate 10.8a–c).

• PHFs of GNE-h-IBM (where GNE is UDP-N-acetylglucosamine-2 epimerase/N-acetylmannosamine kinase) express fewer p-tau epitopes than PHFs of s-IBM, as detailed previously [12]. However, in GNE-h-IBM, light-microscopic immunohistochemistry with p62 antibody highlights clusters of PHFs rather distinctively, although they appear definitely smaller and less frequent than those in s-IBM muscle fibers (Plate 10.8d). Since in s-IBM muscle fibers p62 closely colocalizes with various p-tau epitopes, we postulate that its less abundant immunoreactivity in GNE-h-IBM might be attributed to the paucity of inclusions containing p-tau epitopes in those fibers.

• TDP-43 is expressed in GNE-h-IBM muscle fibers [27]; however, in our hands, the staining is not very pronounced, and it is present in very few fibers on a given transverse section.

• Amyloid, identified by fluorescence-enhanced Congo red technique, is usually not present, but in some older GNE-h-IBM patients it can be detected within rare muscle fibers.

h-IBM due to *VCP* gene mutation (VCP-h-IBM)

Clinical and some pathologic features of this h-IBM are described in Chapter 15. VCP-h-IBM patients

(where VCP is valosin-containing-peptide), have: (a) vacuolated muscle fibers on Engel trichrome staining (Plate 10.9a); (b) large plaque-like amyloid inclusions by Congo red, and (c) clusters of PHFs by electron microscopy [38]. In the family we studied, the most characteristic feature was the presence of numerous large bulging nuclei with large clumps of amyloid deposits by Congo red fluorescence [38]. Those clumps of amyloid corresponded to large clusters of PHFs within the nuclei, which were immunopositive with antibodies directed to various epitopes of p-tau [38, 39]. Also in VCP-h-IBM very prominent are TDP-43-immunoreactive inclusions (Plate 10.9b) [29]. p62 is immunopositive mainly in nuclei of several muscle fibers, in a squiggly configuration (Plate 10.9c).

References

1 Engel WK, Askanas V. (2006) Inclusion-body myositis: clinical, diagnostic, and pathologic aspects. *Neurology* **66**, S20–S29.

2 Griggs RC. (2006) The current status of treatment for inclusion-body myositis. *Neurology* **66**, S30–S32.

3 Engel WK, Cunningham GG. (1963) Rapid examination of muscle tissue and improved trichrome method for fresh-frozen biopsy sections. *Neurology* **13**, 919–923.

4 Engel WK. (1962) The essentiality of histo- and cytochemical studies of skeletal muscle in the investigation of neuromuscular disease. *Neurology* **12**, 778–794.

5 Mendell JR, Sahenk Z, Gales T et al. (1991) Amyloid filaments in inclusion body myositis. Novel findings provide insight into nature of filaments. *Arch Neurol* **48**, 1229–1234.

6 Askanas V, Engel WK, Alvarez RB. (1993) Enhanced detection of congo-red-positive amyloid deposits in muscle fibers of inclusion body myositis and brain of Alzheimer's disease using fluorescence technique. *Neurology* **43**, 1265–1267.

7 Askanas V, Engel WK. (2001) Inclusion-body myositis: newest concepts of pathogenesis and relation to aging and Alzheimer disease. *J Neuropathol Exp Neurol* **60**, 1–14.

8 Vattemi G, Nogalska A, King Engel W et al. (2009) Amyloid-beta42 is preferentially accumulated in muscle fibers of patients with sporadic inclusion-body myositis. *Acta Neuropathol* **117**, 569–574.

9 De Bleecker JL, Engel AG, Ertl BB. (1996) Myofibrillar myopathy with abnormal foci of desmin positivity. II. Immunocytochemical analysis reveals accumulation of multiple other proteins. *J Neuropathol Exp Neurol* **55**, 563–577.

10 Nogalska A, Terracciano C, D'Agostino C et al. (2009) p62/SQSTM1 is overexpressed and prominently accumulated in inclusions of sporadic inclusion-body myositis muscle fibers, and can help differentiating it from polymyositis and dermatomyositis. *Acta Neuropathol* **118**, 407–413.

11 Ksiezak-Reding H, Dickson DW, Davies P et al. (1987) Recognition of tau epitopes by anti-neurofilament antibodies that bind to Alzheimer neurofibrillary tangles. *Proc Natl Acad Sci USA* **84**, 3410–3414.

12 Mirabella M, Alvarez RB, Bilak M et al. (1996) Difference in expression of phosphorylated tau epitopes between sporadic inclusion-body myositis and hereditary inclusion-body myopathies. *J Neuropathol Exp Neurol* **55**, 774–786.

13 Askanas V, Alvarez RB, Mirabella M et al. (1996) Use of anti-neurofilament antibody to identify paired-helical filaments in inclusion-body myositis. *Ann Neurol* **39**, 389–391.

14 Askanas V, Serdaroglu P, Engel WK et al. (1992) Immunocytochemical localization of ubiquitin in inclusion body myositis allows its light-microscopic distinction from polymyositis. *Neurology* **42**, 460–461.

15 Prayson RA, Cohen ML. (1997) Ubiquitin immunostaining and inclusion body myositis: study of 30 patients with inclusion body myositis. *Hum Pathol* **28**, 887–892.

16 Engel WK, Cunningham GG. (1970) Alkaline phosphatase-positive abnormal muscle fibers of humans. *J Histochem Cytochem* **18**, 55–57.

17 Askanas V, Engel WK. (1998) Sporadic inclusion-body myositis and hereditary inclusion-body myopathies: current concepts of diagnosis and pathogenesis. *Curr Opin Rheumatol* **10**, 530–542.

18 Morosetti R, Mirabella M, Gliubizzi C et al. (2006) MyoD expression restores defective myogenic differentiation of human mesoangioblasts from inclusion-body myositis muscle. *Proc Natl Acad Sci USA* **103**, 16995–167000.

19 Askanas V, Alvarez RB, Engel WK. (1993) Beta-amyloid precursor epitopes in muscle fibers of inclusion body myositis. *Ann Neurol* **34**, 551–560.

20 Mikol J, Engel AG. (2004) Inclusion body myositis. In: Engel AG (ed.), *Myology*, 3rd edn. McGraw-Hill Book Co, New York, pp. 1367–1388.

21 Askanas V, Engel WK. (1998) Newest approaches to diagnosis and pathogenesis of sporadic inclusion-body myositis and hereditary inclusion-body myopathies, including molecular-pathologic similarities to Alzheimer disease. In: Askanas V, Serratrice G, Engel WK (eds), *Inclusion-Body Myositis and Myopathies*, 1st edn. Cambridge University Press, Cambridge, pp. 3–78.

22 Needham M, Mastaglia FL. (2007) Inclusion body myositis: current pathogenetic concepts and diagnostic and therapeutic approaches. *Lancet Neurol* **6**, 620–631.

23 Dalakas MC. (2006) Sporadic inclusion body myositis–diagnosis, pathogenesis and therapeutic strategies. *Nat Clin Pract Neurol* **2**, 437–447.

24 Benveniste O, Hilton-Jones D. (2010) International Workshop on Inclusion Body Myositis held at the Institute of Myology, Paris, on 29 May 2009. *Neuromuscul Disord* **20**, 414–421.

25 Chen-Plotkin AS, Lee VM, Trojanowski JQ. (2010) TAR DNA-binding protein 43 in neurodegenerative disease. *Nat Rev Neurol* **6**, 211–220.

26 Gendron TF, Josephs KA, Petrucelli L. (2010) Review: transactive response DNA-binding protein 43 (TDP-43): mechanisms of neurodegeneration. *Neuropathol Appl Neurobiol* **36**, 97–112.

27 Küsters B, van Hoeve B, Schelhaas H et al. (2009) TDP-43 accumulation is common in myopathies with rimmed vacuoles. *Acta Neuropathol* **117**, 209–211.

28 Olive M, Janue A, Moreno D et al. (2009) TAR DNA-Binding protein 43 accumulation in protein aggregate myopathies. *J Neuropathol Exp Neurol* **68**, 262–273.

29 Weihl CC, Temiz P, Miller SE et al. (2008) TDP-43 accumulation in inclusion body myopathy muscle suggests a common pathogenic mechanism with frontotemporal dementia. *J Neurol Neurosurg Psychiatry* **79**, 1186–1189.

30 Salajegheh M, Pinkus JL, Taylor JP et al. (2009) Sarcoplasmic redistribution of nuclear TDP-43 in inclusion body myositis. *Muscle Nerve* **40**, 19–31.

31 D'Agostino C, Nogalska A, Engel WK et al. (2011) In sporadic inclusion-body myositis muscle fibres TDP-43-positive inclusions are less frequent and robust than p62-inclusions, and are not associated with paired helical filaments. *Neuropathol Appl Neurobiol* **37**, 315–320.

32 Oldfors A, Moslemi AR, Jonasson L et al. (2006) Mitochondrial abnormalities in inclusion-body myositis. *Neurology* **66**, S49–S55.

33 Engel WK. (1971) "Ragged-red fibers" in opthamoplegia syndromes and their differential diagnosis. *Excerpta Med Inter Cong Series* **237**, 28.

34 Askanas V, Engel WK. (1993) New advances in inclusion-body myositis. *Curr Opin Rheumatol* **5**, 732–741.

35 Amouri R, Driss A, Murayama K et al. (2005) Allelic heterogeneity of GNE gene mutation in two Tunisian families with autosomal recessive inclusion body myopathy. *Neuromuscul Disord* **15**, 361–363.

36 Askanas V, Engel WK. Hereditary inclusion body myopathies. In: Rosenberg RN, Di Mauro S, Paulson HL et al. (eds), *The Molecular and Genetic Basis of Neurologic and Psychiatric Disease*, 4th edn. Wolters Kluver, Lippincott Williams & Wilkins, Philadelphia, pp. 524–531.

37 Krause S, Schlotter-Weigel B, Walter MC et al. (2003) A novel homozygous missense mutation in the GNE gene of a patient with quadriceps-sparing hereditary inclusion body myopathy associated with muscle inflammation. *Neuromuscul Disord* **13**, 830–834.

38 Alvarez RB, Simmons Z, Engel WK et al. (1998) New autosomal-dominant inclusion-body myopathy (AD-IBM) with many congophilic muscle nuclei that contain paired-helical filaments composed of phosphorylated tau. *Neurology* **50**, A204.

39 Askanas V, Engel WK. (2006) Inclusion-body myositis: a myodegenerative conformational disorder associated with Abeta, protein misfolding, and proteasome inhibition. *Neurology* **66**, S39–S48.

PART 3
Hereditary Inclusion-Body Myopathies

CHAPTER 11

Function and mutations of the *GNE* gene leading to distal myopathy with rimmed vacuoles/hereditary inclusion-body myopathy, animal models, and potential treatment

May Christine V. Malicdan, Satoru Noguchi, and Ichizo Nishino

Department of Neuromuscular Research, National Institute of Neuroscience,
National Center of Neurology and Psychiatry, Tokyo, Japan

Introduction

Distal myopathy with rimmed vacuoles (DMRV) [1, 2] is an autosomal recessive disorder that affects young adults. It is characterized clinically by weakness involving muscles of the distal limbs, and preferential involvement of the tibialis anterior muscles during the early stage of the disease. It is also known as quadriceps-sparing myopathy, because of the peculiar relative sparing of these muscles even in the advanced stages of the illness. Characteristic findings, although not exactly pathognomonic, are seen in muscle pathology, and generally regarded as myodegenerative. These include the presence of scattered atrophic fibers and several fibers with rimmed vacuoles. These rimmed vacuoles are believed to possess some autophagic activity, adjudged from the intense acid phosphatase activity reflecting the presence of acidic compartments in cells, reactivity with various lysosomal markers, and the electron-microscopic findings of autophagic vacuoles with various cellular debris and multilamellar bodies [3, 4]. Within the fibers, with or without rimmed vacuoles, several inclusions were identified to be immunoreactive to amyloid, phosphorylated tau, neurofilament, myosin heavy chain, endoplasmic reticulum-related markers, and others. In addition, 15–20 nm tubulofilamentous inclusions on the nucleus or cytoplasm have been noted on electron-microscopic observation. The presence of these intramyofiber inclusions gave rise to the nosology hereditary inclusion-body myopathy (h-IBM), as comparisons were made with the seemingly nonhereditary type of a similar myopathy, sporadic inclusion-body myositis. As opposed to sporadic inclusion-body myositis, DMRV/h-IBM muscle pathology is generally devoid of inflammatory cell infiltrates, but also presents with similar degenerative features in the muscle, although anecdotally some patients have presented with some inflammatory component in their myofibers [5].

Mutations in the GNE gene cause DMRV/h-IBM

The causative gene has been mapped to chromosome 9p12–13 by two separate groups [6, 7], and later was identified to be the UDP-N-acetylglucosamine-2 epimerase/N-acetylmannosamine kinase (*GNE*) gene [8]. The protein product, GNE, is mainly known to be a bifunctional enzyme that catalyzes the critical steps in sialic acid synthesis in the cytosol. The initial substrate involved in this pathway is UDP *N*-acetylglucosamine (UDP-GlcNAc), the endproduct of hexosamine biosynthesis, and synthesis starts with the release of UDP from UDP-GlcNAc in a two-stage process catalyzed by the bifunctional GNE enzyme [9, 10] (Figure 11.1). GlcNAc is

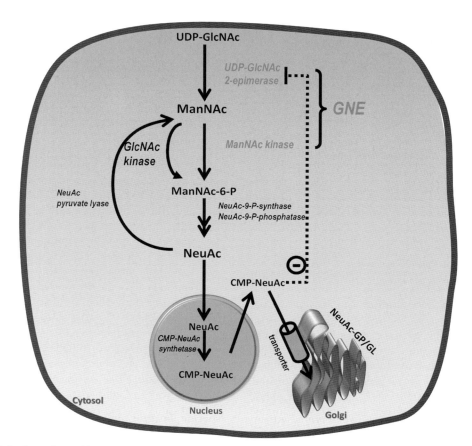

Figure 11.1 The sialic acid biosynthetic pathway. Sialic acid biosynthesis occurs within the cytosol and is governed by the bifunctional enzyme GNE, which has two domains that possess enzymatic activities: UDP-GlcNAc 2-epimerase and ManNAc kinase. Synthesis starts with the epimerization of UDP-GlcNAc to ManNAc by UDP-GlcNAc 2-epimerase after the release of UDP in a two-stage process. Phosphorylation of ManNAc is catalyzed by ManNAc kinase, but in some hyposialylated cells this can be done by GlcNAc kinase. Subsequent steps lead to formation of free NeuAc and its activation to CMP-NeuAc, which is the nucleotide substrate for all sialic acids. After transport to the Golgi apparatus, CMP-NeuAc is then transferred to various oligosaccharide chains of gangliosides or sialoglycoproteins. NeuAc can also be degraded by NeuAc pyruvate lyase into ManNAc. Note that all the enzymes required for completion of the sialic acid biosynthesis are found in the cytosol, except for CMP-NeuAc synthetase, which is found in the nucleus. GL, glycolipid; GP, glycoprotein.

epimerized by UDP-GlcNAc-2-epimerase into *N*-acetyl-D-mannosamine (ManNAc), and then ManNAc kinase catalyzes the phosphorylation of ManNAc into ManNAc-6-phosphate, which is then condensed with phosphoenoylpyruvate to form *N*-acetyl-D-neuraminic acid-9-phosphate (NeuAc-9-P). Dephosphorylation of NeuAc-9-P produces NeuAc, the most abundant sialic acid among mammals. Free NeuAc is then transported into the nucleus and activated into CMP-NeuAc, a donor substrate for sialyltransferase, by CMP-NeuAc synthase. CMP-NeuAc is then transported to the Golgi apparatus and pumped across its membranes using a specific transporter. CMP-NeuAc is ultimately transferred to oligosaccharide chains by a large family of sialyltransferase enzymes; this process allows sialylation of gangliosides or sialoglycoproteins. UDP-GlcNAc 2-epimerase has been demonstrated to be the rate-limiting enzyme in sialic acid synthesis as its activity is feedback-inhibited by CMP-NeuAc [11]. Interestingly, the loss of this feedback inhibition by CMP-NeuAc due to heterozygous missense mutations within the allosteric site of UDP-GlcNAc 2-epimerase (in the region of codons 263–266) has been demonstrated to cause sialuria, resulting in cytoplasmic accumulation and urinary excretion of large quantities of free sialic acid [12]. Sialic acids are N-acylated derivatives of neuraminic acids, composed of nine carbon α-keto aldonic acids, and are the most abundant monosaccharides found in the terminal ends of glycans of eukaryotic cells. Sialic acids serve a variety of biological and cellular functions, including cell–cell adhesion and interaction, cell migration, inflammation, wound healing, and metastasis [13, 14]. Its importance in development, at least in mice, is highlighted by the finding that inactivation of the gene leads to embryonic lethality. Other functions of GNE not directly related to sialic acid biosynthesis have also been identified [15].

In DMRV/h-IBM, most of the mutations that have been identified are missense mutations, with the exception of a few null mutations, and are scattered throughout the open reading frame of *GNE*. Mutations are noted to occur in homozygous or compound heterozygous situations (for a list of reported mutations, see Huizing et al. [16]). To date, no individual has been found to be homozygous for a null mutation, as probably this type of mutation would render the organism unable to survive. Nonetheless, there are reports of single-allele null mutations and nonsense or frameshift mutations. So far, a clear genotype–phenotype correlation has not been reported, as clearly there are some variations in the clinical presentation of patients. Interestingly, GNE mutations have been found in clusters all round the world, with two large groups identified: Japanese and Iranian Jewish patients. The most common among the Japanese population is p.V572L, followed by p.D176V. Among Jewish Iranian patients, the common founder mutation, p.M712T, has been identified. After identification of the causative gene, one essential question has remained unanswered: is DMRV/h-IBM a metabolic disease due to reduced or a lack of sialic acid production?

The GNE protein: isoforms, expression, enzymatic activities, and structure

GNE isoforms and expression

GNE protein is predicted to have three isoforms which are created by four transcript variants. GNE1, consisting of 722 amino acids, is encoded by GNE transcripts I and IV [10, 17, 18]. GNE2 and GNE3 have modified N-termini with the addition of another exon (A1; encodes the first 17 amino acids) and are encoded by two other splice variants [17]. The GNE2 N-terminus is longer by 31 additional amino acids and is encoded by transcript II. GNE3 lacks exon 2 and thus it does not have the first 55 amino acids of GNE1; it is encoded by transcript III. The tissue expression of three isoforms seems tissue-specific, but the roles of these isoforms in disease causation have not been clarified.

GNE1 is a ubiquitously expressed protein with the highest expression levels found in the liver and placenta [10, 19]. In addition, GNE1 is the only isoform with mRNA expression identified in skeletal muscles. GNE2 mRNA expression is highest in placenta, followed by liver, kidney, lung, brain, colon, and pancreas. GNE3 mRNA expression is highest in colon, followed by kidney, liver, and placenta. Analysis of murine GNE revealed that they have at least two isoforms homologous to GNE1 and 2. The murine Gne1 isoform was amplified from cDNA of five tissues examined (brain, colon, kidney, liver, and skeletal muscle). Murine Gne2 was also expressed in all of these tissues, except the liver [17].

GNE enzymatic activities

GNE is comprised mainly of two domains – UDP-GlcNAc 2-epimerase and ManNAc kinase – with activities of both enzymes mapped to different regions of the polypeptide. Human GNE1 possesses both epimerase and kinase activities, implying that it is the major isoform involved in sialic acid production. The analysis of recombinant human GNE2 displayed selective reduction of UDP-GlcNAc 2-epimerase activity by the loss of its tetrameric state [20], while recombinantly expressed human GNE3 only possessed kinase activity. In contrast, murine Gne1 and Gne2 do not show notable differences in terms of activity.

In early studies, site-directed mutagenesis on different conserved amino acid residues was employed to check the function of GNE protein. Histidine mutants of the epimerase domain showed a drastic loss of epimerase activity with almost unchanged kinase activity. Kinase mutants, on the other hand, lost their kinase activity but retained their epimerase activity. Noguchi et al. [21] measured the enzymatic activity of GNE recombinant proteins (expressed in COS7 cells) harboring mutations found in both domains of the *GNE* gene identified in DMRV patients. Epimerase mutants had decreased GlcNAc epimerase activity by about 70–80% and led to a variable reduction of ManNAc kinase activity. On the other hand, the kinase mutants preferably reduced ManNAc kinase activities with a slight reduction in epimerase activities, with an exception of a single mutant, A524V, which decreased epimerase activity more significantly than kinase activity. Penner et al. [22] also analyzed enzymatic activities of human GNE mutants expressed in insect cells and, in general, found a preferential reduction of kinase enzymatic activities in kinase mutants. However, epimerase mutants had decreased activities of both domains, indicating that mutation in GNE may reduce activity of either the epimerase or kinase enzymes regardless of the location the mutation;

certain mutants led to the marked reduction (G576E) or almost total ablation (C303X) of enzymatic activities in both domains. What can be surmised from these data is the notion that the defect in DMRV is due to partial loss of function of GNE, and that GNE mutants may lead to a variable reduction of enzymatic activities. It should be noted that patients can have mutations in either or both epimerase and kinase domains.

GNE protein structure

As a monomer, GNE does not exhibit any activity, but as a dimer the ManNAc kinase shows activity. It is only when monomers are formed into a hexamer that activities of both enzymes are detected [23]. To estimate the structural perturbation effect due to site-directed mutagenesis, the oligomeric state of all mutants was determined by gel filtration analysis. Because GNE is known to oligomerize into hexamers, Noguchi et al. [21] and Penner et al. [22] checked the influence of mutations on GNE protein. The findings from both groups are consistent with an earlier study [24] which showed that mutant proteins (made by site-directed mutagenesis using conserved amino acid residues) are able to make hexameric structures, indicating that there is no influence of amino acid mutations on protein oligomerization. This is, of course, with the exception of specific DMRV/h-IBM mutants, A524V and C303X. This is further supported by the finding that secondary structure of the GNE protein is preserved except in two mutants (G576E, which forms trimers, and N519S, which showed alteration in secondary structure) [22]. Attempts to correlate enzyme activity and enzyme structure by three-dimensional modeling did not give any clue as to what specifically decreases activity [22].

Another three-dimensional model was proposed by Kurochkina et al. [25], which depicted putative active sites in the epimerase and kinase domains of the GNE. Most reported *GNE* mutations appear to have a proximal (in the active sites and their vicinity) and distal (at the interfaces of secondary structures) effects on the structure and function of the enzyme. Further precise modeling may be needed to predict the effect of mutations on GNE structure.

Influence of GNE mutations on overall cellular sialylation

GNE has been demonstrated to be important in regulating cell-surface sialylation [26]. Naturally, the working hypothesis in DMRV/h-IBM is that *GNE* mutations can lead to reduced sialylation. This concept of reduced sialylation and its role on disease pathogenesis has been difficult to comprehend as most of studies that were done using cellular models showed conflicting results. Noguchi et al. [21] measured the level of sialic acid in muscle and primary cultured cells from DMRV patients and showed a 60–75% reduction as compared to controls. Similar results were shown by Saito et al. [27], who identified a DMRV/h-IBM patient with hyposialylation of muscle glycoproteins, and Huizing et al. [28], who showed that α-dystroglycan is hyposialylated in DMRV/h-IBM patients. Also on the same line, Brocollini et al. demonstrated the probable hyposialylation of NCAM [29] and neprilysin [30, 31] in patients. On the other hand, Salama et al. and Hinderlich et al. found no abnormalities in sialylation of patient-derived lymphoblastoid cell lines [32] and myoblasts [33] with the M712T mutation.

The inconsistencies of findings from various groups may be influenced by a variety of factors, including the type of tissue or sample being analyzed and the methodology being employed. Obviously, the status and association of sialylation in DMRV/h-IBM can only be clarified by using the appropriate animal model.

Other studies also add to the controversy of the involvement of hyposialylation in disease pathogenesis, and these were seen in naturally occurring hyposialylated cells. The cells in the human B-lymphoma cell line BJAB K20 are hyposialylated because they lack GNE mRNA as well as epimerase activity [34]. Supplementation with *N*-acetylmannosamine allowed cells to synthesize sialic acid on glycoproteins, indicating that the presence of additional cellular kinases like GlcNAc kinase allows cells to synthesize sialic acid. Similarly, Lec3 Chinese hamster ovary (CHO) cell glycosylation mutants had no detectable UDP-GlcNAc 2-epimerase activity [35] due to a compound heterozygous mutation (E35X and G135E). Hyposialylation in these Lec3 CHO cells was rescued by exogenously added *N*-acetylmannosamine or mannosamine but not by the same concentrations of *N*-acetylglucosamine, glucosamine, glucose, or mannose. Interestingly, however, only transfection with wild-type GNE cDNA or GNE cDNA with a kinase mutation (D413K) restored *in vitro* UDP-GlcNAc 2-epimerase activity and cell-surface polysialic acid expression; on the other hand, cDNA with an epimerase-deficient mutation (H132A or new Lec3 G135E) did not rescue the Lec3 phenotype.

GNE and its role outside sialoglycobiology

GNE is involved in a complex but fascinating sialic acid biosynthetic pathway and its activity is tightly regulated by well-characterized negative-feedback inhibition by CMP-NeuAc, in addition to tetramerization promoted by the substrate UDP-GlcNAc, DNA methylation [36], and phosphorylation by protein kinase C [37]. Recent reports, however, allude to its function outside sialic acid synthesis. In attempts to study how mutations reduce enzymatic activities, it was discovered that GNE interacts with other proteins, like the collapsin-response mediator protein 1, promyelocytic leukemia zinc finger protein [38], and skeletal muscle α-actinin 1 [39]. Indeed, further studies are needed to understand the mechanisms that regulate GNE and its interaction with other proteins, and these are essential to understand the disease pathomechanism completely and thus merit in-depth investigation.

Animal models

To generate animal models for DMRV/h-IBM, several strategies using genetic manipulation of the *GNE* gene have been tried. Genetic ablation of *Gne* in mice by a simple knockout strategy resulted to embryonic lethality by 8.5 dpc [40] to 9.5 dpc (Noguchi et al., unpublished work), suggesting the importance of sialic acid in early embryogenesis. Supplementing embryonic stem cells with ManNAc showed that sialylation can be recovered [40], demonstrating that ManNAc itself is a putative substrate for sialic acid synthesis. Mice that are heterozygous for deficiency were vital. Using the heterozygous Gne-deficient mice, Gagiannis et al. [41] quantified the amount of membrane-bound sialic acid in different organs of mice as compared to wild-type mice, and showed 25% organ-specific reduction of membrane-bound sialic acids in heterozygous Gne-deficient mice.

Galeano et al. [42] generated a knockin mouse carrying the M712T mutation, which is the most common *GNE* mutation among Jewish patients, on the murine C57BL/6J background and on the FVB background. Most homozygous mutant mice died perinatally and could not survive after the third postnatal day (P3). Upon further analysis, it was shown that the M712T mice exhibited a severe renal phenotype comprised of glomerulonephropathy, hematuria, severe proteinuria, and podocytopathy with segmental splitting of the glomerular basement membrane and effacement of podocyte foot processes. This phenomenon was apparently caused by an anomaly in morphogenesis of glomerular tissues due to the remarkable desialylation of podocalyxin, a major glycoprotein found in podocyte foot processes. Interestingly, the survival of homozygous mice was increased to 50% by administration of ManNAc to pregnant mice because of the reversal of podocytopathy. ManNAc supplementation was continued until weaning age (about P21). In the M712T mice that were able to survive beyond P3, however, a phenotype suggesting skeletal-muscle weakness or abnormalities in muscle pathology was not found. From these results it was concluded that the M712T Gne-knockin mice provide a novel animal model of hyposialylation-related podocytopathy and segmental splitting of the glomerular basement membrane, demonstrating the significance of sialic acid synthesis in kidney development and function.

Malicdan et al. [43] took another strategy to generate an animal model, and have taken into consideration the following points. First, completely knocking out the gene was lethal to mice [40] (Noguchi et al., unpublished data), strongly suggesting that the requirement for sialic acid is very high, at least in mice, and that a simple knockin strategy may not allow survival of mice for complete analysis

(DMRV/h-IBM is an early-adult-onset myopathy). Second, the activity of GNE in mammalian muscles is quite low and almost undetectable, implying the possibility that the skeletal muscles may actually tolerate some levels of decreased GNE activity or sialylation. With these points in mind, they decided to create a model whereby the endogenous murine Gne is replaced by a mutated human GNE. The authors then proceeded to generate a transgenic mice that harbored the D176V mutant human GNE cDNA (hGNED176VTg), using a promoter that ensures high expression in all tissues. The hGNED176VTg mice were born normally and had a normal lifespan; all throughout their lives, these mice did not manifest muscle or any other symptoms. The hGNED176VTg mice were later crossed with mice that are heterozygous for Gne deficiency ($Gne^{+/-}$), resulting to $Gne^{-/-}$hGNED176VTg (DMRV/h-IBM mouse): a mouse knocked-out of endogenous Gne but expressing mutated human GNE. Analysis of mRNA GNE expression revealed a high expression of the transgenic GNE in most organs, and the absence of murine Gne expression.

The DMRV/h-IBM mice were born in almost Mendelian proportions and appeared normal, although they were slightly smaller than control littermates. Analysis of overall tissue sialylation revealed that blood and several organs were hyposialylated. As the mice aged, they gradually revealed several myopathic phenotypes seen in human DMRV/h-IBM patients. After 20 weeks of age, the mice started to exhibit some muscle weakness, seen as impaired motor performance of the mouse during treadmill examination [44]. *Ex vivo* analysis of isolated muscles showed physiologic muscle weakness as revealed by reduced force generation in skeletal muscles [44]. This reduction of the force was attributed to muscle atrophy, as twitch and tetanic forces normalized with cross-sectional area were maintained at normal values. Muscle atrophy was accompanied by an increase in the number of small angular fibers in muscle histology and mild elevation of serum creatine. When the mice reached 30 weeks of age, subpar muscle performance in treadmill exercises was more apparent as compared with unaffected control littermates. On analysis of muscle physiology, specific force generation in gastrocnemius and tibialis anterior muscles was notably reduced and was associated with intracellular deposition of amyloid as seen in gastrocnemius muscle cryosections and more discernible variation in fiber size together with the presence of small angular and atrophic myofibers. At about 40 weeks of age, DMRV/h-IBM mice obviously could not run as fast as their littermates. Muscle histology showed the characteristic rimmed vacuoles and accumulation of autophagic vacuoles [3] (Figure 11.2) and inclusion bodies that were immunoreactive to various neurodegenerative markers. Measurement of the muscle force generation showed increasing worsening of tetanic more than isometric contractions, and increasing twitch/tetanic ratio, which could be explained by the increasing number of structural intramyofiber abnormalities that can impair the contractile system of the muscle.

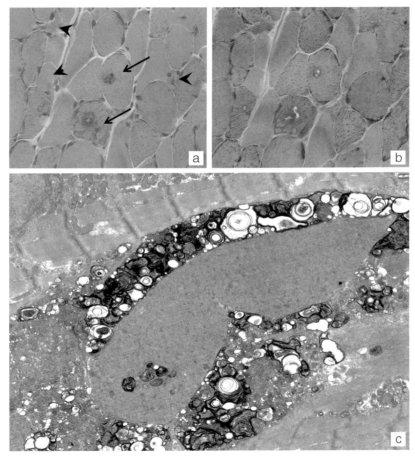

Figure 11.2 Muscle pathology of Gne$^{-/-}$ hGNED176VTg mice. Hematoxylin and eosin (a) shows moderate to severe variation in fiber size with minimal endomysial fibrosis, absence of necrotic or regenerating fibers, and scattered small angular and atrophic fibers (arrowheads). Scattered fibers have rimmed vacuoles (arrows). On modified Gomori trichrome stain, fibers with rimmed vacuoles (shown by arrows in a) are shown to be spaces surrounded by reddish granules that appear like a "rim." This electron micrograph (c) shows an intracytoplasmic area that is composed of autophagic vacuolar structures that surround some large areas of inclusions. The autophagic vacuoles are also interspersed with various intracellular debris. Note that in the areas of such autophagic vacuoles, z-line and myofibrillar structures are completely abolished. Scale bar in (b) denotes 20 μm for (a) and (b).

Intriguingly, some mice died after 20 weeks of age, invariably affecting the survival rate of the cohort, but the reason for the demise could not be clarified. Nonetheless, the Gne$^{-/-}$hGNED176VTg mouse is the only existing pathogenic model for DMRV/h-IBM at the moment. Moreover, the presence of hyposialylation suggests some metabolic impairment that could have other implications.

Perspectives for therapy

At the time of writing, there are no therapies currently available for DMRV/h-IBM. In designing therapeutic strategies for DMRV/h-IBM, several factors need to be considered, foremost of which are the genetic nature of the disease and potentially correctable metabolic impairments. Other important factors are the clinical characteristics of the myopathy, including the onset, slowly progressive course of the disease, and main symptoms involved. General approaches to therapy, with these factors considered, may include pharmacologic therapy (for the metabolic impairment) and gene therapy (for the genetic impairment).

Pharmacologic treatment: compounds for increasing cellular sialylation

The main target for pharmacologic treatment is to address the issue of hyposialylation, which may be a factor that leads to the development of disease. The main theory is that increasing the influx of sialic acid from exogenous sources could be beneficial and could provide cure. Based on this hypothesis, an open-label, nonrandomized trial on four DMRV/h-IBM patients was done using intravenous immunoglobulin G (IVIG) therapy, with the proof of concept that IgG contains about 8 μmol of sialic acid per gram [45]. The patients were given IVIG initially as a loading dose (1 g/kg) on two consecutive days, followed by three single 400 mg/kg doses every week. Functional analysis of muscle in patients showed minimal and transient improvement in strength after IVIG administration (loading and follow-up doses). Analysis of glycoproteins in muscle (NCAM and dystroglycan) and plasma (transferrin) gave inconsistent results. Overall, evaluation of the response to treatment was complicated as it is difficult to show a drastic improvement on a severe and progressive myopathy after a short trial period.

Natural compounds: ManNAc and NeuAc

Another pharmacologic option is the use of metabolites involved in the sialic acid biosynthetic pathway. This is theoretically possible as the function of other enzymes involved in sialic acid synthesis is not affected in cells with *GNE* mutations, suggesting that metabolite supplementation may be an effective option in increasing sialic acid levels. This possibility is further supported by studies on the recovery of cellular sialylation after supplementation with ManNAc or sialic acid [26, 40].

Although all metabolites found downstream of GNE could possibly be used to increase cellular sialylation, only ManNAc and NeuAc may be considered, as the other compounds are mainly nucleotide derivatives, which are thought to be rarely incorporated into cells and phosphorylated compounds, and which can be dephosphorylated before being incorporated into the cell. ManNAc is a natural compound that is uncharged and enters the sialic acid pathway after GNE catalysis. It is known that DMRV/h-IBM patients can have residual ManNAc kinase activities and this can be used by cells to synthesize sialic acid. Furthermore, the presence of other kinases, such as GlcNAc 6-kinase, can phosphorylate exogenously administered ManNAc and allow its incorporation into the pathway. NeuAc, on the other hand, is also a natural compound but is previously thought to be poorly absorbed and incorporated into cells because of its charged (acidic) nature; however, this theory was challenged by a study showing that NeuAc can actually be taken up by eukaryotic cells [46].

The ability of cells to incorporate both ManNAc and NeuAc to possibly a comparable degree is also suggested by culture experiments using DMRV/h-IBM cells. The addition of ManNAc and NeuAc in the medium of primary cells from DMRV/h-IBM led to the recovery of cellular sialylation to a similar level [21]. Nonetheless, this speculation needs to be carefully interpreted, as other factors found in the disease condition itself may influence the choice of agent. In other words, it has to be considered that the target tissue for therapy in DMRV/h-IBM – that is, skeletal muscle – is atrophied and the presence of probable defects in endocytosis, as attested by the presumably arrested autophagic state, can impair full delivery of drug into myofibers. It is likewise important to note that ManNAc and NeuAc reportedly use different routes for the entry into cells [47]. ManNAc is believed to enter the cells either by (passive) diffusion or via a specific transporter (Figure 11.3), although diffusion is more probable

as the cellular incorporation rate is enhanced when the hydrophobicity of ManNAc is increased upon modification by O-acylation. Exogenous free sialic acid (NeuAc) is incorporated by macropinocytosis (Figure 11.3) and is subsequently transported from the endosomes to the lysosomes, and finally into the cytosol via the specific transporter, sialin.

Another issue worth considering that may influence choice of compounds for therapy is the source of such molecules. Both ManNAc and NeuAc are natural compounds. ManNAc is found in trace amounts and only occurs as a free molecule, as

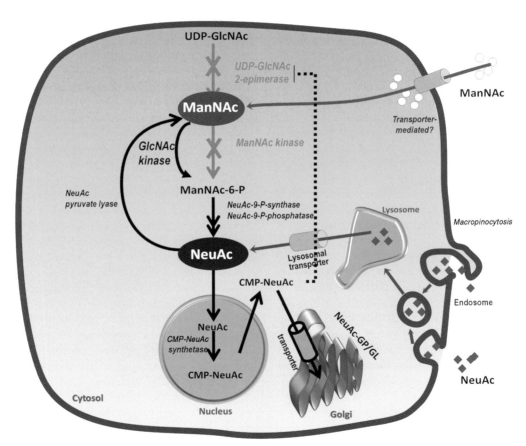

Figure 11.3 Incorporation of exogenous sialic acid metabolites into the pathway for sialic acid synthesis. Mutations in the *GNE* gene cause reduced GlcNAc epimerase and ManNAc kinase enzymatic activities, which can be rescued by supplementation with sialic acid metabolites. ManNAc or NeuAc can be incorporated into the cells by two distinct mechanisms. ManNAc is thought to be absorbed by an active, transporter-mediated mechanism. NeuAc, on the other hand, is shown to be absorbed through macropinocytosis. GL, glycolipid; GP, glycoprotein.

neither glycoconjugate that includes ManNAc residues nor specific glycosyltransferase for ManNAc residues has ever been demonstrated among vertebrates. In contrast, NeuAc is present almost always as a glycoconjugate in glycoproteins and gangliosides, and is almost never found as a free molecule. Notwithstanding that both compounds are natural, large-scale production for drug synthesis by pharmaceutical companies is possible [48].

Pharmacokinetics of sialic acid and its influence on designing therapeutic trials

One of the potential difficulties that may challenge therapeutic design is the fact that extrinsically administered sialic acid is rapidly excreted to urine. Using radioisotope-labeled NeuAc and sialyllactose mice and rats, 90% of orally administered NeuAc was absorbed from the intestine at 4 h but 60–90% was excreted in the urine within 6 h, and less than 6% NeuAc was incorporated into tissues and metabolized into ManNAc and pyruvate [49]. Intravenously administered NeuAc led to more rapid excretion within 10 min. Oral administration of sialyllactose led to longer retention of sialic acid in tissues, but almost all was excreted within 24 h. Approximately half of the total amount administered was retained and metabolized into NeuAc, and eventually excreted. Sialyllactose injected intravenously into rats was rapidly excreted, similar to NeuAc.

Supplementation of NeuAc both by oral and intraperitoneal routes given for 8 days resulted in the increased incorporation of NeuAc in brain gangliosides and glycoproteins after oral dosing [50] as compared to the intraperitoneal route. Further, when compared to a study done in older mammals, these experiments suggest that older animals did not show significant incorporation of sialic acid.

Acute dosing of unlabeled NeuAc via the intraperitoneal route also resulted in rapid excretion of 90% of the compound into the urine within 5–30 min [51]. When given intragastrically, 70% of NeuAc was found in the urine in 30–60 min. A similar pattern of excretion was seen after a single dose of ManNAc was given. These results, together with other studies, suggest that NeuAc and ManNAc are rapidly excreted and that the intragastric route

may be more advantageous in increasing in the blood levels of sialic acid, and imply the need for a frequent and prolonged administration of sialic acid compounds in order to attain a maintained increase of sialic acid in tissues.

Unnatural compounds

The use of other compounds or modified sugars is permitted by the sialic acid biosynthetic pathway due to its promiscuous nature. Modified N-acylmannosamine derivatives have been shown to be effectively metabolized into corresponding N-acyl-modified neuraminic acid and incorporated into sialylglycoconjugates [52–54]. As possible as this may seem, it should be noted that these are actually "unnatural" and may be associated with as-yet-unknown consequences.

Increasing cellular sialylation in DMRV/h-IBM mice

The findings in the DMRV/h-IBM mouse model, especially the reduction in overall sialylation of serum and other organs before the onset of symptoms, led to the hypothesis that hyposialylation may be related to the phenotype seen in DMRV/h-IBM muscles. To prove this hypothesis, there is a need to increase the sialylation status in DMRV/h-IBM mouse tissue and evaluate the response to such a phenomenon in terms of muscle phenotype; in theory, maximum efficacy of treatment can only be shown by preventing the onset of muscle weakness [51].

Initial studies involved determining the lowest effective dose in preventing the onset of myopathy by giving ManNAc in drinking water of the mouse amounting to 20 mg (low dose), 200 mg (medium dose), and 2000 mg (high dose) per kilogram of body weight per day. Analysis revealed no clear dose–response correlation in terms of clinical, pathological, and biochemical response to administered sialic acid metabolites. Hence, low-dose therapy using three agents (NeuAc, ManNAc, and sialyllactose) was implemented in DMRV/h-IBM mice before the onset of disease (10–20 weeks of age). The sialic acid metabolites were dissolved into the drinking water of mice, to try to give the drug as frequently as possible, taking advantage of the fact that mice drink around 11 times during waking hours.

The treatment was continued every day, with the dose adjusted according to the weight of the mice, until the mice reached the age (54–57 weeks of age) when they were expected to show full-blown symptoms of myopathy, i.e., the presence of myodegenerative features as seen in muscle pathology.

During the treatment period, survival rate was remarkably improved as compared with control treated mice with all three compounds. At the end of treatment, the phenotypes of DMRV/h-IBM mouse were evaluated and compared with nonaffected littermates. All compounds seemed to be tolerated by mice in terms of kidney and renal metabolism. In all compounds, serum creatine kinase activity, motor performance of mice, physiological contractile properties of isolated skeletal muscles, as well as muscle pathology were notably improved to a level almost similar to nonaffected littermates. Intracellular protein deposits and rimmed vacuoles were rarely seen in the skeletal muscles of treated mice. Sialic acid levels in the blood and the tissues were elevated, and more importantly the levels of sialic acid in the muscle were recovered to almost normal levels after treatment, providing evidence that prophylactic oral administration of sialic acid to the DMRV/h-IBM mice was remarkably effective. These results further suggest that the three compounds are equally good options for treatment. These data invariably support the notion that hyposialylation is one of the key factors in the DMRV/h-IBM pathogenesis.

Although the results from the above studies are encouraging, it has to be reiterated that the methodology employed involved a therapy designed for prevention, something is not applicable for most patients, as patients at the moment are identified only because they are symptomatic. The issues of which compound should be preferred and the efficacy of such compounds in different stages of the disease can only be answered by further studies that will focus on systematic treatment in various and later ages of DMRV/h-IBM mice.

Other treatment modalities
Other modalities that can be used for therapy include gene and cell therapies. The delivery of a *GNE* gene is possible because of its relatively small size. Gene-delivery systems are now being developed and can be evaluated using the DMRV/h-IBM mice or patient's cells in the near future. The factors that will pose some challenge would be the delivery of gene into the mucle, in addition to the usual safety issues in gene therapy. Jay et al. [55] attempted to deliver wild-type *GNE* and mutant *GNE* using lipoplex delivery systems in Lec3 CHO cells devoid of epimerase activity, and showed that epimerase and kinase activities were recovered in these cells. One may question, however, how an epimerase mutant can recover its enzymatic activity [55], whereas previous studies using similar cells but different epimerase mutants failed to do so [35]; future studies would require clarification of such issues.

One potential but clear benefit of gene therapy is that it may provide the chance to understand GNE itself, as this protein has been implicated to have roles outside glycobiology [15, 38, 39, 56, 57]. Indeed, the application of gene-/cell-based therapies will not only give a definite cure, but also provide insights necessary to elucidate the precise mechanism of how the *GNE* gene defect causes this devastating myopathy.

Acknowledgment

This study is supported partly by the "Research on Psychiatric and Neurological Diseases and Mental Health" from the Japanese Health Sciences Foundation; the Program for Promotion of Fundamental Studies in Health Sciences of the National Institute of Biomedical Innovation (NIBIO); "Research Grant (22-5) for Nervous and Mental Disorders" from the Ministry of Health, Labour and Welfare; the Kato Memorial Trust for Nambyo Research; and the Neuromuscular Disease Foundation.

References

1 Nonaka I, Sunohara N, Ishiura S, Satoyoshi E. (1981) Familial distal myopathy with rimmed vacuole and lamellar (myeloid) body formation. *J Neurol Sci* **51**, 141–155.

2 Kumamoto T, Fukuhara N, Nagashima M et al. (1982) Distal myopathy. Histochemical and ultrastructural study. *Arch Neurol* **39**, 367–371.

3 Malicdan MC, Noguchi S, Nishino I. (2007) Autophagy in a mouse model of distal myopathy with rimmed vacuoles or hereditary inclusion bidy myopathy. *Autophagy* **3**, 396–398.

4 Kumamoto T, Ito T, Horinouchi, H et al. (2000) Increased lysosome-related proteins in the skeletal muscles of distal myopathy with rimmed vacuoles. *Muscle Nerve* **23**, 1686–1693.

5 Yabe I, Higashi T, Kikuchi S et al. (2003) GNE mutations causing distal myopathy with rimmed vacuoles with inflammation. *Neurology* **61**, 384–386.

6 Mitrani-Rosenbaum S, Argov Z, Blumenfeld A et al. (1996) Hereditary inclusion body myopathy maps to chromosome 9p1-q1. *Hum Mol Genet* **5**, 159–163.

7 Ikeuchi T, Asaka T, Saito M et al. (1997) Gene locus for autosomal recessive distal myopathy with rimmed vacuoles maps to chromosome 9. *Ann Neurol* **41**, 432–437.

8 Eisenberg I, Avidan N, Potikha T et al. (2001) The UDP-N-acetylglucosamine 2-epimerase/N-acetylmannosamine kinase gene is mutated in recessive hereditary inclusion body myopathy. *Nat Genet* **29**, 83–87.

9 Brooks SA, Dwek MV, Schumacher U. (2002) *Functional and Molecular Gycobiology*. BIOS Scientific Publishers, Oxford.

10 Stasche R, Hinderlich S, Weise C et al. (1997) A bifunctional enzyme catalyzes the first two steps in N-acetylneuraminic acid biosynthesis of rat liver. Molecular cloning and functional expression of UDP-N-acetyl-glucosamine 2-epimerase/N-acetylmannosamine kinase. *J Biol Chem* **272**, 24319–24324.

11 Schauer R. (2004) Sialic acids: fascinating sugars in higher animals and man. *Zoology* **107**, 49–64.

12 Leroy JG, Seppala R, Huizing M et al. (2001) Dominant inheritance of sialuria, an inborn error of feedback inhibition. *Am J Hum Genet* **68**, 1419–1427.

13 Varki A. (1997) Sialic acids as ligands in recognition phenomena. *FASEB J* **11**, 248–255.

14 Hynes RO, Lander AD. (1992) Contact and adhesive specificities in the associations, migrations, and targeting of cells and axons. *Cell* **68**, 303–322.

15 Wang Z, Sun Z, Li AV, Yarema KJ. (2006) Roles for GNE outside of sialic acid biosynthesis: modulation of sialyltransferase and BiP expression, GM3 and GD3 biosynthesis, proliferation and apoptosis, and ERK1/2 phosphorylation. *J Biol Chem* **281**, 27016–27028.

16 Huizing M, Krasnewich DM. (2009) Hereditary inclusion body myopathy: a decade of progress. *Biochim Biophys Acta* **1792**, 881–887.

17 Reinke SO, Hinderlich S. (2007) Prediction of three different isoforms of the human UDP-N-acetylglucosamine 2-epimerase/N-acetylmannosamine kinase *FEBS Lett* **581**, 3327–3331.

18 Watts GDJ, Thorne M, Kovach MJ et al. (2003) Clinical and genetic heterogeneity in chromosome 9p associated hereditary inclusion body myopathy: exclusion of GNE and three other candidate genes. *Neuromuscul Disord* **13**, 559–567.

19 Hortskorte R, Nöhring S, Wiechens N et al. (1999) Tissue expression and amino acid sequence of murine UDP-N-acetylglucosamine-2-epimerase/N-acetylmannosamine kinase. *FEBS J* **260**, 923–927.

20 Reinke SO, Eidenschink C, Jay CM, Hinderlich S. (2009) Biochemical characterization of human and murine isoforms of UDP-N-acetylglucosamine 2-epimerase/N-acetylmannosamine kinase (GNE). *Glycoconj J* **26**, 415–422.

21 Noguchi S, Keira Y, Murayama K et al. (2004) Reduction of UDP-N-acetylglucosamine 2-epimerase/N-acetylmannosamine kinase activity and sialylation in distal myopathy with rimmed vacuoles. *J Biol Chem* **279**, 11402–11407.

22 Penner J, Mantey LR, Elgavish S et al. (2006) Influence of UDP-GlcNAc 2-Epimerase/ManNAc kinase mutant proteins on hereditary inclusion body myopathy. *Biochemistry* **45**, 2968–2977.

23 Hinderlich S, Stäsche R, Zeitler R, Reutter W. (1997) A bifunctional enzyme catalyzes the first two steps in N-acetylneuraminic acid biosynthesis of rat liver. Purification and characterization of UDP-N-acetylglucosamine 2-epimerase/N-acetylmannosamine kinase. *J Biol Chem* **272**, 24313–24318.

24 Effertz K, Hinderlich S, Reutter W. (1999) Selective loss of either the epimerase or kinase activity of UDP-N-acetylglucosamine 2-epimerase/N-acetylmannosamine kinase due to site-directed mutagenesis based on sequence alignments. *J Biol Chem* **274**, 28771–28778.

25 Kurochkina N, Yardeni T, Huizing M. (2010) Molecular modeling of the bifunctional enzyme UDP-GlcNAc 2-epimerase/ManNAc kinase and predictions of structural effects of mutations associated with HIBM and sialuria. *Glycobiology* **20**, 322–337.

26 Keppler T, Hinderlich S, Langner J et al. (1999) UDP-GlcNAc 2-epimerase: a regulator of cell surface sialylation. *Science* **284**, 1372–1376.

27 Saito F, Tomimitsu H, Arai K et al. (2004) A Japanese patient with distal myopathy with rimmed vacuoles: missense mutations in the epimerase domain of the UDP-N-acetylglucosamine 2-epimerase/N-acetylmannosamine kinase (GNE) gene accompanied by hyposialylation of skeletal muscle glycoproteins. *Neuromuscul Disord* **14**, 158–161.

28 Huizing M, Rakocevic G, Sparks SE et al. (2004) Hypoglycosylation of alpha-dystroglycan in patients with hereditary IBM due to GNE mutations. *Mol Genet Metab* **81**, 196–202.

29 Ricci E, Broccolini A, Gidaro T et al. (2006) NCAM is hyposialylated in hereditary inclusion body myopathy due to GNE mutations. *Neurology* **66**, 755–758.

30 Broccolini A, Gidaro T, Morosetti R et al. (2006) Neprilysin participates in skeletal muscle regeneration and is accumulated in abnormal muscle fibres of inclusion body myositis. *J Neurochem* **96**, 777–789.

31 Broccolini A, Gidaro T, De Cristofaro R et al. (2008) Hyposialylation of neprilysin possibly affects its expression and enzymatic activity in hereditary inclusion-body myopathy muscle. *J Neurochem* **105**, 971–981.

32 Salama I, Hinderlich S, Shlomai Z et al. (2005) No overall hyposialylation in hereditary inclusion body myopathy myoblasts carrying the homozygous M712T GNE mutation. *Biochem Biophys Res Commun* **328**, 221–226.

33 Hinderlich S, Salama I, Eisenberg I et al. (2004) The homozygous M712T mutation of UDP-N-acetylglucosamine 2-epimerase/N-acetylmannosamine kinase results in reduced enzyme activities but not in altered overall cellular sialylation in hereditary inclusion body myopathy. *FEBS Lett* **566**, 105–109.

34 Hinderlich S, Berger M, Keppler OT et al. (2001) Biosynthesis of N-acetylneuraminic acid in cells lacking UDP-N-acetylglucosamine 2-epimerase/N-acetyl-mannosamine kinase. *Biol Chem* **382** 291–297.

35 Hong Y, Stanley P. (2003) Lec3 Chinese hamster ovary mutants lack UDP-N-acetylglucosamine 2-epimerase activity because of mutations in the epimerase domain of the Gne gene. *J Biol Chem* **278**, 53045–53054.

36 Oetke C, Hinderlich S, Reutter W, Pawlita M. (2003) Epigenetically mediated loss of UDP-GlcNAc 2-epimerase/ManNAc kinase expression in hyposialylated cell lines. *Biochem Biophys Res Commun* **308**, 892–898.

37 Horstkorte R, Nöhring S, Danker K et al. (2000) Protein kinase C phosphorylates and regulates UDP-N-acetylglucosamine-2-epimerase/N-acetylmannosamine kinase. *FEBS Lett* **470**, 315–318.

38 Weidemann W, Stelzl U, Lisewski U et al. (2006) The collapsin response mediator protein 1 (CRMP-1) and the promyelocytic leukemia zinc finger protein (PLZF) bind to UDP-N-acetylglucosamine 2-epimerase/N-acetylmannosamine kinase (GNE), the key enzyme of sialic acid biosynthesis. *FEBS Lett* **580**, 6649–6654.

39 Amsili S, Zer H, Hinderlich S et al. (2008) UDP-N-acetylglucosamine 2-epimerase/N-acetylmannosa-mine kinase (GNE) binds to alpha-actinin 1: novel pathways in skeletal muscle? *PLoS One* **3**, e2477.

40 Schwarzkopf M, Knobeloch KP, Rohde E et al. (2002) Sialylation is essential for early development in mice. *Proc Natl Acad Sci USA* **99**, 5267–5270.

41 Gagiannis D, Orthmann A, Danssmann I et al. (2007) Reduced sialylation status in UDP-N-acetylglucosamine-2-epimerase/N-acetylmannosamine kinase (GNE)-deficient mice. *Glycoconj J* **24**, 125–130.

42 Galeano B, Klootwijk R, Manoli I et al. (2007) Mutation in the key enzyme of sialic acid biosynthesis causes severe glomerular proteinuria and is rescued by *N*-acetylmannosamine. *J Clin Invest* **117**, 1585–1594.

43 Malicdan MC, Noguchi S, Nonaka I et al. (2007) A Gne knockout mouse expressing human GNE D176V mutation develops features similar to distal myopathy with rimmed vacuoles or hereditary inclusion body myopathy. *Hum Mol Genet* **16**, 2669–2682.

44 Malicdan MC, Noguchi S, Hayashi YK, Nishino I. (2008) Muscle weakness correlates with muscle atrophy and precedes the development of inclusion body or rimmed vacuoles in the mouse model of DMRV/hIBM. *Physiol Genomics* **17**, 106–115.

45 Sparks S, Rakocevic G, Joe G et al. (2007) Intravenous immune globulin in hereditary inclusion body myopathy: a pilot study. *BMC Neurol* **7**, 3.

46 Oetke C, Hinderlich S, Brossmer R et al. (2001) Evidence for efficient uptake and incorporation of sialic acid by eukaryotic cells. *Eur J Biochem* **268**, 4553–4561.

47 Bardor M, Nguyen DH, Diaz S, Varki A. (2005) Mechanism of uptake and incorporation of the non-human sialic acid N-glycolylneuraminic acid into human cells. *J Biol Chem* **280**, 4228–4237.

48 Yamaguchi S, Ohnishi J, Maru I, Ohta Y. (2006) Simple and large-scale production of N-acetylneuraminic acid and N-acetyl-D-mannosamine. *Trends Glycosci Glycotechnol* **18**, 245–252.

49 Nöule U, Schauer R. (1981) Uptake, metabolism and excretion of orally and intravenously administered, 14C- and 3H-labeled N-acetylneuraminic acid mixture in the mouse and rat. *Hoppe Seylers Z Physiol Chem* **362**, 1495–1506.

50 Carlson SE, House SG. (1986) Oral and intraperitoneal administration of N-acetylneuraminic acid: effect in rat cerebral and cerebellar N-acetylneuraminic acid. *J Nutr* **116**, 881–886.

51 Malicdan MC, Noguchi S, Hayashi YK et al. (2009) Prophylactic treatment with sialic acid metabolites preclude the development of a myopathic phenotype in the DMRV-hIBM mouse model. *Nat Med* **15**, 690–695.

52 Luchansky SJ, Yarema KJ, Takahashi S, Bertozzi CR. (2003) GlcNAc 2-epimerase can serve a catabolic role in sialic acid metabolism. *J Biol Chem* **278**, 8035–8042.

53 Charter NW, Mahal LK, Koshland Jr., DE, Bertozzi CR. (2000) Biosynthetic incorporation of unnatural sialic acids into polysialic acid on neural cells. *Glycobiology* **10**, 1049–1056.

54 Gagiannis D, Gossrau R, Reutter W et al. (2007) Engineering the sialic acid in organs of mice using N-propanoylmannosamine. *Biochem Biophys Acta* **1770**, 297–306.

55 Jay C, Nemunaitis G, Nemunaitis J et al. (2008) Preclinical assessment of wt GNE gene plasmid for management of hereditary inclusion body myopathy 2 (HIBM2). *Gene Regul Syst Bio* **2**, 243–252.

56 Krause S, Hinderlich S, Amsili S et al. (2005) Localization of UDP-GlcNAc 2-epimerase/ManAc kinase (GNE) in the Golgi complex and the nucleus of mammalian cells. *Exp Cell Res* **304**, 365–379.

57 Amsili S, Shlomai Z, Levitzki R et al. (2007) Characterization of hereditary inclusion body myopathy myoblasts: possible primary impairment of apoptotic events. *Cell Death Differ* **14**, 1916–1924.

CHAPTER 12

GNE myopathy (hereditary inclusion-body myopathy/ distal myopathy with rimmed vacuoles): clinical features and epidemiology

Zohar Argov[1], Ichizo Nishino[2], and Ikuya Nonaka[3]

[1]Department of Neurology, Hadassah-Hebrew University Medical Center, Jerusalem, Israel
[2]Department of Neuromuscular Research, National Institute of Neuroscience, National Center of Neurology and Psychiatry, Tokyo, Japan
[3]National Institute of Neuroscience, National Center of Neurology and Psychiatry, Tokyo, Japan

Introduction

About three decades ago, two types of unique hereditary myopathy were described. The first was reported by Nonaka et al. [1] and was termed distal myopathy with rimmed vacuoles (DMRV). That report emphasized the new recognition (at that time) that distal muscle weakness can be caused by a primary myopathy and not solely by neurogenic disorders. The second, reported by Argov and Yarom [2], highlighted a very unusual clinical feature and accordingly was called quadriceps-sparing myopathy (QSM). Both conditions shared similar histological and ultrastructural features of cytoplasmic 'rimmed' vacuoles and inclusions composed of clusters of tubular filaments [1, 3]. This histological picture was reminiscent of the findings in sporadic inclusion-body myositis (although inflammation was absent in the hereditary conditions). Thus, the term hereditary inclusion-body myopathy (h-IBM) was given to the QSM [4, 5].

It was initially not clear that the two conditions were similar, despite the common histopathological features; however, in the past 15 years accumulating scientific data have indicated that this may be the case. In 1996 Mitrani-Rosenbaum et al. [6] linked h-IBM to chromosome 9p1–q1 and DMRV was found to be linked to the same region in 1997 [7]. The identification of defects in the gene encoding UDP-N-acetylglucosamine-2 epimerase/N-acetyl-mannosamime kinase (*GNE*) in h-IBM [8], followed by the identification of different mutations in this gene in DMRV [9], has set the final basis for unification of these two conditions.

We now recognize that h-IBM (IBM2 in the McKusick classification) and DMRV are the same disorder and use the term GNE myopathy throughout this collaborative chapter. First of its kind, it compiles the clinical features of both h-IBM and DMRV to present the full spectrum of the GNE myopathy. In addition we summarize the epidemiology of this worldwide *GNE*-related recessive

Muscle Aging, Inclusion-Body Myositis and Myopathies, First Edition. Edited by Valerie Askanas and W. King Engel.
© 2012 Blackwell Publishing Ltd. Published 2012 by Blackwell Publishing Ltd.

disorder and indicate where initial therapeutic ideas could be implemented in this condition.

Diagnostic criteria

Table 12.1 lists the current suggestions for diagnostic features of GNE myopathy. Histology is not mandatory for diagnosis, since with typical clinical pattern molecular diagnosis suffices and biopsy can be avoided. Some patients may, however, present with phenotypic variations (as will be discussed below) or as 'isolates' (a single patient in an unrecognized ethnic background) that require diagnostic biopsy before embarking on genetic identification. We suggest not including the electron-microscopic finding of inclusions or the immunohistochemical demonstration of various upregulated proteins as a diagnostic criterion since these techniques are available only in selected (usually research-oriented) places. We also group the criteria into definite, most probable, and possible categories to enable better epidemiological assessment of the prevalence of this condition.

Clinical phenotypic features

The age of onset is typically in early adulthood. In the Middle Eastern Jewish population (based on data from about 140 patients, all homozygous for the kinase mutation M712T and all examined personally by ZA) the age of first symptom was estimated to be 30 ± 6 years (mean $\pm$ SD). It should be

Table 12.1   Diagnostic criteria for DMRV/h-IBM.

1   Adult-onset distal myopathy beginning in the legs
2   Typical weakness distribution with quadriceps being spared
3   Mild creatine kinase elevation and nonspecific ("mixed") EMG
4   Rimmed vacuolar myopathy
5   Identification of mutations in GNE
Definite: 1 + 5
Most probable: 1 + 2 + 4
Probable: 1 + 2 + 3

recognized that this estimate is based in many cases on patients' recall and thus could be subject to bias. In the Middle Eastern population the earliest recorded onset is 17 years and the latest is around 48 years [2, 10, 11]. Mean onset in Japanese patients is earlier, at 26 ± 8 years, and this is the case for a recently reported series of patients from India, with a calculated mean age of onset of 26 years [12]. It should be noted that the mutational status of the patients in this series is not yet fully established.

It is important to note that there are three identified elderly persons that are homozygous for the GNE "classical" mutation who are clinically unaffected. One is a 75-year-old Persian Jewish female, belonging to a family with several affected members who are homozygous for the M712T mutation. She is clinically unaffected despite having the same genotype. Another subject is in his mid-fifties, also homozygous for M712T, who was reported to us by his affected sibs as being completely normal (he was not examined). The third is a Japanese patient who harbors the D176V mutation and is unaffected at the end of the seventh decade of life. It is unclear if these subjects will ever develop disease signs and what has protected them for so long a period.

Weakness at onset is typically in the anterior compartment of the leg (mainly tibialis anterior) leading to bilateral foot-drop. This mode of onset led to the early definition of this condition as a distal myopathy. Since this pattern of onset is similar to that of the hereditary neuropathies grouped under the term Charcot-Marie-Tooth (CMT) disease, several of our patients were initially diagnosed as such before the correct diagnosis was made. The posterior calf muscles become involved later and sometimes are spared until the more advanced stages of the disease. Very rarely one may encounter patients in whom the onset of weakness is in the proximal musculature of the leg without distal weakness [13], which appeared about 7 years later. Similarly, in Japanese patients, tibialis anterior muscles are also preferentially involved. The initial symptoms include gait disturbance and difficulty in climbing stairs and running, in addition to foot-drop. The gastrocnemius, hamstrings, and paraspinal and sternocleidomastoid muscles are also involved from an early stage when examined by muscle imaging.

Usually, the iliopsoas is the first and most affected of the hip muscles with a lesser degree of weakness in the glutei, hamstrings, and adductors as the disorder evolves in the lower limbs. The quadriceps muscle remains strong (normal power or minimal reduction) despite the continuous weakening of all other proximal lower limb muscles and this feature is usually preserved through the course of the disease in most patients, even in wheelchair-bound or bedridden patients. This unique pattern of QSM is observed in the vast majority of patients with *GNE* mutations reported worldwide and facilitates the clinical recognition of this condition. However, in a minority of patients (less than 5% in the Middle Eastern cluster) the quadriceps may also become very weak even in the earlier phase of the disease [11, 14]. In other communities the quadriceps was sometimes reported to be "partially" spared.

The reason why the quadriceps is unaffected (both clinically and histologically) is unclear. Biochemical evaluation of the quadriceps in few patients did not show any difference between this and the other muscles [15], so the protective mechanism (clearly important for potential therapy approaches and understanding the disease pathophysiology) currently remains unknown.

The disease progresses slowly to affect the upper limbs, mainly the scapular musculature. This has led in the past to a false classification of such patients as having scapuloperoneal syndrome (thought to be a neurogenic disease) [2]. Weakening of the distal muscles of the arm and the hand occurs usually at later stages, affecting also the long finger flexors which are typically affected in the sporadic IBM. Neck flexors (but not the extensors) may become affected too. Mild facial weakness was reported in two families [16], but the vast majority of patients have no facial involvement and ocular musculature was never found to be affected. Respiration seems to be well preserved until the very final stages of the disease.

Ankle tendon reflexes maybe lost and sensory subjective complaints are sometimes reported at the early stages of the disease, but there are no objective signs of neuropathy. Tendon reflexes may be gradually lost as the disease progress. The brain and other organs are not involved in GNE-opathy. However, in the Japanese community there have been anecdotal reports describing patients with some cardiac symptoms, ranging from seemingly benign to even lethal arrhythmia. In one patient with the homozygous V572L mutation, cardiac arrhythmia was fatal. Autopsy revealed that there were prominent vacuoles in cardiac fibers (although there was no histological conformation whether these were indeed similar to the rimmed vacuoles found in the skeletal muscles). The patient's brother, who had the same *GNE* mutation and presented with distal muscle weakness, also subsequently died suddenly due to cardiac arrhythmia. Another DMRV patient also showed severe cardiac involvement; cardiac biopsy was done because atrioventricular block revealed adipose tissue infiltration in the cardiac muscles.

Recently, a mouse model with a knock in M712T mutation resulted in early fatal kidney disease [17] so it should be noted that human patients do not have renal involvement.

Progression rate is variable and many patients of the Middle Eastern Jewish cluster remain ambulatory, even 15–20 years (or more) after disease onset. Complete loss of ambulation occurs early in those patients with marked quadriceps involvement, even after a few years. Loss of ambulation seems to occur earlier in other populations: the average time to the wheelchair-bound state was estimated recently to be 3–9 years in the Indian series [12]. In Japan, however, there seems to be a wider variation, as patients lose their ability to walk independently in the age range of 26–57 years (average of 12 years after disease onset) [1]. Some of Middle Eastern patients reached the eighth decade and several are alive at the seventh decade of life, suggesting the overall longevity is not markedly affected.

Clinical laboratory tests

Routine laboratory tests toward muscle disease are nonspecific. Serum creatine kinase (CK) activity is usually mildly elevated, up to five times the upper maximal normal value, but normal levels may be observed at onset. Rarely levels as high as 1500 IU/L have been recorded and higher levels should alert the physician to an additional cause or mistaken diagnosis.

Conventional concentric needle electromyography (EMG) may be misleading. Spontaneous activity in the early-affected tibialis anterior (mainly fibrillation potentials) may be found, raising the possibility of a neurogenic condition or an inflammatory myopathy. Such spontaneous activity is not present in other muscles [2]. The motor units are small and polyphasic in most muscles, but reduced recruitment with prolonged, large, and even polyphasic units were also recorded in some affected muscles, again suggesting some neurogenic involvement. However, when quantitative EMG was applied to several Persian Jewish patients the myopathic nature of this condition became apparent [10]. Nerve conductions are normal even in those patients with sensory complaints and reduced tendon reflexes.

In muscle histology, myopathic changes with variation in size in both type 1 and 2 fibers are seen. Rimmed vacuoles are present mostly in fibers which are atrophic, and, on occasions, these fibers with rimmed vacuoles appear to form small groups. Rimmed vacuoles are thought to be clusters of autophagic vacuoles, as these are viewed on electron microscopy to be areas of double-membraned vacuoles, in addition to myeloid whorls and cellular debris. On light microscopy these rimmed vacuoles are positively stained with acid phosphatase fibers, indicating that acidic organelles are present, and autophagic markers like LC3-II may be demonstrated. Other findings on muscle biopsy, including necrotic and regenerating fibers, and inflammatory infiltrates, can rarely be seen.

Differential diagnosis

In institutions where staff are not familiar with GNE myopathy the correct diagnosis may sometimes be delayed. When faced with clinical and histological data the differential diagnosis may be one of the following.
1 Sporadic inclusion-body myositis: the main distinctive points of this condition from the GNE myopathy are the later onset and the presence of diffuse inflammatory infiltrates in the muscle sample. Also, in the sporadic condition the quadriceps is usually the first muscle to be involved.

2 Other distal myopathies with rimmed vacuoles [18]: these other conditions are at times very hard to distinguish from DMRV/h-IBM especially in the early phase, where quadriceps sparing is not apparent. Molecular analysis maybe mandatory for correct diagnosis.
3 CMT and other peroneal muscular atrophies: the early weakness of the peroneal muscles in DMRV/h-IBM mimics these neurogenic conditions. The peripheral neuropathic forms of CMT are easily distinguishable by clinical examination (showing sensory impairment) and nerve-conduction studies. More difficult differential diagnosis is distal spinal muscular atrophy (SMA). EMG may show a nondistinctive mixed pattern and serum CK is either not elevated or only modestly raised in both conditions. Biopsy showing grouping and other neurogenic features without vacuoles may make the SMA diagnosis more plausible.
4 Scapuloperoneal syndromes: patients at a more advanced stage, with upper-limb and scapular involvement, may look similar to those with a scapuloperoneal syndrome [2]. Even before GNE sequencing one may recognize the typical distribution of weakness which is different in these conditions.
5 Limb girdle muscular dystrophy (LGMD): some DMRV/h-IBM patients with proximal weakness beginning in the legs may be clinically indistinguishable from adult-onset LGMD. The distal onset and lack of quadriceps sparing make the diagnosis easier as this is not the case in most LGMD syndromes. Very high serum CK levels and a biopsy with necrotizing myopathy usually lead to the correct diagnosis. One should remember that in LGMD type 2G rimmed vacuoles may be abundant.

Epidemiology

This is a worldwide disorder and patients were diagnosed in many countries, including Europe, North and Middle America, and Africa (see below). Interestingly, the identification of patients with GNE myopathy comes mainly from two sources: a Middle Eastern cluster with a single founder mutation and a "concentration" of cases in Japan which is composed

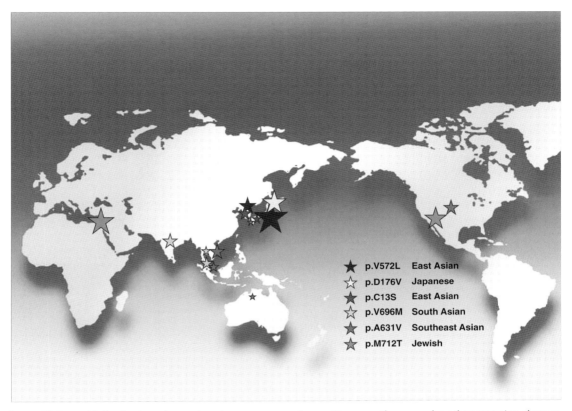

Figure 12.1 World distribution of mutation clusters. The largest mutations clusters are p.M712T and p.V572L. The former is found in Jewish patients mainly in Israel and the USA. The latter is found in East Asia including Japan. However, there are also other mutation clusters. Note that p.A631V in the USA was actually found in Vietnamese patients. The same mutation is found in Southeast Asian patients.

of numerous mutations with two founder mutations and several single-occurrence mutations (Figure 12.1).

The Middle Eastern cluster was first recognized in Persian Jews, mostly originating from present-day Iran [2]. The vast majority of these Jews left Iran around 1948 (immigrating to Israel). A second wave of immigration occurred after 1978 and many of them arrived to the USA, creating two strong communities: in Los Angeles, California, and in Long Island, New York. Also, Jews from Iran's neighboring countries (Afghanistan, Iraq, and Uzbekistan), with a very similar ethnic and cultural background to Persian Jews, were found to carry the disorder [13]. A more surprising observation was the identification of three families from the Karaite sect (a group of Jews that separated from mainstream

Judaism in the Middle Ages on religious grounds) who immigrated to Israel from Egypt. Even more intriguing was the finding of three Muslim Arab families with the same disorder. The six Muslim patients are of Bedouin origin (two families) and twin brothers of Palestinian origin (the Palestinians are thought to be of different historical and ethnic background from the nomad Bedouins). All these families were found not only to have the same homozygous *GNE* mutation (M712T), but were homozygous carriers of a similar haplotype (about 700 kb) around the *GNE* gene. One of the families described from Tunisia [19] is also Muslim Arab, carrying the homozygous M712T mutation, but there are no haplotype data for these patients. This is the basis of our definition of the Middle Eastern cluster of h-IBM. Preliminary unpublished results indicate that the age of this mutation is about 2500 years. In Israel, 119 patients from 62 families were diagnosed by molecular tests to have a M712T homozygous mutation and there are other patients who have refused molecular testing but who have been diagnosed clinically over the past 25 years (Argov et al., unpublished work). There is no central registry of Persian Jewish patients residing in the USA (or elsewhere), but 23 patients from 10 families were tested in Jerusalem and found also to have the Middle Eastern mutation. We estimated (conservatively) that there are another 50–70 patients in this community dispersed across several countries around the world (especially in the USA), some of whom were diagnosed using molecular testing in other laboratories. The calculated mutation carrier frequency in this community was 6.8% [8], compatible with our estimation of prevalence of 1 in 1500 adults who have both of their parents of Persian Jewish origin.

In Japan, two founder mutations have been identified: V572L and D176V. To date, V572L accounts for 54% of mutated alleles identified, while D176V accounts for 22%. The exact prevalence of DMRV to date, nonetheless, has not been calculated, but in the NCNP Institute (Tokyo, Japan) the number of cases from 1978 to 2009 was about 108 (Momma et al., unpublished results). As NCNP serves as the main referral center for the diagnosis of muscle diseases in Japan, the most practical method for estimating the present prevalence of DMRV is by a calculation based on the prevalence of Duchenne muscular dystrophy (DMD). The prevalence of DMD is approximated to be 1.9–3.4 per 100 000 population, and is believed to be similar from country to country. From 1979 to 2006 NCNP had a total of 536 DMD cases, bringing the total number of cases in Japan to about 1500–4000. At this same period about 50 cases of DMRV were diagnosed. Thus, the number of GNE myopathy cases in Japan should be about 150–400 cases, with a prevalence of 1.71–3.05 per 1 000 000 Japanese population.

Several reports have surfaced describing the mutation spectrum of GNE myopathy elsewhere in Asia. In Korea, it has been found that the most common mutation is V572L, which is seen in 11 out of 16 cases, and further implicating a common founder mutation with Japan [20]. In Thailand there was a report of four cases, three of which have a common mutation, V696M [21]. In Taiwan, two patients from the same family were confirmed to have *GNE* mutations [22]. A series of patients from a single region of India was also recently presented [12]. Because of increased awareness of this disease, we expect further reports of mutational analysis in other Asian countries, particularly China.

There are numerous GNE myopathy patients identified from other European and North American countries, and not all have been reported in the literature. All the published Italian, Spanish, Greek, German, Irish, Mexican, white, and African American patients from the USA, and North African patients, have confirmed GNE mutations [8, 19, 21, 23–31]. There are a few more families who have been tested in our laboratories but whose data remains unpublished.

Therapy

There are two general approaches to potential therapy for GNE-associated myopathy: metabolic and genetic.

Since the myopathy is associated with defects in the GNE enzymatic activity, affecting the sialic acid synthetic pathway, the assumption is that reduced sialylation is a major part of the pathogenesis of this condition. Thus, attempts were made to increase the levels of sialic acid in humans by infusing intravenous immunoglobulin (IVIG; which contains high sialic acid levels) to very few patients. This short-term open trial showed mainly a subjective improvement [32].

A more obvious approach is to supplement the deficient sialic acid pathway with one of its intermediates. The use of *N*-acetylmannosamine (ManNAc) is based on the recent findings in the transgenic Gne$^{-/-}$ hGNED176VTg mouse model, in which feeding with ManNAc led to improved muscle function as well as biochemical measurements [33]. Also, feeding ManNAc to pregnant mice with a knockin M712T mutation led to improved outcome in the newborn pups [17]. The dose and mode of oral administration of this sugar compound in humans is still undetermined. A planned ManNAc trial at the US National Institutes of Health awaits toxicology studies before approval. However, we are aware of several patients taking high doses of ManNAc (produced by a nonpharmaceutical company) unsupervised for a few months. In the transgenic animal model other compounds were tried with a similar positive therapeutic effects [33] and thus any compound (preferably natural) with high sialic acid content could be considered as a potential therapeutic agent. This is discussed in detail elsewhere in this book (see Chapter 11).

A more complicated therapeutic intervention in GNE-opathy is gene therapy. The whole field of genetic therapy in myology is evolving but in this disorder there is one advantage and this is the relatively small size of the *GNE* gene, which can fit several vectors. One approach is to deliver the normal gene via a special delivery system (lipoplex). A compassionate trial in one patient with GNE-associated myopathy is currently taking place [34].

Genetic counseling

Counseling in GNE-opathies is similar to that for any other recessively inherited disorder. The counselor should be aware of the variable severity of this myopathy while trying to predict the outcome for a homozygous or compound heterozygous person. Even in the same family we observed different severities of the myopathy. The three known elderly subjects with confirmed homozygous *GNE* mutations but with a normal phenotype (see above) make genetic counseling even more complicated.

References

1 Nonaka I, Sunohara N, Ischiura S, Satayoshi E (1981) Familial distal myopathy with rimmed vacuole and lamellar (myeloid) body formation. *J Neurol Sci* **51**, 141–155.

2 Argov Z, Yarom R (1984) "Rimmed vacuole myopathy" sparing the quadriceps: a unique disorder in Iranian Jews. *J Neurol Sci* **64**, 33–43.

3 Argov Z, Soffer D (2002) Hereditary inclusion body myopathies. In Karpati G (ed.), *Structural and Molecular Basis of Skeletal Muscle Disease*. ISN Neuropath Press, Basel, pp. 274–276.

4 Askanas V, Engel WK (1993) New advances in inclusion-body myositis. *Curr Opin Rheumatol* **5**, 732–741.

5 Askanas V, Engel WK (1998) Newest approaches to diagnosis of sporadic inclusion-body myositis and hereditary inclusion-body myopathies, including molecular-pathologic similarities to Alzheimer disease. In Askanas V, Serratrice G, Engel WK (eds), *Inclusion-Body Myositis and Myopathies*, Cambridge University Press, Cambridge, pp. 3–78.

6 Mitrani-Rosenbaum S, Argov Z, Blumenfeld A et al. (1996) Hereditary inclusion body myopathy maps to chromosome 9p1-q1. *Hum Mol Genet* **5**, 159–163.

7 Ikeuchi T, Asaka T, Saito M et al. (1997) Gene locus for autosomal recessive distal myopathy with rimmed vacuoles maps to chromosome 9. *Ann Neurol* **41**, 432–437.

8 Eisenberg I, Avidan N, Potikha T et al. (2001) The UDP-N -Acetylglucosamine 2-epimerase/N-acetylmanno-samine kinase is mutated in recessive hereditary inclusion body myopathy. *Nat Genet* **29**, 83–87.

9 Nishino I, Noguchi S, Murayama K et al. (2002) Distal myopathy with rimmed vacuoles is allelic to hereditary inclusion body myopathy. *Neurology* **59**, 1689–1693.

10 Sadeh M, Gadoth M, Hadar H, Ben David E (1993) Vacuolar myopathy sparing the quadriceps. *Brain* **116**, 217–232.

11 Sadeh M, Argov Z (1998) Hereditary inclusion body myopathy in Jews of Persian origin: clinical and laboratory data. In Askanas V, Serratrice G, Engel WK (eds), *Inclusion-Body Myositis and Myopathies*, Cambridge University Press, Cambridge, pp. 191–199.

12 Nalini A, Gayathri N (2009) Distal myopathy with rimmed vacuoles (DMRV): Experience of a rare disorder (abstract). *Neuromuscl Disord* **19**, 568.

13 Argov Z, Eisenberg I, Grabov, Nardini G et al. (2003) Hereditary inclusion body myopathy: the Middle Eastern genetic cluster. *Neurology* **60**, 1519–1523.

14 Neufeld MY, Sadeh M, Assa B et al. (1995) Phenotypic heterogeneity in familial inclusion body myopathy. *Muscle Nerve* **18**, 546–548.

15 Salama I, Hinderlich S, Shlomai Z et al. (2005) No overall hyposialylation in hereditary inclusion body myopathy myoblasts carrying the homozygous M712T GNE mutation. *Biochem Biophys Res Commun* **328**, 221–226.

16 Argov Z, Sadeh M, Eisenberg I et al. (1998) Facial involvement in hereditary inclusion body myositis. *Neurology* **50**, 1925–1926.

17 Galeano B, Klootwijk R, Manoli I et al. (2007) Mutation in the key enzyme of sialic acid biosynthesis causes severe glomerular proteinuria and is rescued by N-acetylmannosamine. *J Clin Invest* **117**, 1585–1594.

18 Udd B (2009) 165th ENMC International Workshop: Distal myopathies 6–8th 2009 Naarden, The Netherlands. *Neuromuscul Disord* **19**, 429–438.

19 Amouri R, Driss A, Muruyama K et al. (2005) Allelic heterogeneity of GNE gene mutation in two Tunisian families with autosomal recessive inclusion body myopathy. *Neuromuscul Disord* **15**, 361–363.

20 Kim BJ, Ki CS, Kim JW et al. (2006) Mutation analysis of the GNE gene in Korean patients with distal myopathy with rimmed vacuoles. *J Hum Genet* **51**, 137–140.

21 Liewluck T, Pho-Iam T, Limwongse C et al. (2006) Mutation analysis of the *GNE* gene in distal myopathy with rimmed vacuoles (DMRV) patients in Thailand. *Muscle Nerve* **34**, 775–778.

22 Chu C, Kuo H, Yeh T, et al. (2007) Heterozygous mutations affecting the epimerase domain of the GNE gene causing distal myopathy with rimmed vacuoles in a Taiwanese family. *Clinic Neurol Neurosurg* **109**, 250–256.

23 Eisenberg I, Grabov-Nardini G, Hochner H et al. (2003) Mutations spectrum of the GNE gene in hereditary inclusion body myopathy sparing the quadriceps. *Hum Mutat* **21**, 99.

24 Broccolini A, Pescatori M, D'Amico A et al. (2002) An Italian family with autosomal recessive inclusion-body myopathy and mutations in the GNE gene. *Neurology* **59**, 1808–1809.

25 Darvish D, Vahedifar P, Huo Y (2002) Four novel mutations associated with autosomal recessive inclusion body myopathy (MIM: 600737). *Mol Gen Metab* **77**, 252–256.

26 Vasconcelos OM, Raju R, Dalakas MC (2002) GNE mutations in an American family with quadriceps-sparing IBM and lack of mutations in s-IBM. *Neurology* **59**, 1776–1779.

27 Del Bo R, Baron P, Prelle A et al. (2003) Novel missense mutation and large deletion of GNE gene in autosomal-recessive inclusion-body myopathy. *Muscle Nerve* **28**, 113–117.

28 Krause S, Schlotter-Weigel B, Walter MC et al. (2003) A novel homozygous missense mutation in the GNE gene in a patient with quadriceps-sparing hereditary inclusion body myopathy associated with muscle inflammation. *Neuromuscl Disord* **13**, 830–834.

29 Broccolini A, Ricci E, Cassandrini D et al. (2004) Novel GNE mutations in Italian families with autosomal recessive hereditary inclusion-body myopathy. *Hum Mutat* **23**, 632.

30 Huizing M, Rakocevic G, Sparks et al. (2004) Hypoglycosylation of alpha-dystroglycan in patients with hereditary IBM due to GNE mutations. *Mol Genet Metab* **81**, 196–202.

31 Ro LS, Lee-Chen GJ, Wu YR et al. (2005) Phenotypic variability in a Chinese family with rimmed vacuolar distal myopathy. *J Neurol Neurosurg Psychiatry*. **76**, 752–755.

32 Sparks S, Rakocevic G, Joe G et al. (2007) Intravenous immune globulin in hereditary inclusion body myopathy: a pilot study. *BMC Neurol* **7**, 3.

33 Malicdan MC, Noguchi S, Hayashi YK et al. (2009) Prophylactic treatment with sialic acid metabolites precludes the development of the myopathic phenotype in the DMRV-hIBM mouse model. *Nat Med* **15**, 690–695.

34 Nemunaitis G, Jay CM, Maples PB et al. (2011) Hereditary inclusion body myopathy: single patient response to intravenous dosing of GNE gene Lipoplex. *Hum Gene Ther* (April 25 Epub ahead of print).

CHAPTER 13

Consequences of the hereditary inclusion-body myopathy-characteristic *GNE* mutations on muscle proteins *in vivo* and *in vitro*

Aldobrando Broccolini and Massimiliano Mirabella
Department of Neuroscience, Catholic University School of Medicine, Rome, Italy

Introduction

Autosomal recessive hereditary inclusion-body myopathy (GNE myopathy, h-IBM; MIM 600737) is due to mutations of the UDP-N-acetylglucosamine-2 epimerase/N-acetylmannosamine kinase (*GNE*) gene [1]. *GNE* codes for a bifunctional enzyme, the UDP-N-acetylglucosamine-2 epimerase/N-acetyl-mannosamine kinase (GNE/MNK), with independent epimerase and kinase activities, that is expressed in different tissues and has a critical role in the biosynthesis of sialic acid. Sialic acid is normally present on the distal ends of *N*- and *O*-glycans and is involved in many biological functions including cellular adhesion, stabilization of glycoprotein structure, and signal transduction [2, 3]. Although mutations of the *GNE* gene responsible for h-IBM result in the reduction of both epimerase and kinase activities [4], the cellular pathogenic cascade responsible for the progressive degeneration of muscle fibers has not been fully elucidated. Moreover, the selective involvement of skeletal muscle is particularly perplexing in consideration of the fact that this tissue expresses relatively low levels of the enzyme in comparison to other tissues, like liver, lung, and kidney [5], that remain unaffected. This suggests the existence of putative susceptibility factors of skeletal muscle to a generalized metabolic impairment.

An object of controversy is whether *GNE* mutations lead to reduced sialylation of muscle glycoproteins and this has a pivotal role in h-IBM pathogenesis. Although numerous lines of evidence corroborate this hypothesis, other investigators believe that hyposialylation of muscle glycoproteins represents only a minor by-product of a metabolic impairment that may instead crucially affect other subcellular compartments. Below are summarized the main experimental data available that support each hypothesis.

GNE mutations result in impaired sialylation of muscle glycoproteins *in vivo* and *in vitro*

It has been shown that two independent lines of Lec3 Chinese hamster ovary cell glycosylation mutants carrying homozygous mutations of the *Gne* gene have a reduced level of cellular sialic acid. This is reflected by a reduced amount of polysialic acid (PSA) on the neural cell adhesion molecule

Muscle Aging, Inclusion-Body Myositis and Myopathies, First Edition. Edited by Valerie Askanas and W. King Engel.
© 2012 Blackwell Publishing Ltd. Published 2012 by Blackwell Publishing Ltd.

(NCAM) [6], a sensitive indicator of any perturbation occurring in the sialic acid metabolic pathway [7, 8]. Coincident throughout this experimental indication is the fact that a transgenic mouse model expressing the human *GNE* gene with the p. D176V mutation on a *Gne*-knockout background is characterized by a reduced level of sialic acid in serum and other tissues and develops a myopathy that resembles h-IBM [9]. Moreover, in this animal model the prophylactic supplementation of sialic acid metabolites prevents the development of the myopathic phenotype [10], thus strengthening the hypothesis that a reduced amount of cellular sialic acid underlies disease pathogenesis. However, to date few clues are available regarding specific proteins or cellular processes whose function becomes impaired following this metabolic defect. Muscle sialoglycoproteins presumed to have a role in h-IBM pathogenesis will be discussed below.

α-Dystroglycan

The identification of a gene defect resulting in impaired production of sialic acid within the cell has initially placed h-IBM in the group of myopathies arising from disturbed glycosylation of muscle glycoproteins such as Fukuyama congenital muscular dystrophy (FCMD) and muscle-eye-brain disease (MEB). These disorders are caused by mutations of specific glycosyltransferases that result in abnormal glycosylation of α-dystroglycan (α-DG) [11]. α-DG is a member of the dystrophin–glycoprotein complex that undergoes post-translational N-linked and O-linked glycosylation and provides a connection between proteins of the extracellular matrix (i.e., laminin, perlecan, neurexin, and agrin) and the cellular cytoskeleton. In particular, sialylated O-linked glycans appear to have a critical role in ligand binding [12]. In FCMD and MEB an abnormally glycosylated α-DG shows a reduced laminin-binding capability and this is likely responsible for the muscle and brain pathology observed in these disorders [11]. Despite an early report showing a reduced glycosylation of α-DG in h-IBM muscle [13], later studies have shown that α-DG is only and inconstantly hyposialylated and, more importantly, its capacity for binding laminin is never hampered [14]. Provided that this functional aspect is crucial in maintaining

cellular homeostasis, we believe that α-DG does not have a relevant role in the pathogenic cascade activated in h-IBM muscle.

NCAM

NCAM is a member of the immunoglobulin superfamily of adhesion molecules and physiologically binds long linear homopolymers of α-2,8-sialic acid residues thus forming PSA-NCAM. In skeletal muscle PSA-NCAM plays a role during muscle-fiber development and regeneration whereas in mature muscle fibers its expression is restricted to the neuromuscular junction (NMJ) [15, 16]. As stated above, NCAM is a sensitive indicator of the level of sialic acid within the cell [7, 8]. Accordingly, in h-IBM muscle we have found that NCAM is consistently hyposialylated and this results in increased electrophoretic mobility of the protein by SDS/PAGE. Indeed, by Western-blot analysis NCAM appears as a sharp band of approximately 130 kDa rather than a broader band with a molecular weight ranging between 150 and 200 kDa as observed in all other myopathies [17]. This abnormality has been confirmed also by other investigators and used to monitor the efficacy of therapeutic attempts aimed to restore the normal level of sialic acid within the muscle of h-IBM patients [18]. The possible pathogenic role of hyposialylated NCAM in h-IBM muscle fibers is not known. PSA-NCAM has a role in NMJ physiology, as mice lacking NCAM show structural and functional abnormalities of the NMJ [16]. *In vitro*, cultured h-IBM myotubes cannot be properly innervated by neurites of rat spinal cord explants thus suggesting a mechanism of "myogenous dysreception to innervation" [19]. It can be speculated that in h-IBM muscle fibers the underlying metabolic defect results in abnormal sialylation of NCAM and therefore in impairment of NMJ, as these fibers are initially properly innervated but later probably lose their contact with the nerve terminal. However, our more recent immunochemical studies (see Plate 13.10; Broccolini and Mirabella, personal observation 2009), using both anti-NCAM and anti-PSA-NCAM antibodies, have shown that in h-IBM muscle the NCAM protein present along the NMJ is normally sialylated (Plate 13.10a,b), whereas the protein expressed by nonregenerating abnormal fibers (which probably represents the majority of NCAM expressed by h-IBM muscle) is not (Plate 13.10c). Likewise, the NCAM that is expressed by the rare regenerating muscle fibers of h-IBM muscle appears to be normally sialylated (Plate 13.10d). The mechanism underlying such difference in sialylation of NCAM within h-IBM muscle needs further explanation. The presence of PSA-NCAM in regenerating h-IBM muscle fibers is in keeping with the fact that primary cultured h-IBM myotubes show NCAM with an apparently normal molecular weight by Western blot and are immunolabeled by both anti-NCAM and anti-PSA-NCAM antibodies (Plate 13.10e,f). This is in agreement with a previous report showing no significant difference in sialic acid content between h-IBM and normal control muscle cells in culture [20].

The significance of this evidence is 2-fold. First, h-IBM muscle is still able to produce some amount of sialic acid but mainly during its developmental/ regenerative stage and, to a lesser extent, in the mature muscle fiber as reflected by the PSA-NCAM that is present postsynaptically at the NMJ. A plausible explanation for such a difference between h-IBM adult muscle and cultured myotubes is that the latter express a higher level of *GNE* mRNA, and possibly of the corresponding protein, that can compensate for the functional impairment of the gene (Broccolini and Mirabella, personal observation 2009). Moreover, it has been shown that *GNE*-defective B-lymphoma cell lines are still capable of synthesizing sialic acid through N-acetylglucosamine kinase (NAGK), which acts as a rescue enzyme phosphorylating *N*-acetylmannosamine in place of N-acetylmannosamine kinase [21]. Similarly to *GNE* mRNA, *NAGK* mRNA expression is higher in aneurally cultured myotubes than in the mature skeletal muscle (Broccolini and Mirabella, personal observation 2009). Therefore the possibility exists that increased *NAGK* can efficiently compensate for deficient *GNE* in h-IBM myotubes, thus warranting a normal level of sialic acid. Of course we cannot rule out the possibility that, within h-IBM myotubes and regenerating muscle fibers, sialic acid is synthesized by other as-yet-unknown metabolic pathway(s) specifically activated in the immature fiber and then progressively shut down

as muscle differentiation progresses. If hyposialylation of glycoproteins indeed plays a role in h-IBM pathophysiology, then to better understand and possibly modulate the molecular mechanism(s) underlying the biosynthesis of sialic acid in cultured myotubes and regenerating muscle fibers would potentially offer a therapeutic avenue for this disorder.

Second, it is advisable to exercise great prudence when analyzing data obtained from h-IBM aneurally cultured muscle cells as possible consequences arising from *GNE* mutations in such an experimental setting do not automatically recapitulate the pathologic changes taking place in the mature h-IBM muscle.

Finally, despite the lack of a conclusive evidence of hyposialylated NCAM playing a role in h-IBM muscle degeneration, such an abnormal level of sialylation of NCAM, as evidenced by Western-blot analysis, can be used as a pre-genetic cellular marker to identify patients with a GNE myopathy in the routine diagnostic workup of muscle biopsy in the laboratory. This can be helpful especially when encountering h-IBM patients with uncommon clinical or pathologic features. Indeed, it has been recently shown that, out of a cohort of 84 patients with an uncharacterized muscle disorder, in three patients the NCAM protein showed increased electrophoretic mobility on Western blot, suggesting its abnormal sialylation. The subsequent genetic study demonstrated that they all carried pathogenic mutations of the *GNE* gene [22].

Neprilysin

h-IBM muscle shares many similarities with that of sporadic inclusion-body myositis (s-IBM), including the abnormal accumulation of amyloid β (Aβ). Accumulated Aβ possibly participates in the pathologic cascade that leads to muscle degeneration, as has been previously demonstrated for s-IBM [23]. However, the functional relationship between *GNE* defects, sialic acid metabolism, and the accumulation of Aβ in h-IBM muscle is still elusive. Very recently, attention has been given to neprilysin, a zinc metallopeptidase known to cleave Aβ at multiple sites [24], that plays a role in the pathogenesis of Alzheimer disease through the regulation of Aβ levels in the brain [25–27]. Neprilysin contains a large amount of sialic acid and changes in the sugar moieties of the protein can affect its stability and enzymatic activity [28, 29]. Interestingly, we have shown that neprilysin is hyposialylated in h-IBM muscle and this is associated with a significant reduction in its expression and enzymatic activity. The link between abnormal sialylation and functional impairment of neprilysin is provided by the evidence that, *in vitro*, the enzymatic removal of sialic acid from glycoproteins of cultured human normal myotubes results in reduced neprilysin activity. This is likely caused by a reduced expression of the protein, secondary to its reduced stability, rather than an impairment of the catalytic properties. Moreover, provided that the experimental desialylation of muscle glycoproteins results in impairment of neprilysin, we have found that this is associated with the appearance of Aβ cytoplasmic inclusions within cultured normal myotubes [30]. We do not know whether this functional defect of neprilysin is in itself sufficient to trigger Aβ accumulation. In fact, h-IBM muscle is also characterized by increased expression of the Aβ precursor protein [31, 32], conceivably promoted by abnormal cellular mechanisms connected with mutations of the *GNE* gene. However, in the complex and still undisclosed abnormal milieu of h-IBM muscle, it is possible that hyposialylated and dysfunctional neprilysin has a role in hampering the cellular Aβ-clearing system, thus contributing to its accumulation within vulnerable fibers. How hyposialylation of neprilysin affects its stability is not known, although interference with the correct processing of the protein in the endoplasmic reticulum (ER), leading to a more rapid degradation, can be hypothesized. In general terms, the possibility exists that, in h-IBM, hyposialylation of glycoproteins may perturb their proper folding and trafficking through the ER and Golgi network and the translocation to the plasma membrane. This would activate a mechanism of ER stress that is intended to manage the accumulation of abnormal proteins [33, 34]. Once ER stress conditions are established, the misfolded and unfolded protein-strapped in the ER are retrotranslocated to the cytoplasm and degraded by either the ubiquitin-proteasome system or the autophagic process [33].

Nevertheless further studies are necessary to verify this hypothesis.

Other possible consequences of h-IBM-associated *GNE* mutations on muscle function outside of the sialic acid biosinthetic pathway

An alternative hypothesis is that *GNE* mutations may significantly affect other cellular mechanisms independent from the synthesis of sialic acid. This has arisen from the recent identification of proteins that physically interact with GNE/MNK or whose expression is modulated by GNE/MNK.

Collapsin response mediator protein 1, promyelocytic leukemia zinc-finger protein, and α-actinin 1: new molecular partners of GNE/MNK

In vitro studies have shown that GNE/MNK is able to interact with factors such as the collapsin response mediator protein 1 and the promyelocytic leukemia zinc-finger protein [35], but none of these molecular partners has been proven so far to be involved in the pathogenic cascade of h-IBM muscle. More recently, GNE/MNK has been demonstrated to physically interact also with α-actinin 1, and these two proteins partially colocalize in the sarcomere of mature muscle fibers. However, *in vitro*, no gross difference has been observed between the interaction of α-actinin 1 with wild-type GNE/MNK and mutated GNE/MNK [36]. Although this line of evidence provides novel interesting clues on additional roles of GNE/MNK outside of the sialic acid biosynthetic pathway, it remains to be determined how even a minor impairment of the interaction between α-actinin 1 and GNE/MNK, as hypothesized in h-IBM, may impact the viability of muscle fibers.

Possible role of mutated GNE/MNK in activating the apoptotic cascade

In h-IBM the terminating cellular process, either necrotic or apoptotic, that is primarily responsible for the progressive reduction of muscle bulk, has not been unequivocally elucidated. Indeed, h-IBM muscle fiber necrosis is an infrequent feature found in association with endomysial inflammation [37], and cellular abnormalities ascribable to the activation of the apoptotic cascade have been described in only an isolated report [38]. Nonetheless, recent studies have pointed out a new and unpredicted role of mutated GNE/MNK in the activation of the apoptotic cascade, mainly based on data arising from *in vitro* analysis. Accordingly, it has been shown that after exposure to staurosporine cultured primary h-IBM muscle cells have increased expression of the active forms of caspase 3 and 9 and diminished phosphorylated Akt [39]. This suggests impairment of the apoptotic cascade and possibly of the insulin-like growth factor-I/Akt signaling pathway.

Mitochondria are considered central players in the apoptotic cascade [40]. Although no major mitochondrial abnormalities have been ever described in h-IBM muscle, a recent study has shown dysregulation of genes involved in various mitochondrial processes, including modulation of apoptosis. In addition, primary h-IBM myoblasts display slightly abnormal mitochondria that appear more branched than in control cells [41]. These mitochondrial abnormalities are different from those observed in s-IBM muscle where cytochrome *c* oxidase-deficient muscle fibers and large-scale mitochondrial DNA deletions are encountered, possibly secondary to Aβ overexpression and increased oxidative stress in the cellular milieu of aged muscle [42–44]. On the contrary, in h-IBM it is not exactly known how mutated GNE/MNK can influence mitochondrial function. A report by Wang and coworkers has convincingly demonstrated that GNE/MNK regulates the expression of the ST3Gal5 and ST8Sia1 sialyltransferases that control the cellular levels of the GM3 and GD3 gangliosides, respectively [45]. Interestingly, GM3 and GD3 gangliosides regulate the mRNA level of BiP, a master regulator protein involved in ER stress that has also a role in diverse cellular processes such as proliferation, senescence and apoptosis [46–48]. GD3 elicits production of reactive oxygen species from complex III of the mitochondrial electron transport chain that leads to the opening of the mitochondrial permeability transition pore and the activation of cytochrome *c*-dependent caspase 3 [49]. Nevertheless, the molecular mechanisms through which GNE/MNK influences the level of expression of GM3 and GD3 gangliosides are not

understood and, more importantly, no studies have been conducted on how this functional relationship becomes modified by mutations of the *GNE* gene.

If future studies prove that GNE/MNK has a role in cellular pathways other than that of sialic acid and possibly more relevant for maintaining skeletal muscle homeostasis, then this will also provide valuable clues to understanding the specific susceptibility of muscle to a generalized metabolic impairment that is peculiar to h-IBM.

References

1 Eisenberg I, Avidan N, Potikha T et al. (2001) The UDP-N-acetylglucosamine 2-epimerase/N-acetylmannosamine kinase gene is mutated in recessive hereditary inclusion body myopathy. *Nat Genet* **29**(1), 83–87.

2 Hinderlich S, Stasche R, Zeitler R, Reutter W. (1997) A bifunctional enzyme catalyzes the first two steps in N-acetylneuraminic acid biosynthesis of rat liver. Purification and characterization of UDP-N-acetylglucosamine 2-epimerase/N-acetylmannosamine kinase. *J Biol Chem* **272**(39), 24313–24318.

3 Keppler OT, Hinderlich S, Langner J et al. (1999) UDP-GlcNAc 2-epimerase: a regulator of cell surface sialylation. *Science* **284**(5418), 1372–1376.

4 Penner J, Mantey LR, Elgavish S et al. (2006) Influence of UDP-GlcNAc 2-epimerase/ManNAc kinase mutant proteins on hereditary inclusion body myopathy. *Biochemistry* **45**(9), 2968–2977.

5 Horstkorte R, Nohring S, Wiechens N et al. (1999) Tissue expression and amino acid sequence of murine UDP-N-acetylglucosamine-2-epimerase/N-acetylmannosamine kinase. *Eur J Biochem* **260**(3), 923–927.

6 Hong Y, Stanley P. (2003) Lec3 Chinese hamster ovary mutants lack UDP-N-acetylglucosamine 2-epimerase activity because of mutations in the epimerase domain of the Gne gene. *J Biol Chem* **278**(52), 53045–53054.

7 Bork K, Reutter W, Gerardy-Schahn R, Horstkorte R. (2005) The intracellular concentration of sialic acid regulates the polysialylation of the neural cell adhesion molecule. *FEBS Lett* **579**(22), 5079–5083.

8 Gagiannis D, Orthmann A, Danssmann I et al. (2007) Reduced sialylation status in UDP-N-acetylglucosamine-2-epimerase/N-acetylmannosamine kinase (GNE)-deficient mice. *Glycoconj J* **24**(2–3) 125–130.

9 Malicdan MC, Noguchi S, Nonaka I et al. (2007) A Gne knockout mouse expressing human GNE D176V mutation develops features similar to distal myopathy with rimmed vacuoles or hereditary inclusion body myopathy. *Hum Mol Genet* **16**(22), 2669–2682.

10 Malicdan MC, Noguchi S, Hayashi YK et al. (2009) Prophylactic treatment with sialic acid metabolites precludes the development of the myopathic phenotype in the DMRV-hIBM mouse model. *Nat Med* **15**(6), 690–695.

11 Michele DE, Barresi R, Kanagawa M et al. (2002) Post-translational disruption of dystroglycan-ligand interactions in congenital muscular dystrophies. *Nature* **418** (6896), 417–422.

12 Michele DE, Campbell KP. (2003) Dystrophin-glycoprotein complex: post-translational processing and dystroglycan function. *J Biol Chem* **278**(18), 15457–15460.

13 Huizing M, Rakocevic G, Sparks SE et al. (2004) Hypoglycosylation of alpha-dystroglycan in patients with hereditary IBM due to GNE mutations. *Mol Genet Metab* **81**(3), 196–202.

14 Broccolini A, Gliubizzi C, Pavoni E et al. (2005) alpha-Dystroglycan does not play a major pathogenic role in autosomal recessive hereditary inclusion-body myopathy. *Neuromuscul Disord* **15**(2), 177–184.

15 Rafuse VF, Landmesser L. (1996) Contractile activity regulates isoform expression and polysialylation of NCAM in cultured myotubes: involvement of Ca^{2+} and protein kinase C. *J Cell Biol* **132**(5), 969–983.

16 Rafuse VF, Polo-Parada L, Landmesser LT. (2000) Structural and functional alterations of neuromuscular junctions in NCAM-deficient mice. *J Neurosci* **20** (17), 6529–6539.

17 Ricci E, Broccolini A, Gidaro T et al. (2006) NCAM is hyposialylated in hereditary inclusion body myopathy due to GNE mutations. *Neurology* **66**(5), 755–758.

18 Sparks S, Rakocevic G, Joe G et al. (2007) Intravenous immune globulin in hereditary inclusion body myopathy: a pilot study. *BMC Neurol* **7**, 3.

19 McFerrin J, Engel WK, Askanas V. (1998) Impaired innervation of cultured human muscle overexpressing betaAPP experimentally and genetically: relevance to inclusion-body myopathies. *Neuroreport* **9** (14), 3201–3205.

20 Salama I, Hinderlich S, Shlomai Z et al. (2005) No overall hyposialylation in hereditary inclusion body myopathy myoblasts carrying the homozygous M712T GNE mutation. *Biochem Biophys Res Commun* **328**(1), 221–226.

21 Hinderlich S, Berger M, Keppler OT et al. (2001) Biosynthesis of N-acetylneuraminic acid in cells lacking UDP-N-acetylglucosamine 2-epimerase/N-acetylmannosamine kinase. *Biol Chem* **382**(2), 291–297.

22 Broccolini A, Gidaro T, Tasca G et al. (2010) Analysis of NCAM helps identify unusual phenotypes of hereditary inclusion-body myopathy. *Neurology* **75**(3), 265–272.

23 Askanas V, Engel WK. (2002) Inclusion-body myositis and myopathies: different etiologies, possibly similar pathogenic mechanisms. *Curr Opin Neurol* **15**(5), 525–531.

24 Howell S, Nalbantoglu J, Crine P. (1995) Neutral endopeptidase can hydrolyze beta-amyloid(1–40) but shows no effect on beta-amyloid precursor protein metabolism. *Peptides* **16**(4), 647–652.

25 Akiyama H, Kondo H, Ikeda K et al. (2001) Immunohistochemical localization of neprilysin in the human cerebral cortex: inverse association with vulnerability to amyloid beta-protein (Abeta) deposition. *Brain Res* **902**(2), 277–281.

26 Iwata N, Tsubuki S, Takaki Y et al. (2001) Metabolic regulation of brain Abeta by neprilysin. *Science* **292** (5521), 1550–1552.

27 Leissring MA, Farris W, Chang AY et al. (2003) Enhanced proteolysis of beta-amyloid in APP transgenic mice prevents plaque formation, secondary pathology, and premature death. *Neuron* **40**(6), 1087–1093.

28 Johnson AR, Skidgel RA, Gafford JT, Erdos EG. (1984) Enzymes in placental microvilli: angiotensin I converting enzyme, angiotensinase A, carboxypeptidase, and neutral endopeptidase ("enkephalinase"). *Peptides* **5**(4), 789–796.

29 Lafrance MH, Vezina C, Wang Q et al. (1994) Role of glycosylation in transport and enzymic activity of neutral endopeptidase-24.11. *Biochem J* **302**(2), 451–454.

30 Broccolini A, Gidaro T, De Cristofaro R et al. (2008) Hyposialylation of neprilysin possibly affects its expression and enzymatic activity in hereditary inclusion-body myopathy muscle. *J Neurochem* **105** (3), 971–981.

31 Askanas V, Engel WK, Alvarez RB. (1992) Light and electron microscopic localization of beta-amyloid protein in muscle biopsies of patients with inclusion-body myositis. *Am J Pathol* **141**(1), 31–36.

32 Sarkozi E, Askanas V, Johnson SA et al. (1993) beta-Amyloid precursor protein mRNA is increased in inclusion-body myositis muscle. *Neuroreport* **4**(6), 815–818.

33 Ding WX, Ni HM, Gao W et al. (2007) Linking of autophagy to ubiquitin-proteasome system is important for the regulation of endoplasmic reticulum stress and cell viability. *Am J Pathol* **171**(2), 513–524.

34 Ni M, Lee AS. (2007) ER chaperones in mammalian development and human diseases. *FEBS Lett* **581**(19), 3641–3651.

35 Weidemann W, Stelzl U, Lisewski U et al. (2006) The collapsin response mediator protein 1 (CRMP-1) and the promyelocytic leukemia zinc finger protein (PLZF) bind to UDP-N-acetylglucosamine 2-epimerase/N-acetylmannosamine kinase (GNE), the key enzyme of sialic acid biosynthesis. *FEBS Lett* **580**(28–29) 6649–6654.

36 Amsili S, Zer H, Hinderlich S et al. (2008) UDP-N-acetylglucosamine 2-epimerase/N-acetylmannosamine kinase (GNE) binds to alpha-actinin 1: novel pathways in skeletal muscle? *PLoS One* **3**(6), e2477.

37 Motozaki Y, Komai K, Hirohata M et al. (2007) Hereditary inclusion body myopathy with a novel mutation in the GNE gene associated with proximal leg weakness and necrotizing myopathy. *Eur J Neurol* **14**(9): e14–5.

38 Yan C, Ikezoe K, Nonaka I. (2001) Apoptotic muscle fiber degeneration in distal myopathy with rimmed vacuoles. *Acta Neuropathol* **101**(1), 9–16.

39 Amsili S, Shlomai Z, Levitzki R et al. (2007) Characterization of hereditary inclusion body myopathy myoblasts: possible primary impairment of apoptotic events. *Cell Death Differ* **14**, 1916–1924.

40 Wasilewski M, Scorrano L. (2009) The changing shape of mitochondrial apoptosis. *Trends Endocrinol Metab* **20**(6), 287–294.

41 Eisenberg I, Novershtern N, Itzhaki Z et al. (2008) Mitochondrial processes are impaired in hereditary inclusion body myopathy. *Hum Mol Genet* **17**(23), 3663–3674.

42 Askanas V, McFerrin J, Baque S et al. (1996) Transfer of beta-amyloid precursor protein gene using adenovirus vector causes mitochondrial abnormalities in cultured normal human muscle. *Proc Natl Acad Sci USA* **93**(3), 1314–1319.

43 Moslemi AR, Lindberg C, Oldfors A. (1997) Analysis of multiple mitochondrial DNA deletions in inclusion body myositis. *Hum Mutat* **10**(5), 381–386.

44 Oldfors A, Larsson NG, Lindberg C, Holme E. (1993) Mitochondrial DNA deletions in inclusion body myositis. *Brain* **116**(2), 325–336.

45 Wang Z, Sun Z, Li AV, Yarema KJ. (2006) Roles for UDP-GlcNAc 2-epimerase/ManNAc 6-kinase outside of sialic acid biosynthesis: modulation of sialyltransferase and BiP expression, GM3 and GD3 biosynthesis, proliferation, and apoptosis, and ERK1/2 phosphorylation. *J Biol Chem* **281**(37), 27016–27028.

46 Malisan F, Testi R. (2005) The ganglioside GD3 as the Greek goddess Hecate: several faces turned towards as many directions. *IUBMB Life* **57**(7), 477–482.

47 Pilkington GJ. (2005) Cancer stem cells in the mammalian central nervous system. *Cell Prolif* **38**(6), 423–433.

48 Tessitore A, del Pilar Martin M, Sano R et al. (2004) GM1-ganglioside-mediated activation of the unfolded protein response causes neuronal death in a neurodegenerative gangliosidosis. *Mol Cell* **15**(5), 753–766.

49 Garcia-Ruiz C, Colell A, Paris R, Fernandez-Checa JC. (2000) Direct interaction of GD3 ganglioside with mitochondria generates reactive oxygen species followed by mitochondrial permeability transition, cytochrome c release, and caspase activation. *FASEB J* **14**(7), 847–858.

CHAPTER 14

Function and structure of *VCP* mutations leading to inclusion-body myopathy associated with Paget disease of bone and frontotemporal dementia

Cezary Wójcik

Department of Anatomy and Cell Biology, Indiana University School of Medicine Evansville Center for Medical Education Evansville, IN, USA

Introduction

Autosomal dominant inclusion-body myopathy associated with Paget disease of bone and frontotemporal dementia (IBMPFD) is a multisystem disorder caused by missense mutations of the valosin-containing protein (*VCP*/p97) gene on chromosome 9p13.3 (OMIM 167320) [1, 2]. IBMPFD is characterized by a triad of: (a) inclusion-body myopathy (IBM), which clinically presents as a progressive proximal myopathy; (b) Paget disease of bone; and (c) premature frontotemporal dementia (FTD) with neuronal nuclear inclusions containing ubiquitin, VCP, and TAR DNA-binding protein 43 (TDP-43) [3–6]. However, only a minority of patients (12%) show the complete triad of symptoms [1, 6], whereas some patients manifest additional symptoms such as dilated cardiomyopathy with heart failure [7, 8], hepatic fibrosis, or cataracts [9].

Endoplasmic reticulum, endoplasmic reticulum-associated degradation, and the unfolded protein response

VCP was originally purified as a major ATPase associated with endoplasmic reticulum (ER)-derived microsomes, but is also ubiquitous in the cytoplasm and the nucleus [10–12]. The ER comprises about half of the total membrane area and one-third of the newly translated proteins in a typical eukaryotic cell [13, 14]. Professional secretory cells synthesize 13 million secretory proteins per minute in a crowded environment where ER protein concentrations reach 100 mg/mL [15]. After cotranslational insertion into the ER, new proteins undergo folding, assembly, and post-translational modifications, which are scrutinized by a rigorous quality-control mechanism [16]. Misfolded proteins which fail to

Muscle Aging, Inclusion-Body Myositis and Myopathies, First Edition. Edited by Valerie Askanas and W. King Engel.
© 2012 Blackwell Publishing Ltd. Published 2012 by Blackwell Publishing Ltd.

refold properly are retrotranslocated to the cytosol where they undergo degradation mediated by the ubiquitin-proteasome system (UPS), a process known as ER-associated degradation (ERAD) [16–20]. Besides its quality-control function, ERAD is also exploited in the regulated degradation of properly folded proteins, such as 3-hydroxy-3-methyl-glutaryl-CoA reductase (HMG-CoA reductase) and inositol trisphosphate (IP3) receptors [21, 22]. An increase in protein misfolding within the ER leads to an integrated cellular response, which involves translational attenuation, decreasing the input of new proteins, followed by a transcriptional reaction known as the unfolded protein response (UPR) [23–26]. UPR leads to the upregulation of multiple proteins, including components of ERAD, which counteract at different levels the ER dysfunction caused by protein misfolding. Thus, UPR is an adaptive mechanism which promotes survival. However, prolonged UPR activation eventually triggers apoptosis [14, 15].

Structure and function of VCP

VCP is an abundant and highly conserved ATPase of the AAA family which is essential in yeast, *Drosophila*, and mice [27–29]. It was originally isolated as a factor necessary for the homotypic fusion between membranes of the ER and mitotic Golgi fragments [12, 30–32]. Later it was implicated in UPS-dependent degradation of cytosolic proteins [33–36], ERAD [21, 22, 37, 38], regulated ubiquitin-dependent processing [39, 40], mitotic spindle disassembly [36, 41], replication, and nucleotide excision repair [42, 43], as well as autophagosome maturation [44].

VCP has two adjacent D1 and D2 AAA domains assembling into a hexameric ring [45–47], with the N-terminal domains of the individual subunits free to interact with multiple proteins [48, 49]. Among the more than 30 known proteins which interact with VCP the Ufd1-Npl4 dimer is of particular importance, forming a stable $VCP^{Ufd1-Npl4}$ complex involved in UPS-dependent protein degradation [35, 50–53]. $VCP^{Ufd1-Npl4}$ is involved in recovery of oligo-ubiquitinated substrates, promotion of the

extension of their polyubiquitin chain by the activity of an associated E4 (Ufd2), and then finally transfer of those substrates to Rad23, which delivers them to the 26S proteasome for final degradation [54, 55].

While the role of yeast Cdc48, Ufd1, and Npl4 in ERAD is well established, implication of mammalian $VCP^{Ufd1-Npl4}$ complex in ERAD is based mostly upon reconstitution experiments, with dominant negative VCP mutants inhibiting ERAD of a model quality-control substrate in permeabilized cells [17, 52, 56, 57]. In contrast, more solid evidence exists for the involvement of VCP in the regulated degradation of properly folded ER proteins, such as IP3 receptors upon binding of IP3 [22] and HMG-CoA reductase in the presence of abundant cholesterol [21]. The role of VCP in ERAD is supported by the fact that it interacts with multiple proteins involved in ERAD, including ubiquitin ligases gp78 and HRD1, peptide N-glycanase, and Rad23 [38, 55, 58–61]. RNA interference (RNAi) of VCP, Ufd1, and Npl4 induces accumulation of polyubiquitinated proteins in form of multiple dispersed cytosolic ubiquitin-positive aggregates [36, 62–64]. Moreover, VCP, Ufd1, and Npl4 are required for aggresome formation [36, 65, 66]. Overexpression of dominant negative ATPase mutants of VCP [67, 68] or RNAi of VCP [36, 64] induces formation of ER-derived vacuoles, a process which is enhanced by proteasome inhibition. RNAi of Ufd1 and Npl4 does not induce vacuole formation indicating that this function does not require the $VCP^{Ufd1-Npl4}$ complex [36, 64, 65]. VCP also appears to be involved in the control of protein glycosylation within the ER [69].

The $VCP^{Ufd1-Npl4}$ complex is recruited to the ER membrane through interactions with VCP-interacting membrane protein (VIMP) and derlin-1[38, 57, 70]. While this final stage seems to be common to all substrates, mechanistic differences exist on earlier stages, where ERAD-C, ERAD-M, and ERAD-L is distinguished depending upon the location where the misfolded domain of an ERAD substrate is located: cytosol, the ER membrane, or the ER lumen [71–74]. Retrotranslocation may be mediated through the Sec61 translocon [73, 75] or a novel derlin-1 protein channel [38, 57, 70], while tail-anchored ER proteins may be removed from the membrane directly by the proteasome [75].

Despite the elegance and simplicity of this model derived mostly from studies in yeast, it is known that not all ERAD is UPS-dependent [20, 76, 77]. Even when UPS is involved, ERAD does not always require VCP$^{Ufd1-Npl4}$. While yeast Cdc48, Ufd1, and Npl4 mutants are defective in ERAD and accumulate polyubiquitinated substrates in association with the ER [53, 56, 78–80], even in yeast some substrates are extracted from the ER and degraded without those factors [81, 82]. In mammalian cells the situation is far more complex, since VCP mediates the retrotranslocation of some but not all ERAD substrates, while Ufd1-Npl4 appears to delay retrotranslocation [64, 65]. Moreover, 26S proteasomes bind directly to the retrotranslocation channel formed by Sec61 [83] and are recruited to ER membranes after ER stress [84], most likely directly interacting with the emerging polypeptides [85]. The A1 chain of cholera toxin is known to exploit the ERAD pathway to reach the cytosol [86]; however, VCP does not appear to be required for this process [87, 88]. The extrapolation of the yeast model to mammalian cells was made mostly based on the requirement of VCP for the degradation of a single substrate – the major histocompatibility complex (MHC) class I heavy chain – in permeabilized cells expressing the US11 protein of the cytomegalovirus (CMV) [52, 56, 57]. This is hardly a physiological situation, since the degradation of MHC class I heavy chains relies on viral proteins the expression of which induces UPR [89].

There is reason to believe that the role played by mammalian homologs is quite different from yeast Cdc48p, Ufd1p, and Npl4p. VCP and Cdc48 are 71% identical but VCP fails to rescue yeast *Cdc48* mutations [90], and in mammalian cells, contrary to yeast, an impairment of the VCP ATPase activity reduces the size of polyubiquitin chains synthesized on the MHC class I heavy chains [56].

Ufd1-Npl4 probably performs a regulatory function, preventing the premature retrotranslocation of emerging proteins and their delivery to the 26S proteasome [65, 88, 91]. This is similar to the role of Rad23, another polyubiquitin-binding protein involved in ERAD [55, 92, 93]. Following retrotranslocation most ERAD substrates are normally degraded locally by ER-recruited proteasomes, while heavily misfolded proteins which "choke" proteasomes are delivered by a microtubule-dependent mechanism to a specialized area around the centrosome, called the proteolytic center of the cell [94, 95]. When proteasome activity is inhibited all substrates are diverted to this pathway, forming aggresomes [94–97]. VCP interacts with Ufd1-Npl4 at a later stage following retrotranslocation, securing the delivery of ERAD substrates to the proteolytic center of the cell. Therefore cells deficient in components of the VCP$^{Ufd1-Npl4}$ complex form dispersed aggregates of ubiquitinated proteins rather than single aggresomes at the proteolytic center [36, 65]. Overexpression of two different VCP mutants associated with IBMPFD (R155H and A232E) impairs the degradation of cotransfected ΔF508-CFTR, a polytopic membrane protein mutated in cystic fibrosis, which is degraded by the ERAD pathway. However, at the same time there is a global impairment of the UPS as evidenced by accumulation of polyubiquitinated proteins. Moreover, cystic fibrosis transmembrane conductance regulator (CFTR) is a heavily glycosylated protein and observed changes in its levels may have been secondary to VCP's role in protein glycosylation [2].

Involvement of VCP in human disease

The importance of VCP is highlighted by the fact that its levels and activity must be tightly regulated in order to maintain proper homeostasis. Any departure from the physiological status quo results in pathology. Therefore, increased VCP expression and/or activity is associated with cancer, while impaired VCP function is associated with neurodegenerative disorders. VCP has prosurvival and anti-apoptotic functions which depend on the activation of prosurvival Akt and nuclear factor κB (NFκB) pathways; therefore, loss of function or depletion of VCP triggers apoptosis [36, 64, 65, 68, 98, 99]. However, VCP may also promote apoptosis induced by ER stress [100] and overexpression of poly-Q proteins [101], which may depend on its role in the processing of caspases [99].

Overexpression and increased activity of VCP is associated with poor prognosis in several types of human cancer, including esophageal squamous cell carcinoma [102], non-small-cell lung carcinoma [103], pancreatic ductal adenocarcinoma [104], colorectal adenocarcinoma [105], gastric carcinoma [106], and hepatocellular carcinoma [107]. Poor prognosis in cancer is also associated with increased expression of the gp78 ER-anchored Ubiquitin [108, 109], which directly interacts with VCP [110]. It is likely that upregulation of VCP increases the resistance of cancer cells to ER stress [111]; therefore, development of potential inhibitors of VCP is of great interest for cancer therapy [112].

VCP also plays an important role in the pathogenesis of neurodegenerative diseases. VCP has been observed in ubiquitin-positive intraneuronal inclusions found in common neurodegenerative diseases such as Parkinson disease, Huntington disease, and amyotrophic lateral sclerosis (ALS) [62, 67, 113]. Such inclusions are often regarded as signs of "intracellular indigestion" that is associated with impaired UPS function and can be modeled by protein aggregates induced with proteasome inhibitors or "aggresomes" [94, 96, 114]. While there is some controversy over whether VCP is actually recruited to aggresomes, it is required for efficient aggresome formation [36, 66, 68]. Expression of several pathologic VCP mutants promoted formation of aggregates in cells co-expressing polyglutamine proteins as well as cells treated with proteasome inhibitors [2, 115]. Overexpression of VCP protects the cells against the formation of discrete cytoplasmic aggregates of misfolded proteins [116], while in another system it is associated with a worsening of the neurodegenerative phonotype [101]. The C-terminal tail of VCP interacts with histone deacetylase HDAC6, a mediator for aggresome formation, suggesting that VCP participates in transporting ubiquitinated proteins to aggresomes. This function of VCP is impaired by inhibition of the deacetylase activity of HDAC6 or by overexpression of VCP mutants that do not bind ubiquitinated proteins or HDAC6 [117]. VCP prevents protein aggregation *in vitro* and *in vivo*, mainly through the D1 and D2 domains of VCP [66, 118].

Whenever the UPS is inhibited and aggresomes form at the proteolytic center, they can no longer be removed by the UPS even if proteasome inhibitors are removed. Instead, formation of autophagosomes engulfing dense protein aggregates is observed [94]. Indeed, a recent work has confirmed those early findings, showing that accumulation of polyubiquitin chains constitutes a signal triggering the formation of autophagosomal vacuoles [119]. VCP deficiency by RNAi-mediated knockdown or overexpression of disease-associated VCP mutants (R155H and A232E) VCP results in significant accumulation of immature autophagic vesicles, some of which are abnormally large, acidified, and exhibit cathepsin B activity. VCP was found to be essential to autophagosome maturation under basal conditions and in cells challenged by proteasome inhibition, but not in cells challenged by starvation, suggesting that VCP might be selectively required for autophagic degradation of ubiquitinated substrates. Indeed, a high percentage of the accumulated autophagic vesicles have ubiquitin-positive contents, a feature that is not observed in autophagic vesicles that accumulate following starvation or treatment with bafilomycin A. Finally, we show accumulation of numerous, large lysosomal-associated membrane protein (LAMP)-1- and LAMP-2-positive vacuoles and accumulation of LC3-II in myoblasts derived from patients with IBMPFD. We conclude that VCP is essential for maturation of ubiquitin-containing autophagosomes and that defect in this function may contribute to IBMPFD pathogenesis [44].

VCP mutations associated with IBMPFD

There is no evidence that common variants in VCP confer a strong risk to the development of sporadic FTD [120] or Paget disease of the bone in the absence of myopathy and dementia [121]. Multiple *VCP* mutations associated with IBMPFD have been described. In the first study linking them to IBMPFD six different *VCP* mutations (R155H, R155P, R155C, A232E, R95G, and R191Q) were found in 13 different families [1, 5]. Since then, multiple mutations of the *VCP* gene have been described, most of them affecting the N-terminal region of the CDC48 domain, which is involved in ubiquitin binding, for example: R155C [122, 123], R93C, R155C [9], R159H [124], G157R [125], N387H, L198W [126], R93C [127], and R159C [128]. *VCP* mutations are clustered mostly in exon 5 of the *VCP* gene. They are associated with interfamilial and intrafamilial? variability in terms of severity, distribution of weakness and presence or not of Paget disease or cognitive impairment [127]. The penetrance of the *VCP* mutations is estimated to be 82% for myopathy, 49% for Paget disease, and 30% for frontotemporal dementia [129]. Only a minority of patients (12%) show the complete triad of IBMFD symptoms [1, 6]. It is therefore likely that some mutations affect more one aspect of VCP function than another, which translates into different, yet often overlapping, sets of clinical symptoms [9]. Moreover, other genes could account for decreased penetrance in some cases of the same mutation [130], as has been observed for APOE 4 [129].

Mice expressing mutant *VCP* (R155H or A232E) in all tissues develop pathology that is limited to muscle, brain, and bone, recapitulating the spectrum of disease in humans with IBMPFD. The mice exhibit progressive muscle weakness with IBM including rimmed vacuoles and TDP-43 pathology. The mice exhibit abnormalities in behavioral testing and pathological examination of the brain shows widespread TDP-43 pathology. Furthermore, radiological examination of the skeleton reveals that mutant mice develop severe osteopenia accompanied by focal lytic and sclerotic lesions [131].

Molecular and cellular effects of IBM-associated *VCP* mutations

Based on the known role of VCP in different cell signaling pathways, pathogenesis of each of the major IBMFD symptoms can be analyzed separately. Glutathione S-transferase pull-down experiments showed that all three pathologic *VCP* mutations tested do not affect the binding to Ufd1, Npl4, and ataxin-3 [7]. Moreover, mutated VCPs have preserved ATPase activities as well as elevated binding affinities not only for those VCP cofactors, but also for ubiquitinated proteins [115]. Structural analysis demonstrated that both arginine residues which are

most often mutated (R93 and R155) are both surface-accessible residues located in the center of cavities that may enable ligand binding. Mutations at R93 and R155 are predicted to induce changes in the tertiary structure of the VCP protein. The search for putative ligands to the R93 and R155 cavities identified cyclic sugar compounds with high binding scores [7]. Moreover, depletion of cellular VCP by RNAi significantly alters the profile of N-linked oligosaccharides, further implying this protein in regulation of glycans [69]. Indeed, lysosomal membrane proteins LAMP-1 and LAMP-2 show increased molecular weights in myoblasts from IBMPFD patients due to differential *N*-glycosylation [132]. It remains to be tested how the differential glycosylation patterns of multiple membrane-associated proteins affect their functions contributing to the pathology of IBMPFD.

Expression of several pathologic VCP mutants promoted formation of aggregates in cells coexpressing polyglutamine proteins as well as cells treated with proteasome inhibitors [115]. These findings indicate that the molecular mechanism leading to pathology associated with VCP mutations may involve increased propensity to aggregate formation. Therefore, decreasing aggregate formation-promoting activities and/or increasing unfoldase activities could be of significance for the treatment of IBMPFD [115]. The alteration of cellular processes by mutant VCP is relatively subtle, since it only occurs in postmitotic cells such as neurons and cardiomyocytes, taking many years to develop a phenotype. There is no evidence of any protein aggregates in actively dividing cells of the same paients nor in stably transfected cell lines [7].

Effect on the bone

Mutations that predispose individuals to Paget disease of bone have been identified in four genes related to the RANKL/OPG/RANK/NF-κB signaling pathway including VCP [133]. Upon binding of the receptor activator of NFκB ligand (RANK) ligand produced by osteoblasts to the RANK receptor expressed by osteoclast precursors, a signal transduction cascade is activated which ultimately leads to formation and activation of osteoclasts, and therefore to increased bone resorption. This signaling pathway involves different branches of the UPS [134]. It involves the formation of Lys-63-linked polyubiquitin chains on TRAF6, which are necessary for the recruitment of subsequent factors such as the zinc-finger domain of TAB2 to the complex, necessary for the activation of the TAK1 kinase. Subsequently, TAK1 activates downstream kinases to activate the transcription factor NF-κB. NF-κB is normally inactive by being associated with inhibitory proteins of the inhibitory κB (IκB) family which obliterate the nuclear localization sequence (NLS) of this transcription factor, preventing its transloction to the nucleus. Activation of NF-κB is caused by IκB polyubiquitination, followed by VCP-mediated extraction of polyubiquitinated IκB and its delivery to the 26S proteasome for degradation. Released NF-κB then translocates to the nucleus and initiates the transcription of genes involved in osteoclast activity. VCP has a known role in mediating the degradation of IκBa by the ubiquitin-proteasome pathway [135]. Expression of two different mutant VCPs (R155H or A232E) in transgenic mice leads to increased degradation of IκB and therefore to increased NF-κB activation [131]. However, there is no association between common VCP varaints with sporadic Paget disease of the bone in the absence of myopathy and dementia [121].

Effects on the central nervous system

Expression of several pathologic VCP mutants promoted formation of aggregates in cells coexpressing polyglutamine proteins as well as cells treated with proteasome inhibitors [115]. In the central nervous system IBMPFD is characterized by frontal and temporal lobar atrophy, neuron loss and gliosis, and ubiquitin-positive inclusions, which are distinct from those seen in other sporadic and familial cases of frontotemporal lobal dementia [136]. Formation of such ubiquitin-positive inclusions is a hallmark of neurodegeneration found in different spontaneous and hereditary neurodegenerative disorders, which results from concerted impairment of the UPS [114] and autophagy [137] and leads to cell loss by apoptosis [138].

Ubiquitinated inclusions colocalized with accumulations of TDP-43 in both intranuclear inclusions and dystrophic neuritis from IBMPFD patients sug-gesting that a dominant negative loss or alteration of VCP function results in impaired degradation of TDP-43 [139]. The formation of intraneuronal TDP-43-containing inclusions is the common link between neuronal changes seen in IBMPFD and sporadic ALS, sporadic frontotemporal lobar dementia, and most familial forms of frontotemporal lobar dementia [136, 139, 140]. TDP-43 is a highly conserved, ubiquitously expressed protein, predominantly localized to the nucleus under normal conditions, which participates in transcription, splicing regulation, microRNA biogenesis, apoptosis, cell division, mRNA stabilization, and regulation of neuronal plasticity by acting as a neuronal activity response factor. It undergoes dramatic changes in subcellular distribution from the nucleus to the cytoplasm in affected cells in FTD, ALS, and IBMPFD. However, the exact mechanism of how this leads to pathology remains unknown [141]. Clearence of cellular TDP-43 requires a concerted action of both the UPS and the autophagic pathway [140].

Effects on muscle

The UPS is involved in the degradation of myofibrillar proteins, especially during muscle atrophy associated with states as different as denervation, sepsis, uremia, congestive heart failure, and cachexia associated with cancer. While each of these pathological conditions involves the induction of a slightly different set of genes, they all induce of common set of genes known as atrogenes, which include components of the UPS such as different ubiquitin ligases [142–144]. However, VCP and its direct interactors are not among those atrogenes. Therefore, the role of VCP in degradation of structural proteins in the skeletal muscle remains unknown. It is reasonable to assume that in myofibers VCP also participates in ERAD, which has a very specific function in muscles due to the spatial architecture of the sarcoplasmic reticulum. Pathogenic *VCP* mutations lead to the accumulation of ubiquitinated inclusions and protein aggregates in samples of patient muscle, as well as in muscle from transgenic animals. Formation of those aggresome-like inclusions is most likely a protective mechanism from direct toxic effects of soluble species of misfolded proteins. Nevertheless, mutant VCP may disrupt normal homeostasis through its effect on the structure and function of the sarcoplasmic reticulum, through decreased activity of the UPS by recruitment of its components into aggresomes, and/or by impaired degradation of specific regulatory proteins, resulting in degeneration of skeletal muscle [6].

Expression of several pathologic *VCP* mutants promoted formation of aggregates in cells coexpressing polyglutamine proteins as well as cells treated with proteasome inhibitors [115].

In an animal model of transgenic mice expressing VCP with the R155H mutation under a muscle-specific promoter an increase in the levels of polyubiquitinated proteins and formation of aggresomes preceded the onset of structural changes and measurable associated muscle weakness [145]. Moreover, increasing weakness was paralleled by increased levels of polyubiquitin conjugates. At the same time myofibers displayed vacuolation and disorganized membrane morphology with reduced caveolin-3 expression at the sarcolemma [145]. Similar to the changes found in neurons from patients with IBMPFD, in myofibers the TDP-43 nuclear staining is decreased, while it appears recruited to sarcoplasmic ubiquitinated inclusions [146]. Decreased nuclear content of TDP-43 may alter microRNA, contributing to the pathology [147].

These changes resembled those found in samples of human skeletal muscle from IBMPFD patients bearing three different VCP mutations (R93C, R155H, and R155C). They all had degenerative changes and filamentous VCP- and ubiquitin-positive cytoplasmic and nuclear protein aggregates. Mutant *VCP* leads to a novel form of dilatative cardiomyopathy with inclusion bodies. In contrast to postmitotic striated muscle cells and neurons of IBMPFD patients, evidence of protein aggregate pathology was not detected in primary IBMPFD myoblasts or in transient and stable transfected cells using wild-type VCP and R93C-, R155H-, R155C-VCP mutants. Glutathione S-transferase pull-down experiments showed that all three *VCP* mutations did not affect binding to Ufd1, Npl4, and ataxin-3 [7].

Myoblasts derived from patients with IBMPFD accumulate numerous, large LAMP-1- and LAMP-2-positive vacuoles containing ubiquitin-positive material consistent with immature autophago-

somes. Mutant VCP thus dysregulates autophagy of aggresome-like material in myofibers resulting in the observed pathology. This dysregulation may result from its impaired role in the processing of *N*-glycosylated proteins, since both LAMP-1 and LAMP-2 are hyperglycosylated under those conditions [44, 132]. This further supports the role of VCP in the glycosylation of proteins in the ER [69]. Autophagy is required for cellular survival and for the clearance of damaged proteins and altered organelles. Excessive autophagy activation contributes to muscle loss in different catabolic conditions. However, muscle-specific Atg7-null mice that are deficient in basal autophagy display muscle atrophy, weakness, and features of myofiber degeneration including formation of protein aggregates, abnormal mitochondria, accumulation of membrane bodies, sarcoplasmic reticulum distension, vacuolization, oxidative stress, and apoptosis [148]. All these features strikingly resemble the phenotype observed in mice overexpressing the mutant *VCP* in skeletal muscle, suggesting that impairment of autophagy due to mutant *VCP* may be the main cause of skeletal-muscle pathology in IBMFD patients.

Conclusions and perspectives

Since one of the best studied roles of VCP is its involvement in ERAD, it has been proposed that mutant VCP impairs degradation of proteins extracted from the ER, causing the observed pathology. Indeed, markers of ER stress and impaired ERAD have been reported in cells expressing mutant *VCP* [2, 136]. However, neither patients with IBMPFD nor transgenic mice expressing mutant *VCP* have any pathology involving β cells of the pancreas, B-lymphocytes, or other cell types sensitive to ER stress [6, 131]. This strongly argues against a major role of impaired ERAD in IBMPDFTD pathology. The triad of symptoms observed in patients with IBMPFD can be explained by the selective derangement of the role played by VCP in other biological pathways. Paget disease of the bone results from dysregulation of the RANKL/RANK/NFκB signaling pathway, likely due to increased NFκB activation. Both IBM and frontotemporal dementia result from cell degeneration and death secondary to deficient targeting of polyubiquitinated aggregates of proteins or aggresomes in myofibers to the autophagic vacuoles, which probably results from an altered pattern of protein glycosylation and deficient binding of mutant VCP to oligosaccharide moieties. One of the known important regulatory proteins whose degradation is impaired under these conditions is TDP-43.

Future attempts to treat patients with IBMPTD may involve stimulation of autophagy, use of chemical chaperones minimizing protein aggregation, and increasing the unfoldase activity of VCP. Prevention of Paget disease of the bone should involve inhibition of the NFκB pathway. Unfortunately, proteasome inhibitors such as Velcade™, which directly inhibit IκBa degradation and therefore are one of the strongest available NFκB activation inhibitors, could increase the pathology associated with accumulation of polyubiquitinated proteins in muscle and the central nervous system.

Reference

1 Watts GD, Wymer J, Kovach MJ et al. (2004) Inclusion body myopathy associated with Paget disease of bone and frontotemporal dementia is caused by mutant valosin-containing protein. *Nat Genet* **36**(4), 377–381.

2 Weihl CC, Dalal S, Pestronk A, Hanson PI. (2006) Inclusion body myopathy-associated mutations in p97/VCP impair endoplasmic reticulum-associated degradation. *Hum Mol Genet* **15**(2), 189–199.

3 Schroder R, Watts GD, Mehta SG et al. (2005) Mutant valosin-containing protein causes a novel type of frontotemporal dementia. *Ann Neurol* **57**(3), 457–461.

4 Forman MS, Mackenzie IR, Cairns NJ et al. (2006) Novel ubiquitin neuropathology in frontotemporal dementia with valosin-containing protein gene mutations. *J Neuropathol Exp Neurol* **65**(6), 571–581.

5 Kimonis VE, Watts GD. (2005) Autosomal dominant inclusion body myopathy, Paget disease of bone, and frontotemporal dementia. *Alzheimer Dis Assoc Disord* **19** (Suppl. 1), S44–S47.

6 Weihl CC, Pestronk A, Kimonis VE. (2009) Valosin-containing protein disease: inclusion body myopathy with Paget's disease of the bone and fronto-temporal dementia. *Neuromuscul Disord* **19**(5), 308–315.

7 Hubbers CU, Clemen CS, Kesper K et al. (2007) Pathological consequences of VCP mutations on human striated muscle. *Brain* **130**(2), 381–393.

8 Miller TD, Jackson AP, Barresi R et al. (2009) Inclusion body myopathy with Paget disease and frontotemporal dementia (IBMPFD): clinical features including sphincter disturbance in a large pedigree. *J Neurol Neurosurg Psychiatry* **80**(5), 583–584.

9 Guyant-Marechal L, Laquerriere A, Duyckaerts C et al. (2006) Valosin-containing protein gene mutations: clinical and neuropathologic features. *Neurology* **67**(4), 644–651.

10 Peters JM, Harris JR, Lustig A et al. (1992) Ubiquitous soluble Mg (2 +)-ATPase complex. *A structural study. J Mol Biol* **223**(2), 557–571.

11 Frohlich KU, Fries HW, Peters JM, Mecke D. (1995) The ATPase activity of purified CDC48p from *Saccharomyces cerevisiae* shows complex dependence on ATP-, ADP-, and NADH-concentrations and is completely inhibited by NEM. *Biochim Biophys Acta* **1253**(1), 25–32.

12 Rabouille C, Levine TP, Peters JM, Warren G. (1995) An NSF-like ATPase, p97, and NSF mediate cisternal regrowth from mitotic Golgi fragments. *Cell* **82**(6), 905–914.

13 Voeltz GK, Rolls MM, Rapoport TA. (2002) Structural organization of the endoplasmic reticulum. *EMBO Rep* **3**(10), 944–950.

14 Boyce M, Yuan J. (2006) Cellular response to endoplasmic reticulum stress: a matter of life or death. *Cell Death Differ* **133**(3), 363–373.

15 Wu J, Kaufman RJ. (2006) From acute ER stress to physiological roles of the Unfolded Protein Response. *Cell Death Differ* **13**(3), 374–384.

16 Ellgaard L, Helenius A. (2003) Quality control in the endoplasmic reticulum. *Nat Rev Mol Cell Biol* **4**(3), 181–191.

17 Tsai B, Ye Y, Rapoport TA. (2002) Retro-translocation of proteins from the endoplasmic reticulum into the cytosol. *Nat Rev Mol Cell Biol* **3**(4), 246–255.

18 Kostova Z, Wolf DH. (2003) For whom the bell tolls: protein quality control of the endoplasmic reticulum and the ubiquitin-proteasome connection. *EMBO J* **22**(10), 2309–2317.

19 Sitia R, Braakman I. (2003) Quality control in the endoplasmic reticulum protein factory. *Nature* **426**(6968), 891–894.

20 Ahner A, Brodsky JL. (2004) Checkpoints in ER-associated degradation: excuse me, which way to the proteasome? *Trends Cell Biol* **14**(9), 474–478.

21 Song BL, Sever N, Bose-Boyd RA. (2005) Gp78, a membrane-anchored ubiquitin ligase, associates

with Insig-1 and couples sterol-regulated ubiquitination to degradation of HMG CoA reductase. *Mol Cell* **19**(6), 829–840.

22 Alzayady KJ, Panning MM, Kelley GG, Wojcikiewicz RJ. (2005) Involvement of the p97-Ufd1-Npl4 complex in the regulated endoplasmic reticulum-associated degradation of inositol 1,4, *5-trisphosphate receptors. J Biol Chem* **280**(41), 34530–34537.

23 Harding HP, Calfon M, Urano F et al. (2002) Transcriptional and translational control in the mammalian unfolded protein response. *Annu Rev Cell Dev Biol* **18**, 575–599.

24 Ma Y, Hendershot LM. (2002) The mammalian endoplasmic reticulum as a sensor for cellular stress. *Cell Stress Chaperones* **7**(2), 222–229.

25 Hampton RY. (2003) IRE1: a role in UPREgulation of ER degradation. *Dev Cell* **4**(2), 144–146.

26 Shen X, Zhang K, Kaufman RJ. (2004) The unfolded protein response-a stress signaling pathway of the endoplasmic reticulum. *J Chem Neuroanat* **28**(1–2) 79–92.

27 Moir D, Stewart SE, Osmond BC, Botstein D. (1982) Cold-sensitive cell-division-cycle mutants of yeast: isolation, properties, and pseudoreversion studies. *Genetics* **100**(4), 547–563.

28 Leon A, McKearin D. (1999) Identification of TER94, an AAA ATPase protein, as a Bam-dependent component of the *Drosophila* fusome. *Mol Biol Cell* **10**(11), 3825–3834.

29 Mouse Genome Informatics (MGI). (2005) Lexicon Genetics Data Submission to MGI via the NIH Knockout Project MGI, 3609573 J, 103485. http://www.informatics.jax.org/external/ko/lexicon/3468.html

30 Latterich M, Frohlich KU, Schekman R. (1995) Membrane fusion and the cell cycle: Cdc48p participates in the fusion of ER membranes. *Cell* **82**(6), 885–893.

31 Roy L, Bergeron JJ, Lavoie C et al. (2000) Role of p97 and syntaxin 5 in the assembly of transitional endoplasmic reticulum. *Mol Biol Cell* **11**(8), 2529–2542.

32 Hetzer M, Meyer HH, Walther TC et al. (2001) Distinct AAA-ATPase p97 complexes function in discrete steps of nuclear assembly. *Nat Cell Biol* **3**(12), 1086–1091.

33 Ghislain M, Dohmen RJ, Levy F, Varshavsky A. (1996) Cdc48p interacts with Ufd3p, a WD repeat protein required for ubiquitin-mediated proteolysis in *Saccharomyces cerevisiae. EMBO J* **15**(18), 4884–4899.

34 Dai RM, Chen E, Longo DL et al. (1998) Involvement of valosin-containing protein, an ATPase Co-purified with IkappaBalpha and 26 S proteasome, in ubiquitin-proteasome-mediated degradation of IkappaBalpha. *J Biol Chem* **273**(6), 3562–3573.

35 Dai RM, Li CC. (2001) Valosin-containing protein is a multi-ubiquitin chain-targeting factor required in ubiquitin-proteasome degradation. *Nat Cell Biol* **3**(8), 740–744.

36 Wojcik C, Yano M, DeMartino GN. (2004) RNA interference of valosin-containing protein (VCP/p97) reveals multiple cellular roles linked to ubiquitin/proteasome-dependent proteolysis. *J Cell Sci* **117**(2), 281–292.

37 Bays NW, Hampton RY. (2002) Cdc48-Ufd1-Npl4: stuck in the middle with Ub. *Curr Biol* **12**(10), R366–R371.

38 Ye Y, Shibata Y, Kikkert M et al. (2005) Inaugural article: recruitment of the p97 ATPase and ubiquitin ligases to the site of retrotranslocation at the endoplasmic reticulum membrane. *Proc Natl Acad Sci USA* **102**(40), 14132–14138.

39 Rape M, Hoppe T, Gorr I et al. (2001) Mobilization of processed, membrane-tethered SPT23 transcription factor by CDC48 (UFD1/NPL4), a ubiquitin-selective chaperone. *Cell* **107**(5), 667–677.

40 Hitchcock AL, Krebber H, Frietze S et al. (2001) The conserved npl4 protein complex mediates proteasome-dependent membrane-bound transcription factor activation. *Mol Biol Cell* **12**(10), 3226–3241.

41 Cao K, Nakajima R, Meyer HH, Zheng Y. (2003) The AAA-ATPase Cdc48/p97 regulates spindle disassembly at the end of mitosis. *Cell* **115**(3), 355–367.

42 Zhang H, Wang Q, Kajino K, Greene MI. (2000) VCP, a weak ATPase involved in multiple cellular events, interacts physically with BRCA1 in the nucleus of living cells. *DNA Cell Biol* **19**(5), 253–263.

43 Yamada T, Okuhara K, Iwamatsu A et al. (2000) p97 ATPase, an ATPase involved in membrane fusion, interacts with DNA unwinding factor (DUF) that functions in DNA replication. *FEBS Lett* **466**(2–3) 287–291.

44 Tresse E, Salomons FA, Vesa J et al. (2010) VCP/p97 is essential for maturation of ubiquitin-containing autophagosomes and this function is impaired by mutations that cause IBMPFD. *Autophagy* **6**(2), 217–227.

45 Zhang X, Shaw A, Bates PA et al. (2000) Structure of the AAA ATPase p97. *Mol Cell* **6**(6), 1473–1484.

46 DeLaBarre B, Brunger AT. (2003) Complete structure of p97/valosin-containing protein reveals communication between nucleotide domains. *Nat Struct Biol* **10**(10), 856–863.

47 DeLaBarre B, Brunger AT. (2005) Nucleotide dependent motion and mechanism of action of p97/VCP. *J Mol Biol* **347**(2), 437–452.

48 Wang Q, Song C, Li CC. (2004) Molecular perspectives on p97-VCP: progress in understanding its structure and diverse biological functions. *J Struct Biol* **146**(1–2) 44–57.

49 Dreveny I, Pye VE, Beuron F et al. (2004) p97 and close encounters of every kind: a brief review. *Biochem Soc Trans* **32**(5), 715–720.

50 Meyer HH, Shorter JG, Seemann J et al. (2000) A complex of mammalian ufd1 and npl4 links the AAA-ATPase, p97, to ubiquitin and nuclear transport pathways. *EMBO J* **19**(10), 2181–2192.

51 Meyer HH, Wang Y, Warren G. (2002) Direct binding of ubiquitin conjugates by the mammalian p97 adaptor complexes, p47 and Ufd1-Npl4. *EMBO J* **21**(21), 5645–5652.

52 Ye Y, Meyer HH, Rapoport TA. (2003) Function of the p97-Ufd1-Npl4 complex in retrotranslocation from the ER to the cytosol: dual recognition of nonubiquitinated polypeptide segments and polyubiquitin chains. *J Cell Biol* **162**(1), 71–84.

53 Bays NW, Wilhovsky SK, Goradia A et al. (2001) HRD4/NPL4 is required for the proteasomal processing of ubiquitinated ER proteins. *Mol Biol Cell* **12**(12), 4114–4128.

54 Richly H, Rape M, Braun S et al. (2005) A series of ubiquitin binding factors connects CDC48/p97 to substrate multiubiquitylation and proteasomal targeting. *Cell* **120**(1), 73–84.

55 Doss-Pepe EW, Stenroos ES, Johnson WG, Madura K. (2003) Ataxin-3 interactions with rad23 and valosin-containing protein and its associations with ubiquitin chains and the proteasome are consistent with a role in ubiquitin-mediated proteolysis. *Mol Cell Biol* **23**(18), 6469–6483.

56 Ye Y, Meyer HH, Rapoport TA. (2001) The AAA ATPase Cdc48/p97 and its partners transport proteins from the ER into the cytosol. *Nature* **414**(6864), 652–656.

57 Ye Y, Shibata Y, Yun C et al. (2004) A membrane protein complex mediates retro-translocation from the ER lumen into the cytosol. *Nature* **429**(6994), 841–847.

58 Kim I, Mi K, Rao H. (2004) Multiple interactions of rad23 suggest a mechanism for ubiquitylated substrate delivery important in proteolysis. *Mol Biol Cell* **15**(7), 3357–3365.

59 Kim I, Ahn J, Liu C et al. (2006) The Png1-Rad23 complex regulates glycoprotein turnover. *J Cell Biol* **172**(2), 211–219.

60 Medicherla B, Kostova Z, Schaefer A, Wolf DH. (2004) A genomic screen identifies Dsk2p and Rad23p as essential components of ER-associated degradation. *EMBO Rep* **5**(7), 692–697.

61 Biswas S, Katiyar S, Li G et al. (2004) The N-terminus of yeast peptide: N-glycanase interacts with the DNA repair protein Rad23. *Biochem Biophys Res Commun* **323**(1), 149–155.

62 Ishigaki S, Hishikawa N, Niwa J et al. (2004) Physical and functional interaction between Dorfin and Valosin-containing protein that are colocalized in ubiquitylated inclusions in neurodegenerative disorders. *J Biol Chem* **279**(49), 51376–51385.

63 Nan L, Wu Y, Bardag-Gorce F et al. (2005) RNA interference of VCP/p97 increases Mallory body formation. *Exp Mol Pathol* **78**(1), 1–9.

64 Wojcik C, Rowicka M, Kudlicki A et al. (2006) Valosin-containing protein (p97) is a regulator of ER stress and of the degradation of N-end rule and ubiquitin-fusion degradation pathway substrates in mammalian cells. *Mol Biol Cell* **17**(11), 4606–4618.

65 Nowis D, McConnell E, Wojcik C. (2006) Destabilization of the VCP-Ufd1-Npl4 complex is associated with decreased levels of ERAD substrates. *Exp Cell Res* **312**(15), 2921–2932.

66 Kitami MI, Kitami T, Nagahama M et al. (2006) Dominant-negative effect of mutant valosin-containing protein in aggresome formation. *FEBS Lett* **580**(2), 474–478.

67 Hirabayashi M, Inoue K, Tanaka K et al. (2001) VCP/p97 in abnormal protein aggregates, cytoplasmic vacuoles, and cell death, phenotypes relevant to neurodegeneration. *Cell Death Differ* **8**(10), 977–984.

68 Mimnaugh EG, Xu W, Vos M et al. (2006) Endoplasmic reticulum vacuolization and valosin-containing protein relocalization result from simultaneous hsp90 inhibition by geldanamycin and proteasome inhibition by velcade. *Mol Cancer Res* **4**(9), 667–681.

69 Lass A, McConnell E, Nowis D et al. (2007) A novel function of VCP (valosin-containing protein; p97) in the control of N-glycosylation of proteins in the endoplasmic reticulum. *Arch Biochem Biophys* **462**(1), 62–73.

70 Lilley BN, Ploegh HL. (2004) A membrane protein required for dislocation of misfolded proteins from the ER. *Nature* **429**(6994), 834–840.

71 Taxis C, Hitt R, Park SH et al. (2003) Use of modular substrates demonstrates mechanistic diversity and reveals differences in chaperone requirement of ERAD. *J Biol Chem* **278**(38), 35903–35013.

72 Carvalho P, Goder V, Rapoport TA. (2006) Distinct ubiquitin-ligase complexes define convergent pathways for the degradation of ER proteins. *Cell* **126**(2), 361–373.

73 Wiertz EJ, Tortorella D, Bogyo M et al. (1996) Sec61-mediated transfer of a membrane protein from the endoplasmic reticulum to the proteasome for destruction. *Nature* **384**(6608), 432–438.

74 Zhou M, Schekman R. (1999) The engagement of Sec61p in the ER dislocation process. *Mol Cell* **4**(6), 925–934.

75 Walter J, Urban J, Volkwein C, Sommer T. (2001) Sec61p-independent degradation of the tail-anchored ER membrane protein Ubc6p. *EMBO J* **20**(12), 3124–3131.

76 Mancini R, Aebi M, Helenius A. (2003) Multiple endoplasmic reticulum-associated pathways degrade mutant yeast carboxypeptidase Y in mammalian cells. *J Biol Chem* **278**(47), 46895–46905.

77 Schmitz A, Herzog V. (2004) Endoplasmic reticulum-associated degradation: exceptions to the rule. *Eur J Cell Biol* **83**(10), 501–509.

78 Rabinovich E, Kerem A, Frohlich KU et al. (2002) AAA-ATPase p97/Cdc48p, a cytosolic chaperone required for endoplasmic reticulum-associated protein degradation. *Mol Cell Biol* **22**(2), 626–634.

79 Jarosch E, Taxis C, Volkwein C et al. (2002) Protein dislocation from the ER requires polyubiquitination and the AAA-ATPase Cdc48. *Nat Cell Biol* **4**(2), 134–139.

80 Braun S, Matuschewski K, Rape M et al. (2002) Role of the ubiquitin-selective CDC48 (UFD1/NPL4) chaperone (segregase) in ERAD of OLE1 and other substrates. *EMBO J* **21**(4), 615–621.

81 Lee RJ, Liu CW, Harty C et al. (2004) Uncoupling retro-translocation and degradation in the ER-associated degradation of a soluble protein. *EMBO J* **23**(11), 2206–2215.

82 Mayer TU, Braun T, Jentsch S. (1998) Role of the proteasome in membrane extraction of a short-lived ER-transmembrane protein. *EMBO J* **17**(12), 3251–3257.

83 Kalies KU, Allan S, Sergeyenko T et al. (2005) The protein translocation channel binds proteasomes to the endoplasmic reticulum membrane. *EMBO J* **24**(13), 2284–2293.

84 van Laar T, van der Eb AJ, Terleth C. (2001) Mif1: a missing link between the unfolded protein response pathway and ER-associated protein degradation? *Curr Protein Pept Sci* **2**(2), 169–190.

85 Oyadomari S, Yun C, Fisher EA et al. (2006) Cotranslocational degradation protects the stressed endoplasmic reticulum from protein overload. *Cell* **126**(4), 727–739.

86 Lencer WI, Tsai B. (2003) The intracellular voyage of cholera toxin: going retro. *Trends Biochem Sci* **28**(12), 639–645.

87 Kothe M, Ye Y, Wagner JS et al. (2005) Role of p97 AAA-ATPase in the retrotranslocation of the cholera toxin A1 chain, a non-ubiquitinated substrate. *J Biol Chem* **280**(30), 28127–28132.

88 McConnell E, Lass A, Wojcik C. (2007) Ufd1-Npl4 is a negative regulator of cholera toxin retrotranslocation. *Biochem Biophys Res Commun* **355**(4), 1087–1090.

89 Tirosh B, Iwakoshi NN, Lilley BN et al. (2005) Human cytomegalovirus protein US11 provokes an unfolded protein response that may facilitate the degradation of class I major histocompatibility complex products. *J Virol* **79**(5), 2768–2779.

90 Madeo F, Schlauer J, Frohlich KU. (1997) Identification of the regions of porcine VCP preventing its function in Saccharomyces cerevisiae. *Gene* **204**(1–2) 145–151.

91 Lass A, McConnell E, Fleck K et al. (2008) Analysis of Npl4 deletion mutants in mammalian cells unravels new Ufd1-interacting motifs and suggests a regulatory role of Npl4 in ERAD. *Exp Cell Res* **314**(14), 2715–2723.

92 Raasi S, Pickart CM. (2003) Rad23 ubiquitin-associated domains (UBA) inhibit 26 S proteasome-catalyzed proteolysis by sequestering lysine 48-linked polyubiquitin chains. *J Biol Chem* **278**(11), 8951–8959.

93 Hwang GW, Sasaki D, Naganuma A. (2005) Overexpression of Rad23 confers resistance to methylmercury in *Saccharomyces cerevisiae* via inhibition of the degradation of ubiquitinated proteins. *Mol Pharmacol* **68**(4), 1074–1078.

94 Wojcik C, Schroeter D, Wilk S et al. (1996) Ubiquitin-mediated proteolysis centers in HeLa cells: indication from studies of an inhibitor of the chymotrypsin-like activity of the proteasome. *Eur J Cell Biol* **71**(3), 311–318.

95 Wojcik C. (1997) On the spatial organization of ubiquitin-dependent proteolysis in HeLa cells. *Folia Histochem Cytobiol* **35**(2), 117–118.

96 Johnston JA, Ward CL, Kopito RR. (1998) Aggresomes: a cellular response to misfolded proteins. *J Cell Biol* **143**(7), 1883–1898.

97 Kopito RR, Sitia R. (2000) Aggresomes and Russell bodies. Symptoms of cellular indigestion? *EMBO Rep* **1**(3), 225–231.

98 Wu D, Chen PJ, Chen S et al. (1999) *C. elegans* MAC-1, an essential member of the AAA family of ATPases, can bind CED-4 and prevent cell death. *Development* **126**(9), 2021–2031.

99 Braun RJ, Zischka H. (2008) Mechanisms of Cdc48/VCP-mediated cell death - from yeast apoptosis to human disease. *Biochim Biophys Acta* **1783**(7), 1418–1435.

100 Rao RV, Poksay KS, Castro-Obregon S et al. (2004) Molecular components of a cell death pathway activated by endoplasmic reticulum stress. *J Biol Chem* **279**(1), 177–187.

101 Higashiyama H, Hirose F, Yamaguchi M et al. (2002) Identification of ter94, *Drosophila* VCP, as a modulator of polyglutamine-induced neurodegeneration. *Cell Death Differ* **9**(3), 264–273.

102 Yamamoto S, Tomita Y, Hoshida Y et al. (2004) Expression level of valosin-containing protein (p97) is associated with prognosis of esophageal carcinoma. *Clin Cancer Res* **10**(16), 5558–5565.

103 Yamamoto S, Tomita Y, Hoshida Y et al. (2004) Expression level of valosin-containing protein (p97) is correlated with progression and prognosis of non-small-cell lung carcinoma. *Ann Surg Oncol* **11**(7), 697–704.

104 Yamamoto S, Tomita Y, Hoshida Y et al. (2004) Increased expression of valosin-containing protein (p97) is associated with lymph node metastasis and prognosis of pancreatic ductal adenocarcinoma. *Ann Surg Oncol* **11**(2), 165–172.

105 Yamamoto S, Tomita Y, Hoshida Y et al. (2004) Expression of valosin-containing protein in colorectal carcinomas as a predictor for disease recurrence and prognosis. *Clin Cancer Res* **10**(2), 651–657.

106 Yamamoto S, Tomita Y, Hoshida Y et al. (2003) Expression level of valosin-containing protein is strongly associated with progression and prognosis of gastric carcinoma. *J Clin Oncol* **21**(13), 2537–2544.

107 Yamamoto S, Tomita Y, Nakamori S et al. (2003) Elevated expression of valosin-containing protein (p97) in hepatocellular carcinoma is correlated with increased incidence of tumor recurrence. *J Clin Oncol* **21**(3), 447–452.

108 Hirono Y, Fushida S, Yonemura Y et al. (1996) Expression of autocrine motility factor receptor correlates with disease progression in human gastric cancer. *Br J Cancer* **74**(12), 2003–2007.

109 Timar J, Raso E, Dome B et al. (2002) Expression and function of the AMF receptor by human melanoma in experimental and clinical systems. *Clin Exp Metastasis* **19**(3), 225–232.

110 Zhong X, Shen Y, Ballar P et al. (2004) AAA ATPase p97/valosin-containing protein interacts with gp78, a ubiquitin ligase for endoplasmic reticulum-associated degradation. *J Biol Chem* **279**(44), 45676–45684.

111 Ma Y, Hendershot LM. (2004) The role of the unfolded protein response in tumour development: friend or foe? *Nat Rev Cancer* **4**(12), 966–977.

112 Adams J, Kauffman M. (2004) Development of the proteasome inhibitor Velcade (Bortezomib). *Cancer Invest* **22**(2), 304–311.

113 Mizuno Y, Hori S, Kakizuka A, Okamoto K. (2003) Vacuole-creating protein in neurodegenerative diseases in humans. *Neurosci Lett* **343**(2), 77–80.

114 Sherman MY, Goldberg AL. (2001) Cellular defenses against unfolded proteins: a cell biologist thinks about neurodegenerative diseases. *Neuron* **29**(1), 15–32.

115 Kakizuka A. (2008) Roles of VCP in human neurodegenerative disorders. *Biochem Soc Trans* **36**(1), 105–108.

116 Yamanaka K, Okubo Y, Suzaki T, Ogura T. (2004) Analysis of the two p97/VCP/Cdc48p proteins of Caenorhabditis elegans and their suppression of polyglutamine-induced protein aggregation. *J Struct Biol* **146**(1–2) 242–250.

117 Song C, Xiao Z, Nagashima K et al. (2008) The heavy metal cadmium induces valosin-containing protein (VCP)-mediated aggresome formation. *Toxicol Appl Pharmacol* **228**(3), 351–363.

118 Song C, Wang Q, Li CC. (2007) Characterization of the aggregation-prevention activity of p97/valosin-containing protein. *Biochemistry* **46**(51), 14889–14898.

119 Bjorkoy G, Lamark T, Brech A et al. (2005) p62/SQSTM1 forms protein aggregates degraded by autophagy and has a protective effect on huntingtin-induced cell death. *J Cell Biol* **171**(4), 603–614.

120 Schumacher A, Friedrich P, Diehl J et al. (2009) No association of common VCP variants with sporadic frontotemporal dementia. *Neurobiol Aging* **30**(2), 333–335.

121 Lucas GJ, Mehta SG, Hocking LJ et al. (2006) Evaluation of the role of Valosin-containing protein in the pathogenesis of familial and sporadic Paget's disease of bone. *Bone* **38**(2), 280–285.

122 Guyant-Marechal L, Laquerriere A, Duyckaerts C et al. (2006) Valosin-containing protein gene mutations: clinical and neuropathologic features. *Neurology* **67**(4), 644–651.

123 Gidaro T, Modoni A, Sabatelli M et al. (2008) An Italian family with inclusion-body myopathy and

frontotemporal dementia due to mutation in the VCP gene. *Muscle Nerve* **37**(1), 111–114.

124 Haubenberger D, Bittner RE, Rauch-Shorny S et al. (2005) Inclusion body myopathy and Paget disease is linked to a novel mutation in the VCP gene. *Neurology* **65**(8), 1304–1305.

125 Djamshidian A, Schaefer J, Haubenberger D et al. (2009) A novel mutation in the VCP gene (G157R) in a German family with inclusion-body myopathy with Paget disease of bone and frontotemporal dementia. *Muscle Nerve* **39**(3), 389–391.

126 Watts GD, Thomasova D, Ramdeen SK et al. (2007) Novel VCP mutations in inclusion body myopathy associated with Paget disease of bone and frontotemporal dementia. *Clin Genet* **72**(5), 420–426.

127 Stojkovic T, Hammouda H, Richard P et al. (2009) Clinical outcome in 19 French and Spanish patients with valosin-containing protein myopathy associated with Paget's disease of bone and frontotemporal dementia. *Neuromuscul Disord* **19**(5), 316–323.

128 Bersano A, Del BR, Lamperti C et al. (2009) Inclusion body myopathy and frontotemporal dementia caused by a novel VCP mutation. *Neurobiol Aging* **30**(5), 752–758.

129 Mehta SG, Watts GD, Adamson JL et al. (2007) APOE is a potential modifier gene in an autosomal dominant form of frontotemporal dementia (IBMPFD). *Genet Med* **9**(1), 9–13.

130 van der Zee J, Pirici D, Van LT et al. (2009) Clinical heterogeneity in 3 unrelated families linked to VCP p. Arg159His. *Neurology* **73**(8), 626–632.

131 Custer SK, Neumann M, Lu H et al. (2010) Transgenic mice expressing mutant forms VCP/p97 recapitulate the full spectrum of IBMPFD including degeneration in muscle, brain and bone. *Hum Mol Genet* **19**, 1741–1755.

132 Vesa J, Su H, Watts GD et al. (2009) Valosin containing protein associated inclusion body myopathy: abnormal vacuolization, autophagy and cell fusion in myoblasts. *Neuromuscul Disord* **19**(11), 766–772.

133 Daroszewska A, Ralston SH. (2006) Mechanisms of disease: genetics of Paget's disease of bone and related disorders. *Nat Clin Pract Rheumatol* **2**(5), 270–277.

134 Chiu YH, Zhao M, Chen ZJ. (2009) Ubiquitin in NF-kappaB signaling. *Chem Rev* **109**(4), 1549–1560.

135 Asai T, Tomita Y, Nakatsuka S et al. (2002) VCP (p97) regulates NFkappaB signaling pathway, which is important for metastasis of osteosarcoma cell line. *Jpn J Cancer Res* **93**(3), 296–304.

136 Gitcho MA, Strider J, Carter D et al. (2009) VCP mutations causing frontotemporal lobar degeneration disrupt localization of TDP-43 and induce cell death. *J Biol Chem* **284**(18), 12384–12398.

137 Williams A, Jahreiss L, Sarkar S et al. (2006) Aggregate-prone proteins are cleared from the cytosol by autophagy: therapeutic implications. *Curr Top Dev Biol* **76**, 89–101.

138 Honig LS, Rosenberg RN. (2000) Apoptosis and neurologic disease. *Am J Med* **108**(4), 317–330.

139 Neumann M, Mackenzie IR, Cairns NJ et al. (2007) TDP-43 in the ubiquitin pathology of frontotemporal dementia with VCP gene mutations. *J Neuropathol Exp Neurol* **66**(2), 152–157.

140 Urushitani M, Sato T, Bamba H et al. (2010) Synergistic effect between proteasome and autophagosome in the clearance of polyubiquitinated TDP-43. *J Neurosci Res* **88**(4), 784–797.

141 Neumann M. (2009) Molecular neuropathology of TDP-43 proteinopathies. *Int J Mol Sci* **10**(1), 232–246.

142 Russell AP. (2010) The molecular regulation of skeletal muscle mass. *Clin Exp Pharmacol Physiol* **37**(3), 378–384.

143 Sacheck JM, Hyatt JP, Raffaello A et al. (2007) Rapid disuse and denervation atrophy involve transcriptional changes similar to those of muscle wasting during systemic diseases. *FASEB J* **21**(1), 140–155.

144 Sacheck JM, Ohtsuka A, McLary SC, Goldberg AL. (2004) IGF-I stimulates muscle growth by suppressing protein breakdown and expression of atrophy-related ubiquitin ligases, atrogin-1 and MuRF1. *Am J Physiol Endocrinol Metab* **287**(4), E591–E601.

145 Weihl CC, Miller SE, Hanson PI, Pestronk A. (2007) Transgenic expression of inclusion body myopathy associated mutant p97/VCP causes weakness and ubiquitinated protein inclusions in mice. *Hum Mol Genet* **16**(8), 919–928.

146 Weihl CC, Temiz P, Miller SE et al. (2008) TDP-43 accumulation in inclusion body myopathy muscle suggests a common pathogenic mechanism with frontotemporal dementia. *J Neurol Neurosurg Psychiatry* **79**(10), 1186–1189.

147 Olive M, Janue A, Moreno D et al. (2009) TAR DNA-Binding protein 43 accumulation in protein aggregate myopathies. *J Neuropathol Exp Neurol* **68**(3), 262–273.

148 Masiero E, Sandri M. (2010) Autophagy inhibition induces atrophy and myopathy in adult skeletal muscles. *Autophagy* **6**(2), 307–309.

CHAPTER 15

Clinical spectrum of VCP myopathy, Paget disease, and frontotemporal dementia: experimental models and potential treatments

Virginia E. Kimonis[1], Eric Dec[2], Mallikarjun Badadani[2], Angele Nalbandian[2], Jouni Vesa[2], Vincent Caiozzo[3], Douglas Wallace[2,4], Barbara Martin[5], Charles Smith[5], and Giles D. Watts[6]

[1]Department of Pediatrics, University of California Irvine School of Medicine, Orange, CA, USA
[2]Division of Genetics and Metabolism, Department of Pediatrics and Center for Molecular, and Mitochondrial Medicine and Genetics, University of California, Irvine, CA, USA
[3]Department of Orthopedic Surgery, University of California, Irvine, CA, USA
[4]Department of Biological Chemistry, Departments of Ecology and Evolutionary Biology, University of California, Irvine, CA, USA
[5]Department of Neurology, University of Kentucky Medical School, Lexington, KY, USA
[6]School of Medicine, Cell Biology and Biochemistry, Health Policy and Practice, University of East Anglia, Norwich, Norfolk, UK

Introduction

Clinical features of VCP hereditary inclusion-body myopathy

Hereditary inclusion-body myopathy (h-IBM) is a heterogeneous group of disorders associated with rimmed vacuoles and cytoplasmic and intranuclear inclusions of 15–21-nm filaments [1]. An autosomal recessive quadriceps-sparing form of the disorder with onset in early adulthood prevalent among the Iranian Jewish population is associated with mutations in the UDP-N-acetylglucosamine-2 epimerase/N-acetylmannosamine kinase (*GNE*) gene [2, 3]. Nonaka inclusion-body myopathy is an allelic disorder with a similar phenotype [4].

Inclusion-body myopathy associated with Paget disease of the bone and frontotemporal dementia (IBMPFD; OMIM 167320), first reported in 2000, is an autosomal dominant, progressive, and ultimately lethal condition with onset typically in the 20s to 30s. Physical exam reveals muscle weakness and atrophy of the pelvic and shoulder girdle, marked scapular winging, and difficulty walking up stairs [5–7]. Muscle disease typically progresses to involve other limb and respiratory groups; ultimately, individuals die in their 50s to 60s from progressive muscle weakness, and cardiac and respiratory failure [5, 8]. Electromyography shows both myopathic and neurogenic changes suggestive of myopathy, and serum creatine kinase concentration is usually normal to mildly elevated (range, 40–1145 U/L; normal range, 20–222 U/L).

Histologically, patients show the presence of rimmed vacuoles and inclusion bodies in the muscle fibers (see Plate 15.11). Electron micrographs of affected skeletal muscle demonstrate prominent 15–21-nm tubulofilamentous inclusions within myonuclei. Weihl et al. [9] identified large TAR

Muscle Aging, Inclusion-Body Myositis and Myopathies, First Edition. Edited by Valerie Askanas and W. King Engel.
© 2012 Blackwell Publishing Ltd. Published 2012 by Blackwell Publishing Ltd.

DNA-binding protein 43 (TDP-43)-positive ubiquitinated inclusions in muscle cytoplasm in IBMPFD patients, thus adding h-IBMs to the growing list of TDP-43-positive inclusion diseases. Kimonis et al. [5] reported cardiomyopathy in three out of 11 individuals in the original family. Hubbers et al. [10] reported that mutant valosin-containing protein (*VCP*) leads to a novel form of dilatative cardiomyopathy with inclusion bodies.

Paget disease of the bone in IBMPFD

Paget disease of the bone (PDB) is a common condition characterized by increased and disorganized bone turnover, which can affect one or several skeletal regions (Figure 15.1). These abnormalities disrupt normal bone architecture and lead to various clinical complications such as bone pain, osteoarthritis, pathological fracture, and bone deformity. Genetic mutations play an important role in PDB by disrupting normal signaling in bone remodeling. The nuclear factor κB (NFκB) signaling pathway is one such pathway identified as being important in PDB. To date there are four gene mutations or polymorphisms in the NFκB signaling pathway associated with increased risk of PDB. These include TNFRSF11A, which encodes receptor activator of NFκB ligand (RANK), TNFRSF11B, which encodes osteoprotegerin, VCP, and SQSTM1 [11, 12], the latter of which encodes the signaling adaptor p62, a multidomain protein implicated in the activation of the transcription factor NFκB [13–16]. Recently variants in optineurin (OPTN) was found to be a risk factor for Paget's disease in a genome-wide association study [15]. Interestingly OPTN mutations have also been found in patients with amyotropic lateral sclerosis [16]. Thus these mutations are likely to predispose to PDB by disrupting normal NFκB signaling. NFκB plays a critical role in cell survival, in addition to regulating bone turnover.

Early-onset PDB is seen in 49% of IBMPFD patients [5, 7], and typically begins in the 30s to 40s, the mean age of onset being 42 years. The diagnosis of PDB is based on serum alkaline phosphatase (ALP) concentration, urine concentrations of pyridinoline (PYD) and deoxypyridinoline (DPD), and radionuclide scans or skeletal radiographs. Zoledro-

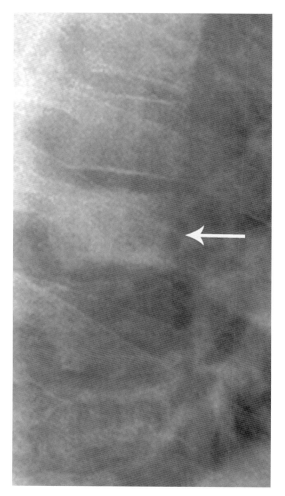

Figure 15.1 Lateral spine X-ray of a 43-year-old man with Paget disease and myopathy shows sclerotic changes of the vertebral body at the level of T7 thoracic vertebral body.

nic acid is a potent bisphosphonate that has recently been licensed for the treatment of established PDB. A single injection results in sustained biochemical remission in over 95% of subjects for up to 2 years [17]. It is therefore feasible and appropriate to identify these patients, since they represent a high-risk group who might gain benefit from early therapy.

Frontotemporal dementia in IBMPFD

Frontotemporal dementia (FTD) is a clinicopathological entity comprising about 3% of all dementias of the elderly [18–20]. Symptoms typically involve personality or mood changes such as depression and withdrawal, and language difficulties. Patients may become disinhibited or exhibit antisocial behavior. Some individuals with asymmetric involvement of the left hemisphere may develop extraordinary visual or musical creativity while experiencing language impairment. In contrast to Alzheimer disease patients who typically develop early symptoms of episodic memory loss, FTD patients exhibit altered behavior or loss of speech or language as initial manifestations. Episodic memory in FTD is relatively preserved. In later stages of FTD, patients may develop Parkinsonism or amyotrophic lateral sclerosis (ALS)-like features.

In the disinhibition-dementia-Parkinsonism-amyotrophy complex, mapping to chromosome 17q21–q22, mutations disrupt the *tau* (microtubule-associated protein tau; *MAPT*) gene. The majority of FTD families, however, have no demonstrable *tau* mutations [21–24]. Recently FTD has been associated with mutations in progranulin [25], which maps very close to the *MAPT* gene on chromosome 17, accounting for early confusion in the designation of FTD-17 families. Progranulin mutations are associated pathologically with ubiquinated neuronal cytoplasmic inclusions positive for TDP-43. In contrast, FTD associated with mutations in the *CHMP2B* gene have ubiquitin-positive but TDP-43-negative inclusions.

In patients with IBMPFD, onset of dementia in affected individuals occurred on average at 54 years (range 39–62 years) with an overall frequency of 33% [26]. The diagnosis of FTD is based on comprehensive neuropsychological assessments that reveal behavioral alteration (e.g. personal/social unawareness, or disinhibition), early expressive language dysfunction or semantic loss, and preservation of memory, orientation, and ideomotor praxis [27].

We performed a systematic analysis of the brain neuropathologic changes in eight patients with *VCP* mutations and identified ubiquitin-positive neuronal intranuclear inclusions and dystrophic neurites [28] (see Plate 15.12), making VCP disease another example of familial frontotemporal lobar degeneration with ubiquitin-positive inclusions (FTLD-U). Neumann et al. [29] found that a hyperphosphory-

lated, ubiquitinated, and cleaved form of TDP-43, known as pathologic TDP-43, is the major disease protein in ubiquitin-positive tau- and α-synuclein-negative FTD (FTLD-U), and in ALS. Accumulations of TDP-43 colocalized with ubiquitin pathology in eight of our patient IBMPFD brains, including both intranuclear inclusions and dystrophic neurites [30]. FTD associated with VCP is now classified under the rubrick of FTLD-U along with disorders such as ALS [31, 32]. Thus our work on the FTD associated with IBMPFD has lent new insights into the common pathogenesis of a spectrum of ubiquitin-related disorders that include FTD alone (progranulin-associated), FTD plus muscle and bone disease (IBMPFD), familial FTD with ALS, and motor-system degeneration without FTD (ALS).

Because of the variable phenotype in inclusion-body myopathy, PDB and FTD modifier genes were evaluated. From a database of 231 members of 15 families, 174 had an apolipoprotein E (*APOE*) genotype available for regression analysis. Analysis of the data suggested a potential link between the *APOE* 4 genotype and the FTD found in IBMPFD. In contrast we observed no association between FTD and the *MAPT* H2 haplotype [33].

Molecular studies of IBMPFD

A genome scan, performed at the Marshfield mammalian genotyping center, revealed linkage to chromosome 9p13.3–p12 in the original family reported [5] and three other families [6]. IBMPFD was subsequently attributed to being caused by mutations in the gene encoding VCP by Watts et al. [26], who identified six missense mutations in *VCP* in 13 families. VCP is highly conserved in evolution, belonging to the family of AAA proteins (ATPases associated with a variety of cellular activities) and has two ATPase domains (D1 and D2) [34–38] and two linker domains (L1 and L2), as well as the N-terminal- and C-terminal domains (Figure 15.2). VCP forms homohexamers and binds to multiple cofactors at both its N-terminal and C-terminal domains. Through binding cofactor molecules, VCP can adapt its function to suit many homeostatic processes important for the cell's life cycle. It has

CDC48/VCP/p97

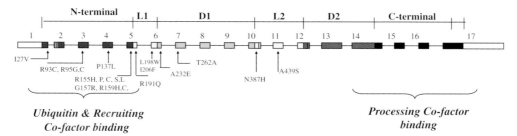

Figure 15.2 Functional domains and disease mutations in VCP. The domains of VCP include the ubiquitin-binding N-terminal domain (CDC48), flexible linker (L1), first AAA ATPase domain (D1), linker region (L2), second AAA ATPase domain (D2), and the C-terminal domains. There are 17 exons and arrows indicate the locations of all 20 mutations. The majority of mutations occur in the ubiquitin-binding N terminal domain.

been reported to be involved in several cellular activities including endoplasmic reticulum (ER)-associated degradation (ERAD) of proteins, homotypic membrane fusion, transcription activation, nuclear envelope reconstruction, postmitotic organelle reassembly, cell-cycle control, and apoptosis [39–41].

BMPFD is increasingly recognized as a distinct disorder although it is still underdiagnosed because of its variable phenotype, which leads to misdiagnoses. Kimonis et al. [8] reviewed data on 49 affected individuals in nine IBMPFD families and identified myopathy among 42 (87%) individuals, diagnoses including limb girdle muscular dystrophy (LGMD), facioscapular humeral muscular dystrophy, scapuloperoneal muscular dystrophy, and ALS, among others. Kimonis and Watts [42, 43] have reviewed clinical results in IBMPFD and summarized findings in 20 families harboring 10 missense mutations [44].

As a result of studies in patients from our North American families with *VCP* mutations [26], families are now being reported from several parts of the world with unique phenotypes: Germany [45, 46], France [47], Austria [48], Italy [49, 50], the UK [51], and other families from the USA [52] and by our group [53]. As a result of increased awareness of VCP disease, and hence accurate reporting of VCP disease, the phenotypic range associated with *VCP* mutations has significantly expanded. Dilated cardiomyopathy,

cataracts, sphincter disturbance, hepatic fibrosis, and features of ALS and Parkinson disease are now a part of the spectrum of IBMPFD manifestations.

At the present time 20 disease mutations have been reported (Figure 15.2, Table 15.1) with many more mutations expected to be identified as recognition of this disorder increases. The majority of the mutations have been found to cluster in the N-terminus of VCP which encompasses a domain that can bind ubiquitin and other substrate-recruiting proteins [54, 55]. In particular, we have identified a mutation hotspot at amino acid residue 155 (R155H/P/C/S/L). Additionally, most of the mutated residues causing IBMPFD are adjacent and potentially interact with each other, suggesting that these residues may have a similar and specific function within the VCP homohexamer [53].

We reviewed clinical features of families with VCP disease in order to perform a genotype/phenotype analysis. Because of the enormous intrafamilial variation, genotype/phenotype analysis was difficult between families. Notable associations, however, included a more severe and early-onset myopathy and dementia in family 6 that had the A232E mutation. Families with the R159C mutation did not develop PDB [57]. Although, none of the mutations had a significant effect on the age of onset for FTD (which was relatively consistent between families with VCP mutations), there was an increase in the incidence of FTD among females.

Table 15.1 List of VCP disease mutations

	Amino acid	c. DNA Base change	Exon	Domain	Number of families	References
1	I27V	79A → G	2	N-terminus	1	[80]
2	R93C	277C → T	3	N-terminus	4	[10, 47, 81]
3	R95G	283C → G	3	N-terminus	2	[26]
4	R95C	283C → T	3	N-terminus	1	[44]
5	P137L	410C → T	4	N-terminus	1	[82]
6	R155C	463C → T	5	N-terminus	5	[12, 26, 45, 47, 83]
7	R155H	464G → A	5	N-terminus	8	[10, 26]
8	R155P	464G → C	5	N-terminus	1	[26]
9	R155S	463C → A	5	N-terminus	1	[69]
10	R155L	N/A	5	N-terminus	1	[84]
11	G157R	469 G → C	5	N-terminus	1	[46]
12	R159H	476G → A	5	N-terminus	2	[48]
13	R159C	476G → A	5	N-terminus	2	[49, 52]
14	R191Q	572G → A	5	Linker 1	1	[26, 52]
15	L198W	593T → G	6	Linker 1	1	[53, 84]
16	I206F	828A → T	6	Linker 1	1	[82]
17	A232E	695C → A	6	Junction (L1–D1)	1	[26]
18	T262A	N/A	7	AAA D1	1	[52]
19	N387H	1159A → C	10	AAA D1	1	[53]
20	A439S	N/A	11	Linker 2	1	[85]

VCP is at the intersection of the ubiquitin-proteasome system and autophagy

The ubiquitin-proteasome system (UPS) is the major extralysosomal pathway responsible for degradation of both structural and regulatory proteins during muscle remodeling in eukaryotes. The UPS comprises a ubiquitin-conjugating system and the 26S proteasome. The ubiquitin-proteasome protein degradation system (UPD) has been shown to involve VCP via its cooperation with a binary Ufd1/Npl4 cofactor, enabling VCP targeting of specific substrates for degradation [54, 56–58]. Protein degradation mediated by the UPS is essential for the elimination of misfolded proteins from the ER in response to ER stress. It has been reported that the AAA ATPase p97/VCP/CDC48 dislocates proteins across the ER membrane allowing subsequent ubiquitin-dependent degradation by the 26S proteasome in the cytosol. Degradation of a prototypical misfolded ERAD substrate, ΔF508 CFTR, is slowed in IBMPFD mutant-expressing cells. Consistent with

this, the undegraded ΔF508CFTR colocalized with IBMPFD mutant p97/VCP in ubiquitinated inclusions. [59]. Hubbers et al. [10] found that transient and stable expression of IBMPFD mutants p97/VCP R93C, R155C, and R155H in HEK293 and C2F3 myoblasts did not result in an increase in ubiquitinated proteins. Genetic studies in *Caenorhabditis elegans* revealed that IBMPFD mutations selectively impair the proteasomal degradation of the myosin chaperone, Unc-45, lending support for the dysregulation of the UPS [60–62].

Alterations in UPS function have been implicated in the pathogenesis of a variety of sporadic and familial neurodegenerative diseases including Parkinson disease, Alzheimer disease, polyglutamine repeat diseases, and ALS [63–65]. Mizuno et al. [66] called VCP "vacuole-creating protein" and demonstrated that VCP was observed in ubiquitin-positive intraneuronal inclusions in both motor neuron disease with dementia, and ballooned neurons in Creutzfeldt–Jakob disease. In Alzheimer disease, VCP has been found in dystrophic neurites while granules of granulovacuolar degeneration and neu-rofibrillary tangles were not positively stained for VCP. In Parkinson's disease, Lewy and Marinesco bodies and Lewy neurites have been found to stain positive for VCP as well. These results indicate that VCP reacts with abnormal or misfolded proteins and plays a role in accelerating the process of degener-ation and cell death.

A gain-of-function concept explains much of the phenotype seen in this disease as indicated by the work by other researchers [67, 68]. The work of our laboratory and that of other researchers suggest that *VCP*-mutation-induced neurodegen-eration is mediated by several mechanisms in-cluding ERAD ubiquitin-proteasome and autop-hagy pathways. IBMPFD thereby joins familial forms of Alzheimer disease, Parkinson disease, Marinesco–Sjögren syndrome, and other neuro-degenerative diseases in which intracellular pro-tein accumulation results from perturbation of ER chaperone function.

Autophagy is a process that degrades long-lived proteins and cytoplasmic components within au-tophagosomes. Proteins and cytoplasmic compo-nents destined for degradation are sequestered and enveloped into vesicles that later mature through a series of steps including membrane fusion with lysosomes. Upon activation of autophagy, the 18 kDa LC3 (LC3-I) protein undergoes proteolytic cleavage followed by lipid modification converting the 18 kDa form into the 16 kDa membrane-bound form (LC3-II). LC3-II is specifically localized to the autophagosomal membranes whereas LC3-I is pri-marily cytosolic. The conversion from LC3-I to LC3-II is used as a marker for autophagic processing in mammalian cells. A buildup of either molecule suggests a disruption in the normal maturation of autophagosomes. Western-blotting analysis has demonstrated that protein lysates extracted from mutant cells have significantly increased amounts of LC3-II when compared to wild-type cell lines [69]. Related research [69] found accumulation of enlarged vacuoles in myoblasts from patients with VCP-associated inclusion-body myopathy. These findings suggest an impairment of autophagosome maturation and hence accumulation of autophago-somes at an immature state which are seen as vacuoles. Further analysis of the enlarged vacuoles via immunological staining revealed positivity for LAMP-1 and LAMP-2 antibodies. LAMP proteins are lysosomal-associated membrane proteins sug-gesting that vacuoles are able to fuse with the endosomal or lysosomal compartments (Figure 15.3). Lysosomal membrane proteins LAMP-1 and LAMP-2, however, showed increased molecular weights in patients' myoblasts due to differential *N*-glycosylation [69].

Ju et al. [70, 71] also identified impaired autop-hagy in cells transfected with *VCP* mutations, and in an overexpressing transgenic mouse model, by dem-onstrating increased ubiquitinated p62/sequesto-some, a marker for autophagy. Sequestosome is a multimeric protein complex that serves as a depot for proteins destined for degradation. p62 has an LIR domain (LC3-interacting region) that recognizes and binds LC3, thereby initiating the first steps in autophagy. It is already known that mutations in the p62/sequestosome is a cause of PDB, seen in ap-proximately 50% of familial and 30% of simplex cases of Paget disease. Similarly, p62 is found to be associated with a number of other diseases associ-ated with cytoplasmic inclusion bodies. In particu-lar, p62 has been identified in neuronal and glial inclusions associated with FTD [72] and mutations have been identified in ALS.

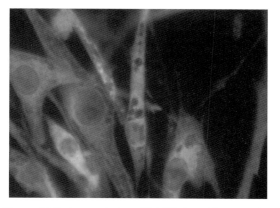

Figure 15.3 Accumulation of LAMP-1-positive vacuoles in cultured myoblasts from an IBMPFD patients with the R155H mutation. Mutant cells are also defective in myotube formation.

Autophagy has also been implicated in the other type of h-IBM, autosomal recessive distal myopathy with rimmed vacuoles (DMRV) or h-IBM. h-IBM is an early adult-onset distal myopathy caused by mutations in the *GNE* gene which encodes a bifunctional enzyme involved in sialic acid biosynthesis. It is pathologically characterized by the presence of rimmed vacuoles, especially in atrophic muscle fibers, which also occasionally contain congophilic materials that are immunoreactive to β-amyloid, lysosomal proteins, ubiquitin, and tau proteins. Hyposialylation plays an important role in the pathogenesis of DMRV/h-IBM. It is uncertain if a similar mechanism may be involved in VCP h-IBM [73]. Disruption of the ER/autophagy pathway thus holds potential for revealing insights into the pathogenesis of VCP muscle, bone, and brain disease.

VCP mouse models

Human and mouse VCP proteins differ by only one amino acid residue at position 684. The targeted homozygous deletion of VCP by Cre-loxP technology was reported to result in early embryonic lethality [74]. In contrast, heterozygous mice lacking one *VCP* allele and having one wild-type allele were apparently indistinguishable from their wild-type littermates. Weihl et al. [75] found that transgenic mice overexpressing the most common human IBMPFD mutation (R155H) under the regulation of a muscle creatine kinase promoter became progressively weaker in a dose-dependent manner starting at 6 months of age. These mutant mice showed muscle pathology including coarse internal architecture, and disorganized membrane morphology and vacuole-like clefts with reduced caveolin-3 expression at the sarcolemma. Even before animals displayed measurable weakness there was an increase in ubiquitin-containing protein inclusions and high-molecular-weight ubiquitinated proteins.

Recently Custer et al. [76] reported a transgenic mouse overexpressing mutant forms of VCP. The mice expressed muscle weakness, and pathology characteristic of inclusion-body myopathy including blue rimmed vacuoles, and TDP-43 pathology.

Radiological examination of the skeleton revealed focal lytic and sclerotic regions in the vertebrae and femur. Additionally the brain revealed widespread TDP-43 lesions and the mice also exhibited abnormalities in behavioral testing. To replicate the human disease associated with VCP mutations our laboratory [77] has generated a knock-in mouse model of the common VCP R155H mutation. Mice demonstrated progressive muscle weakness, vacuolization of myofibrils, and centrally located myonuclei, in addition to TDP-43- and ubiquitin-positive inclusion bodies in quadriceps myofibrils and brain. Additionally, muscle sections showed increased numbers of autophagosomes, elevated caspase-3 activity, and an increased number of TUNEL-positive nuclei supporting involvement of autophagy and apoptosis in the pathogenesis of the disease. Bone histology showed increased osteoclastogenesis suggestive of PDB. The Custer overexpressed mutant VCP transgenic mice and our knock-in mice thus replicate the human disease and represent useful models for trials of novel therapies for diseases with similar pathogenesis.

Treatment

Currently there are no known treatments for the muscle component of VCP disease or the dementia however treatment trials are needed in this disease. PDB, however, is well treated with bisphosphonates and it is hypothesized that progressive disease can be prevented if treated at an early stage of the disease. Autophagy is negatively regulated by the mammalian target of rapamycin (mTOR) and can be induced in all mammalian cell types by mTOR inhibitors such as rapamycin. A number of investigators have reported dramatic effects of rapamycin on the size of renal angiomyolipomas and sub-ependymal giant cell astrocytomas in tuberous sclerosis patients [78, 79], neurofibromatosis, and polycystic kidney disease. Autophagy is a major clearance pathway for the removal of mutant huntington protein associated with Huntington disease, and many other disease-causing, cytoplasmic, aggregate-prone proteins. Research in IBMPFD will likely address important pathophysiologic principles underlying many other common related disorders. Pharmacologic strategies to modify autophagy and other pathways such as proteasomal inhibition, and ER stress modifiers, may hold potential not only in VCP disease but also other disorders such as the vacuolar myopathies including GNE-associated h-IBM, sporadic inclusion-body myositis (s-IBM), oculopharyngeal muscular dystrophy (OPMD), and other proteinopathies such as FTD and ALS. Potential therapeutic strategies can be explored using the available cell and mouse models for preclinical studies.

Acknowledgments

We thank the families and their healthcare providers for their enthusiastic participation, and our numerous collaborators for their contributions. Funding of this study is from the NIAMS, National Institutes of Health (RO1 AR050236 and RO3 AR46869), Muscular Dystrophy Association, and Paget Foundation. This work was also supported by the Muscular Dystrophy Association (grant to VK and development grant to JV), NIH 1K01AR056002-01A2 trainee award (to GW) and the ICTS (Institute of Clinical Translation Science, UC Irvine).

Electronic database information

Kimonis V, Donkervoort S, Watts G. (2011) Inclusion Body Myopathy Associated with Paget Disease of Bone and/or Frontotemporal Dementia Gene GeneTests (wwwgenetestsorg) and University of Washington, Seattle.

Online Mendelian Inheritance in Man (OMIM) http://www3.ncbi.nlm.nih.gov/omim (for inclusion body myopathy, early onset Paget disease of bone, and frontotemporal dementia; IBMPFD, MIM 167320).

References

1 Askanas V, Engel WK. (2002) Inclusion-body myositis and myopathies: different etiologies, possibly similar pathogenic mechanisms. *Curr Opin Neurol* **15**(5), 525–531.

2 Argov Z, Yarom R. (1984) "Rimmed vacuole myopathy" sparing the quadriceps. A unique disorder in Iranian Jews. *J Neurol Sci* **64**(1), 33–43.

3 Eisenberg I, Avidan N, Potikha T et al. (2001) The UDP-N-acetylglucosamine 2-epimerase/N-acetyl-mannosamine kinase gene is mutated in recessive hereditary inclusion body myopathy. *Nat Genet* **29**(1), 83–87.

4 Tomimitsu H, Ishikawa K, Shimizu J et al. (2002) Distal myopathy with rimmed vacuoles: novel mutations in the GNE gene. *Neurology* **59**(3), 451–454.

5 Kimonis VE, Kovach MJ, Waggoner B et al. (2000) Clinical and molecular studies in a unique family with autosomal dominant limb-girdle muscular dystrophy and Paget disease of bone. *Genet Med* **2**(4), 232–241.

6 Kovach MJ, Waggoner B, Leal SM et al. (2001) Clinical delineation and localization to chromosome 9p13.3-p12 of a unique dominant disorder in four families: hereditary inclusion body myopathy, Paget disease of bone, and frontotemporal dementia. *Mol Genet Metab* **74**(4), 458–475.

7 Watts GD, Thorne M, Kovach MJ et al. (2003) Clinical and genetic heterogeneity in chromosome 9p associated hereditary inclusion body myopathy: exclusion of GNE and three other candidate genes. *Neuromuscul Disord* **13**(7–8) 559–567.

8 Kimonis VE, Mehta SG, Fulchiero E.C et al. (2008) Clinical studies in familial VCP myopathy associated with Paget disease of bone and frontotemporal dementia. *Am J Med Genet* **146**(6), 745–757.

9 Weihl CC, Temiz P, Miller SE et al. (2008) TDP-43 accumulation in inclusion body myopathy muscle suggests a common pathogenic mechanism with frontotemporal dementia. *J Neurol Neurosurg Psychiatry* **79**(10), 1186–1189.

10 Hubbers CU, Clemen CS, Kesper K et al. (2007) Pathological consequences of VCP mutations on human striated muscle. *Brain* **130**(2), 381–393.

11 Hocking LJ, Lucas GJ, Daroszewska A et al. (2004) Novel UBA domain mutations of SQSTM1 in Paget's disease of bone: genotype phenotype correlation, functional analysis, and structural consequences. *J Bone Miner Res* **19**(7), 1122–1127.

12 Hocking LJ, Lucas GJ, Daroszewska A et al. (2002) Domain-specific mutations in sequestosome 1 (SQSTM1) cause familial and sporadic Paget's disease. *Hum Mol Genet* **11**(22), 2735–2739.

13 Moscat J, Diaz-Meco MT. (2009) p62 at the crossroads of autophagy, apoptosis, and cancer. *Cell* **137**(6), 1001–1004.

14 Ramesh Babu J, Lamar Seibenhener M, Peng J et al. (2008) Genetic inactivation of p62 leads to accumulation of hyperphosphorylated tau and neurodegeneration. *J Neurochem* **106**(1), 107–120.

15 Albagha OM, Visconti MR, Alonso N et al (2010) Genome-wide association study identifies variants at CSF1, OPTN and TNFRSF11A as genetic risk factors for Paget's disease of bone. *Nat Genet* 42:520–524

16 Maruyama H, Morino H, Ito H et al (2010) Mutations of optineurin in amyotrophic lateral sclerosis. *Nature* 465:223–226

17 Reid IR, Miller P, Lyles K et al. (2005) Comparison of a single infusion of zoledronic acid with risedronate for Paget's disease. *N Engl J Med* **353**(9), 898–908.

18 Arnold SE, Han LY, Clark CM et al. (2000) Quantitative neurohistological features of frontotemporal degeneration. *Neurobiol Aging* **21**(6), 913–919.

19 Turner RS, Kenyon LC, Trojanowski JQ et al. (1996) Clinical, neuroimaging, and pathologic features of progressive nonfluent aphasia. *Ann Neurol* **39**(2), 166–173.

20 Zhukareva V, Vogelsberg-Ragaglia V, Van Deerlin VM et al. (2001) Loss of brain tau defines novel sporadic and familial tauopathies with frontotemporal dementia. *Ann Neurol* **49**(2), 165–175.

21 Hutton M, Lendon CL, Rizzu P et al. (1998) Association of missense and 5'-splice-site mutations in tau with the inherited dementia FTDP-17. *Nature* **393**(6686), 702–705.

22 Spillantini MG, Murrell JR, Goedert M et al. (1998) Mutation in the tau gene in familial multiple system tauopathy with presenile dementia. *Proc Natl Acad Sci USA* **95**(13), 7737–7741.

23 Wilhelmsen KC, Clark LN, Miller BL, Geschwind DH. Tau mutations in frontotemporal dementia. "Dementia and geriatric cognitive disorders." *Dement Geriatr Cogn Disord.* 1999;**10** (Suppl 1):88–92.

24 Rosso SM, Kamphorst W, de Graaf B et al. (2001) Familial frontotemporal dementia with ubiquitin-positive inclusions is linked to chromosome 17q21–22. *Brain* **124**(10), 1948–1957.

25 Baker M, Mackenzie IR, Pickering-Brown SM et al. (2006) Mutations in progranulin cause tau-negative frontotemporal dementia linked to chromosome 17. *Nature* **442**(7105), 916–919.

26 Watts GD, Wymer J, Kovach MJ et al. (2004) Inclusion body myopathy associated with Paget disease of bone and frontotemporal dementia is caused by mutant valosin-containing protein. *Nat Genet* **36**(4), 377–381.

27 Miller BL, Ikonte C, Ponton M et al. (1997) A study of the Lund-Manchester research criteria for frontotemporal dementia: clinical and single-photon emission CT correlations. *Neurology* **48**(4), 937–942.

28 Forman MS, Mackenzie IR, Cairns NJ et al. (2006) Novel ubiquitin neuropathology in frontotemporal dementia with valosin-containing protein gene mutations. *J Neuropathol Exp Neurol* **65**(6), 571–581.

29 Neumann M, Sampathu DM, Kwong LK et al. (2006) Ubiquitinated TDP-43 in frontotemporal lobar degeneration and amyotrophic lateral sclerosis. *Science* **314** (5796), 130–133.

30 Neumann M, Mackenzie IR, Cairns NJ et al. (2007) TDP-43 in the ubiquitin pathology of frontotemporal dementia with VCP gene mutations. *J Neuropathol Exp Neurol* **66**(2), 152–157.

31 Cairns NJ, Bigio EH, Mackenzie IR et al. (2007) Neuropathologic diagnostic and nosologic criteria for frontotemporal lobar degeneration: consensus of the Consortium for Frontotemporal Lobar Degeneration. *Acta Neuropathol* **114**(1), 5–22.

32 Liscic RM, Grinberg LT, Zidar J et al. (2008) ALS and FTLD: two faces of TDP-43 proteinopathy. *Eur J Neurol* **15**(8), 772–780.

33 Mehta SG, Watts GD, Adamson JL et al. (2007) APOE is a potential modifier gene in an autosomal dominant form of frontotemporal dementia (IBMPFD). *Genet Med* **9**(1), 9–13.

34 Confalonieri F, Duguet M. (1995) A 200-amino acid ATPase module in search of a basic function. *Bioessays* **17**(7), 639–650.

35 Neuwald AF, Aravind L, Spouge JL, Koonin EV. (1999) AAA+: A class of chaperone-like ATPases associated with the assembly, operation, and disassembly of protein complexes. *Genome Res* **9**(1), 27–43.

36 Ogura T, Wilkinson AJ. (2001) AAA+ superfamily ATPases: common structure--diverse function. *Genes Cells* **6**(7), 575–597.

37 Patel S, Latterich M. (1998) The AAA team: related ATPases with diverse functions. *Trends Cell Biol* **8**(2), 65–71.

38 Zwickl P, Baumeister W. (1999) AAA-ATPases at the crossroads of protein life and death. *Nat Cell Biol* **1**(4), E97–E98.

39 Rabouille C, Kondo H, Newman R et al. (1998) Syntaxin 5 is a common component of the NSF- and p97-mediated reassembly pathways of Golgi cisternae from mitotic Golgi fragments in vitro. *Cell* **92**(5), 603–10.

40 Hetzer M, Meyer HH, Walther TC et al. (2001) Distinct AAA-ATPase p97 complexes function in discrete steps of nuclear assembly. *Nat Cell Biol* **3**(12), 1086–1091.

41 Rabinovich E, Kerem A, Frohlich KU et al. (2002) AAA-ATPase p97/Cdc48p, a cytosolic chaperone required for endoplasmic reticulum-associated protein degradation. *Mol Cell Biol* **22**(2), 626–634.

42 Kimonis VE, Watts GD. (2005) Autosomal dominant inclusion body myopathy, Paget disease of bone, and frontotemporal dementia. *Alzheimer Dis Assoc Disord* **19** (Suppl. 1), S44–S47.

43 Kimonis V, Watts G. (2007) Inclusion Body Myopathy Associated with Paget Disease of Bone and/or Frontotemporal Dementia Gene GeneTests (wwwgenetests-org) and University of Washington, Seattle.

44 Kimonis VE, Fulchiero E, Vesa J, Watts G. (2008) VCP disease associated with myopathy, paget disease of bone and frontotemporal dementia: Review of a unique disorder. *Biochim Biophys Acta* **1782**(12), 744–748.

45 Schroder R, Watts GD, Mehta SG et al. (2005) Mutant valosin-containing protein causes a novel type of frontotemporal dementia. *Ann Neurol* **57**(3), 457–461.

46 Djamshidian A, Schaefer J, Haubenberger D et al. (2009) A novel mutation in the VCP gene (G157R) in a German family with inclusion-body myopathy with Paget disease of bone and frontotemporal dementia. *Muscle Nerve* **39**(3), 389–391.

47 Guyant-Marechal L, Laquerriere A, Duyckaerts C et al. (2006) Valosin-containing protein gene mutations: clinical and neuropathologic features. *Neurology* **67** (4), 644–651.

48 Haubenberger D, Bittner RE, Rauch-Shorny S et al. (2005) Inclusion body myopathy and Paget disease is linked to a novel mutation in the VCP gene. *Neurology* **65**(8), 1304–1305.

49 Bersano A, Del Bo R, Lamperti C et al. (2009) Inclusion body myopathy and frontotemporal dementia caused by a novel VCP mutation. *Neurobiol Aging* **30**(5), 752–758.

50 Viassolo V, Previtali SC, Schiatti E et al. (2008) Inclusion body myopathy, Paget's disease of the bone and frontotemporal dementia: recurrence of the VCP R155H mutation in an Italian family and implications for genetic counselling. *Clin Genet* **74**, 54–60.

51 Miller TD, Jackson AP, Barresi R et al. (2009) Inclusion body myopathy with Paget disease and frontotemporal dementia (IBMPFD), clinical features including sphincter disturbance in a large pedigree. *J Neurol Neurosurg Psychiatry* **80**(5), 583–584.

52 Spina S, Van Laar A, Murrell JR et al. (2008) Frontotemporal dementia associated with a valosin-containing protein mutation: report of three families. *FASEB J* **22**, 58.4.

53 Watts GD, Thomasova D, Ramdeen SK et al. (2007) Novel VCP mutations in inclusion body myopathy associated with Paget disease of bone and frontotemporal dementia. *Clin Genet* **72**(5), 420–426.

54 Dai RM, Li CC. (2001) Valosin-containing protein is a multi-ubiquitin chain-targeting factor required in ubiquitin-proteasome degradation. *Nat Cell Biol* **3**(8), 740–744.

55 Rape M, Hoppe T, Gorr I et al. (2001) Mobilization of processed, membrane-tethered SPT23 transcription factor by CDC48(UFD1/NPL4), a ubiquitin-selective chaperone. *Cell* **107**(5), 667–677.

56 Jarosch E, Geiss-Friedlander R, Meusser B et al. (2002) Protein dislocation from the endoplasmic reticulum--pulling out the suspect. *Traffic* **3**(8), 530–536.

57 Kondo H, Rabouille C, Newman R et al. (1997) p47 is a cofactor for p97-mediated membrane fusion. *Nature* **388**(6637), 75–78.

58 Meyer HH, Shorter JG, Seemann J et al. (2000) A complex of mammalian ufd1 and npl4 links the AAA-ATPase, p97, to ubiquitin and nuclear transport pathways. *EMBO J* **19**(10), 2181–2192.

59 Weihl CC, Dalal S, Pestronk A, Hanson PI. (2006) Inclusion body myopathy-associated mutations in p97/VCP impair endoplasmic reticulum-associated degradation. *Hum Mol Genet* **15**(2), 189–199.

60 Hoppe T. (2008) Less is more: how protein degradation regulates muscle development. *Ernst Schering Foundation Symposium Proceedings* **1**, 67–73.

61 Hoppe T, Cassata G, Barral JM et al. (2004) Regulation of the myosin-directed chaperone UNC-45 by a novel E3/E4-multiubiquitylation complex in C. elegans. *Cell* **118**(3), 337–349.

62 Janiesch PC, Kim J, Mouysset J et al. (2007) The ubiquitin-selective chaperone CDC-48/p97 links myosin assembly to human myopathy. *Nat Cell Biol* **9**(4), 379–390.

63 Seitelberger F, Lassmann H, Bancher C. (1991) Cytoskeleton pathology in Alzheimer's disease and related disorders. *J Neural Transm Suppl* **33**, 27–33.

64 Sakamoto KM. (2002) Ubiquitin-dependent proteolysis: its role in human diseases and the design of therapeutic strategies. *Mol Genet Metab* **77**(1–2) 44–56.

65 van Leeuwen FW, Hol EM, Fischer DF. (2006) Frameshift proteins in Alzheimer's disease and in other conformational disorders: time for the ubiquitin-proteasome system. *J Alzheimers Dis* **9** (3 Suppl.) 319–325.

66 Mizuno Y, Hori S, Kakizuka A, Okamoto K. (2003) Vacuole-creating protein in neurodegenerative diseases in humans. *Neurosci Lett* **343**(2), 77–80.

67 Halawani D, Leblanc A, Rouiller I et al. (2009) Hereditary inclusion body myopathy-linked p97/VCP mutations in the NH2-domain and the D1 ring modulate p97/VCP ATPase activity and D2 AAA+ ring conformation. *Mol Cell Biol* **29**(16), 4484–4494.

68 Kakizuka A. (2008) Roles of VCP in human neurodegenerative disorders. *Biochem Soc Trans* **36**(1), 105–108.

69 Vesa J, Su H, Watts GD, Krause S et al. (2009) Valosin containing protein associated inclusion body myopathy: abnormal vacuolization, autophagy and cell fusion in myoblasts. *Neuromuscul Disord* **19**(11), 766–772.

70 Ju JS, Fuentealba RA, Miller SE et al. (2009) Valosin-containing protein (VCP) is required for autophagy and is disrupted in VCP disease. *J Cell Biol* **187**(6), 875–888.

71 Ju JS, Weihl CC. (2010) p97/VCP at the intersection of the autophagy and the ubiquitin proteasome system. *Autophagy* **6**(2), 283–285.

72 Pikkarainen M, Hartikainen P, Alafuzoff I. (2008) Neuropathologic features of frontotemporal lobar degeneration with ubiquitin-positive inclusions visualized with ubiquitin-binding protein p62 immunohistochemistry. *J Neuropathol Exp Neurol* **67**(4), 280–298.

73 Malicdan MC, Noguchi S, Nishino I. (2007) Perspectives on distal myopathy with rimmed vacuoles or hereditary inclusion body myopathy: contributions from an animal model. Lack of sialic acid, a central determinant in sugar chains, causes myopathy? *Acta Myol* **26**(3), 171–175.

74 Muller JM, Deinhardt K, Rosewell I et al. (2007) Targeted deletion of p97 (VCP/CDC48) in mouse results in early embryonic lethality. *Biochem Biophys Res Commun* **354**(2), 459–465.

75 Weihl CC, Miller SE, Hanson PI, Pestronk A. (2007) Transgenic expression of inclusion body myopathy associated mutant p97/VCP causes weakness and ubiquitinated protein inclusions in mice. *Hum Mol Genet* **16**(8), 919–928.

76 Custer SK, Neumann M, Lu H et al. (2010) Transgenic mice expressing mutant forms VCP/p97 recapitulate the full spectrum of IBMPFD including degeneration in muscle, brain and bone. *Hum Mol Genet* **19**, 1741–1755.

77 Badadani M, Watts G, Vesa J et al. (2010) VCP associated inclusion body myopathy and Paget disease of bone knock-in mouse model exhibits tissue pathology typical of human disease. *PloS ONE* **5**(10), e13183.

78 Ess KC. (2010) Tuberous sclerosis complex: a brave new world? *Curr Opin Neurol* **23**(2), 189–193.

79 Koenig MK, Butler IJ, Northrup H. (2008) Regression of subependymal giant cell astrocytoma with rapamycin in tuberous sclerosis complex. *J Child Neurol* **23** (10), 1238–1239.

80 Rohrer JD, Warren JD, Reiman D et al. (2011) A novel exon 2 I27V VCP variant is associated with dissimilar clinical syndromes. *J Neurol* Mar 9, epub ahead of print.

81 Krause S, Gohringer T, Walter MC et al. (2007) Brain imaging and neuropsychology in late-onset dementia due to a novel mutation (R93C) of valosin-containing protein. *Clin Neuropathol* **26**(5), 232–240.

82 Peyer AK KJ, Frank S, Fuhr P, Fischmann A, Kneifel S, Thomann S, Camano P, Sinnreich M, Renaud S. Novel valosin containing protein mutation in a Swiss family with hereditary inclusion body myopathy, Paget's disease of the bone and dementia. Abstract. World Federation of Neurology XII International Congress on Neuromuscular Diseases, Naples, Italy. 2010.

83 Gidaro T, Modoni A, Sabatelli M et al. (2008) An Italian family with inclusion-body myopathy and frontotemporal dementia due to mutation in the VCP gene. *Muscle Nerve* **37**(1), 111–114.

84 Kumar KR, Needham M, Mina K, Davis M, Brewer J, Staples C, Ng K, Sue CM, Mastaglia FL. Two Australian families with inclusion-body myopathy, Paget's disease of bone and frontotemporal dementia: novel clinical and genetic findings. *Neuromuscul Disord.* 2010.**20**:330–4.

85 Stojkovic T, Hammouda el H, Richard P, Lopez de Munain A, Ruiz-Martinez J, Gonzalez PC, et al. Clinical outcome in 19 French and Spanish patients with valosin-containing protein myopathy associated with Paget's disease of bone and frontotemporal dementia. Neuromuscul Disord. 2009 May;**19**(5):316–23.

CHAPTER 16

Drosophila and mouse models of hereditary myopathy caused by mutations in *VCP*/p97

Nisha M. Badders and J. Paul Taylor
Department of Developmental Neurobiology, St. Jude Children's Research Hospital, Memphis, TN, USA

Introduction

Inclusion-body myopathy associated with Paget's disease of the bone and frontotemporal dementia (IBMPFD) is an autosomal dominant, multisystem disease, affecting muscle, brain, and bone [1–3]. Symptoms are predominantly manifested as muscle weakness, occurring in approximately 90% of patients, with a mean onset of 45 years [4, 5]. However, 51% of patients also develop Paget's disease of the bone and 32% develop frontotemporal dementia (FTD), with a mean onset of 42 and 54 years, respectively [6, 7]. Other, less commonly reported symptoms include cardiomyopathy, hepatic fibrosis, cataracts, and sensory-motor axonal neuropathy [8–10].

Muscle weakness often initially occurs in the proximal or distal lower extremities, followed by the scapulohumeral, axial, facial, and tongue muscles [3, 11]. Consequently, IBMPFD is often misdiagnosed as limb girdle muscular dystrophy, fascioscapular humeral dystrophy, Welander or Miyoshi distal myopathies, as well as amyotrophic lateral sclerosis (ALS) [11]. Weakness slowly progresses with age, often leading to wheelchair confinement of the patient. IBMPFD ultimately culminates in death, usually by the late 60s, due to respiratory or cardiac failure, or as an indirect result of FTD, such as feeding apraxia [12].

The myopathic features of IBMPFD vary tremendously between patients, but usually encompass the typical characteristics of inclusion-body myopathy (IBM), including the presence of ubiquitin-positive inclusions, centralized nuclei, and an increased prevalence of endomysial connective tissue [3, 10, 13]. In addition, inclusions containing TAR DNA-binding protein-43 (TDP-43), which colocalize with ubiquitin, are often found in the sarcolemma and sarcoplasm of affected muscles [14, 15]. However, TDP-43-positive inclusions are also found in several other myopathies, as well as dominantly inherited and sporadic cases of ALS [16]. Other myopathic characteristics of IBMPFD may include regional variations in muscle-fiber size, as well as the presence of rimmed vacuoles and/or inflammatory infiltrates [3, 10, 11].

Paget's disease of the bone is a metabolic bone disorder in which one or more of the bones undergo continuous dysregulated remodeling [6, 17]. Hyperactivation of osteoclasts in the affected bones leads to improper resorption of bony tissue, followed by a compensatory overproduction of poorly formed bone by osteoblasts. This typically results in both osteoporosis and bone deformation, and can lead to frail, disfigured bones that are prone to fracture [6]. This, coupled with the symptoms of IBM, can lead to greatly diminished mobility of patients with IBMPFD.

Muscle Aging, Inclusion-Body Myositis and Myopathies, First Edition. Edited by Valerie Askanas and W. King Engel.
© 2012 Blackwell Publishing Ltd. Published 2012 by Blackwell Publishing Ltd.

The onset of FTD is characterized by the emergence of language and behavioral abnormalities, resulting from progressive neurodegeneration of the frontotemporal lobes of the brain [18]. The pathology observed in brain tissue from these patients largely resembles that of other tau-negative, ubiquitin-positive FTD cases, including redistribution of TDP-43 protein from the nucleus to the cytoplasm, often within distinct ubiquitin-containing inclusions [19, 20]. Interestingly, TDP-43-positive inclusions can be found in either the cytoplasm or the nucleus of neuronal cells, although the functional significance of this is unclear. Nevertheless, it has been speculated that the localization of both TDP-43 and ubiquitin within these inclusions is the result of impairment in one or more protein-degradation pathways [7, 18, 21].

To date, IBMPFD has been detected in 26 families, and all known cases have been found to result from missense mutations in the valosin-containing protein (*VCP*/p97) gene on chromosome 9p21.1–p12 [9, 22–26]. VCP is a highly conserved, multifunctional chaperone, belonging to the AAA+ (ATPase associated with diverse cellular activities) family of ATPases [27]. The VCP protein contains three functional domains: an N-terminal domain, which mediates substrate and cofactor binding, and two ATPase domains (D1 and D2), which mediate the catalytic activity of VCP (Figure 16.1a). In its active form, VCP exists as a homohexamer, which forms a ring-like structure around a central pore. The N-terminal domains are positioned on the outward edge of the ring, while the D1 and D2 domains are located near the inner pore (Figure 16.1b,c). It is likely that multiple various cofactors are able to direct the specificity of VCP substrate binding and, thus, function by binding the N-terminal domain on the outside surface of the homohexamer, forming a large proteinaceous complex [28–32].

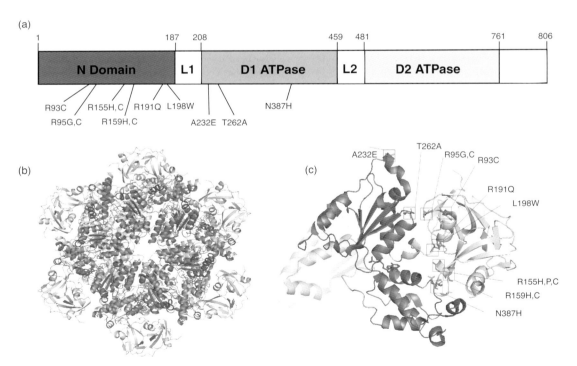

Figure 16.1 Schematic of VCP protein structure. (a) VCP consists of two ATPase domains (D1 and D2) and an N-terminal domain (N). (b) Structure of VCP homohexamer, illustrating barrel shape and central pore. (c) Structure of VCP monomer. N, D1, and D2 domains are indicated by grey shading. Disease-causing mutations are indicated by boxed regions.

VCP has been well characterized to play many roles in a myriad of cellular processes, especially protein degradation via autophagy or the ubiquitin-proteasome system (UPS) [33, 34]. VCP shuttles ubiquitinated substrates to the 26S proteasome and, thus, is a key regulator of both endoplasmic reticulum-associated degradation (ERAD) and the ubiquitin-fusion domain (UFD) pathways. In addition, VCP activity has recently been shown to be required for proper autophagosome maturation, and impaired autophagy has been suggested to contribute to the accumulation of toxic proteins, leading to IBMPFD-associated degeneration [35]. VCP is also an important regulator of sarcomere maintenance, chromatin decondensation following mitosis, nuclear envelope formation, and membrane fusion events leading to the biogenesis of the Golgi and ER [33]. VCP substrates include (although this is certainly not an exhaustive list) inhibitory κB (IκB), cyclinE, Hif1α, ataxin-3, BRCA, and auroraB kinase [14], implicating a role for VCP in varied cellular functions, ranging from the initiation of inflammatory responses to DNA repair.

Since mutations in VCP primarily result in progressive muscle weakness, it is not surprising that VCP plays a critical role in the regulation of sarcomere integrity. In a *Caenorhabditis elegans* model of IBMPFD, VCP was found to indirectly control sarcomere formation by tightly regulating the levels of the mysosin chaperone protein, Unc-45, which is required for myosin assembly during thick filament formation [36]. Interestingly, both attenuated as well as augmented Unc-45 protein levels result in myofibril disorganization, producing extensive sarcomeric defects. VCP controls the available cellular stores of Unc-45 protein by mediating its turnover through ubiquitin-dependent proteolysis. Disease-causing mutations in VCP lead to an over-accumulation of Unc-45 and, thus, myopathic degeneration [37, 38].

Fourteen unique mutations have been detected in patients with IBMPFD [9, 22–26], mostly affecting the N-terminal and D1 domains (Figure 16.1). Of these mutations, R155H is the most common, occurring in approximately 50% of affected families, while the A232E mutation results in the most severe symptoms [1, 13, 26, 39]. In order to glean

insight into the mechanism in which VCP mutations result in the tissue-specific symptoms of IBMPFD, it becomes necessary to utilize robust models of VCP-induced degeneration. Both invertebrate and mammalian systems have proven successful in fully characterizing the mechanisms of disease pathogenesis. The fruit fly has proved to be a powerful and effective tool for elucidating the pathogenesis of disease by detecting genetic modifiers through genetic screens, since flies exhibit both rapid life cycles and generation times, allowing analysis of large numbers of progeny quickly [40]. In contrast, mammalian models, such as the laboratory mouse, are essential to determine the mechanism and extent of pathology in complex tissues, closely replicating human disease states [41]. Here we review the characterization and insights gained from recently developed models of IBMPFD in both *Drosophila melanogaster* and *Mus musculus*.

A model of IBMPFD in *Drosophila melanogaster*

The fruit fly *Drosophila melanogaster* has a long and rich history as an important model organism for biologists and has helped provide the foundation for present-day research in genetics, developmental biology, neurobiology, and cancer research. In recent years, studies using fruit flies have provided important insights into the pathogenesis of neurodegenerative and neuromuscular disorders [40, 42]. Most human genes have a fly counterpart, but the fly genome is much more compact with smaller gene families and less redundancy, fewer and smaller introns and splice variants, and simpler noncoding regulatory regions [43], thus making genes easier to study and their functions easier to understand. The presence of numerous powerful genetic tools developed over the last century has allowed these genes to be manipulated rapidly to allow their *in vivo* function to be investigated. *Drosophila* models of disease have the added advantage of permitting unbiased genetic screens [44, 45], which can lead to unanticipated insights into pathogenesis.

Drosophila has a highly conserved ortholog of human *VCP* encoded by the gene *TER94* [46].

This gene encodes a single protein, referred to as dVCP, that shares 92% sequence similarity with human VCP (hVCP). Moreover, all amino acid residues mutated in association with human disease are conserved in dVCP [47]. To investigate the mechanism by which VCP mutations result in IBMPFD, we generated *Drosophila* that overexpressed wild-type or mutant forms of *TER94* [47]. The mutant versions of *TER94* (dVCP) were designed to replicate the mutations in human *VCP* that cause disease. Overexpression of mutant dVCP, but not wild-type dVCP, resulted in pronounced degeneration in the eye, brain, and muscle when expression was targeted to these tissues. Specifically, mutant dVCP expression in the eye produced a severe external rough eye phenotype with necrotic patches and vacuolar degeneration (Plate 16.13a). Expression of mutant dVCP in the central nervous system resulted in greatly reduced hatch rates and shortened lifespan as a result of neurodegeneration [47]. Interestingly, degeneration associated with the A232E mutation was more pronounced than the R155H mutation, recapitulating the differential levels of symptom severity seen in human cases of IBMPFD (Plate 16.13). This fly model of VCP-related disease promises to be an important tool for future studies of the disease pathogenesis. Indeed, our study provides evidence that mutations in VCP indirectly impact regulation of RNA metabolism, as described below.

To gain insight into which biological pathway(s) are disrupted by disease-causing mutations in VCP, we performed an unbiased, two-stage genetic screen to identify dominant genetic modifiers of mutant VCP-related eye degeneration in the *Drosophila* model [47]. In the first stage, we performed a "deficiency screen" to rapidly identify genomic intervals containing genetic modifiers. This was accomplished by genetic cross of flies expressing mutant VCP with "deficiency strains" that each contain a unique heterozygous deletion in the fly genome. By screening through several hundred deficiency lines, we were able to interrogate over 95% of the entire fly genome for regions of haploinsufficiency that significantly exacerbate or mitigate the degeneration associated with expression of mutant VCP. After filtering and validation, we iden-

tified 10 chromosomal regions containing genes of interest. In the second stage, we identified the specific genes of interest by RNA interference (RNAi)-mediated knockdown. We made use of transgenic flies expressing double-stranded RNA targeting every gene within the chromosomal regions of interest and screened for those that replicated the effect of exacerbating or mitigating VCP-related degeneration. In this way, we were able to define a series of individual genes whose expression level strongly influences VCP-related degeneration. Specifically, we identified three RNA-binding proteins as dominant suppressors of degeneration. Hrb27C, x16, and TDPH are *Drosophila* homologs of DAZAP1, 9G8, and TDP-43, respectively [47]. All three contain RNA recognition motifs (RRMs) and all are multifunctional proteins involved in transcription, mRNA export, splicing, and translation. The genetic interaction observed between VCP and these three RNA-binding proteins strongly suggests an intersection between ubiquitin signaling and control of RNA metabolism.

Of the three RNA-binding proteins identified in this screen, TDP-43 stands out as a particularly interesting finding. Abnormal deposition of TDP-43 in ubiquitin-positive cytoplasmic inclusions is a prominent histopathological feature of familial IBM and sporadic inclusion-body myositis (s-IBM) as well as several human neurodegenerative diseases, including familial and sporadic forms of ALS and FTD. Indeed, TDP-43 pathology is the most sensitive and specific feature of IBM where it is reported to be present in approximately 23% of patient muscle fibers [15]. The importance of TDP-43 in these diseases is underscored by the discovery that mutations in TDP-43 are causative of disease. In diseases characterized by TDP-43 pathology, the immunoreactivity of this protein is shifted from its normal location in the nucleus to multiple discrete, ubiquitin-positive puncta in the cytoplasm [48–50]. To investigate the relationship between VCP and TDP-43, we performed genetic crosses of flies expressing dVCP (wild-type or mutant) with flies expressing TDP-43 (wild-type or mutant) [47]. Coexpression of wild-type TDP-43 and wild-type dVCP did not result in degeneration. In contrast, coexpression of wild-type TDP-43 and mutant dVCP resulted in strong exacerbation of the degenerative phenotype. When examined histologically, it became apparent that as a consequence of expressing mutant VCP, TDP-43 was redistributed to cytoplasm. This phenomenon was enhanced, and degeneration exacerbated further, by introducing a disease-associated mutation into TDP-43. These findings suggested that degeneration initiated by mutations in VCP is mediated by inappropriate cytoplasmic accumulation of TDP-43. To test this idea, we engineered flies expressing TDP-43 that was directed to the cytoplasm by introducing mutations to the nuclear localization sequence. These results revealed that targeting excess TDP-43 to the cytoplasm is sufficient to cause degeneration [47].

The implication of these findings is that VCP plays some role in regulating the activity of RNA-binding proteins and mutations in VCP impair this function. Thus, there may be mechanistic overlap between the pathogenesis of IBM and the vast array of diseases that are characterized by defects in RNA metabolism, including myotonic dystrophy, oculopharyngeal muscular dystrophy, spinal muscular atrophy, and many others [51].

A model of IBMPFD in *Mus musculus*

Muller et al. [52] generated mice with a targeted deletion of VCP. Homozygous deletion of VCP resulted in early embryonic lethality, whereas heterozygous mice were found to be viable, healthy, and otherwise normal. This indicates that VCP activity is essential during development, and that one allele is sufficient for normal function. To model the myopathic features of IBMPFD, Weihl et al. [53] generated transgenic mice that express wild-type VCP(wt) or VCP(R155H) under control of the muscle-specific creatine kinase promoter. Mice expressing VCP (R155H) exhibited muscle weakness that was associated with the presence of ubiquitin-containing inclusions, increased endomysial connective tissue, and variable muscle-fiber sizes. Thus, expression of mutant VCP in mouse muscle was found to recapitulate, at least in part, the myopathy associated with IBMPFD.

In order to more closely model human IBMPFD, we generated transgenic mice expressing human VCP(wt), VCP(R155H), or VCP(A232E) under the ubiquitous chicken β-actin promoter [54]. Expression of mutant VCP in these mice resulted in decreased lifespan and decreased body mass, while expression of VCP(wt) had no effect, compared to nontransgenic (NT) control mice. In addition, mice expressing mutant VCP demonstrated an obvious clasping phenotype (a nonspecific indicator of central nervous system pathology), which first became prevalent at 3–6 months and progressively worsened with age. It is apparent that expression of mutant VCP results in a distinct phenotype that is not observed in response to expression of wild-type VCP. Therefore, transgenic expression of mutant human VCP in the mouse is a useful tool to model the multisystem pathological responses found in IBMPFD.

To assess the extent of myopathic degeneration in response to mutant VCP, we tested muscle strength of wild-type and mutant mice by evaluating their performance in a hanging wire test, which is an assay of limb strength. Both VCP(R155H) and VCP (A232E) mice demonstrated decreased muscle strength, which progressed with age, compared to VCP(wt) and NT mice (Plate 16.14a). Moreover, VCP(A232E) mice displayed greater weakness than VCP(R155H) mice, reproducing the symptom severity observed in human IBMPFD patients carrying the A232E mutation. Histological analysis of skeletal muscle sections from these mice revealed myogenic atrophy characterized by the presence of centralized nuclei, irregular fiber sizes, rimmed vacuoles, and modest inflammatory infiltrates, which were not found in wild-type and NT mice [54]. Thus, the known myopathic features of IBMPFD were fully recapitulated in our transgenic mouse model.

To further investigate the pathological mechanism of muscle weakness and degeneration, we immunostained muscle tissue sections from wild-type and mutant VCP mice with an antibody that recognizes TDP-43. In NT and VCP(wt) mice TDP-43 expression was localized to the nuclei of muscle fibers. However, extensive sarcoplasmic redistribution was observed in degenerating muscle fibers of mutant VCP mice (Plate 16.14b–e). Moreover, sarcoplasmic expression of TDP-43 colocalized with ubiquitin staining, suggesting that mutant VCP results in impaired protein degradation, leading to TDP-43 accumulation in the sarcoplasm. As predicted by our fruit fly model, sarcoplasmic localization of TDP-43 may be a driving force in muscle-fiber degeneration in the mouse [47].

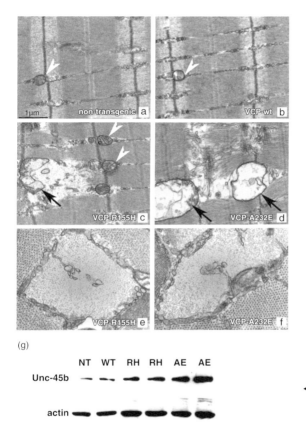

(g)

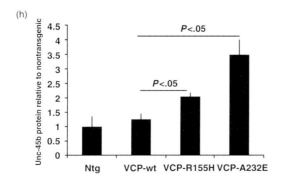

Upon staining of muscle tissue sections with modified trichrome Gomori staining, we found the presence of rimmed vacuoles in the sarcoplasm of affected muscle fibers from VCP(A232E) mice (Plate 16.14f), which is a relatively common pathological feature of IBM in IBMPFD patients [55, 56]. In addition, ultrastructural analysis of muscle tissue from wild-type and mutant VCP mice by transmission electron microscopy also revealed the presence of disrupted sarcomeres and highly disorganized myofibril structure in VCP(R155H) and VCP(A232E) mice. Interestingly, we also found an accumulation of enlarged, abnormally shaped mitochondria in these tissues (Figure 16.2a–f), which were very similar in morphology to the abnormal mitochondria present in the indirect flight muscles of mutant VCP fruit flies (unpublished observation). Since VCP has been shown to be an important mediator in autophagosome maturation during autophagy as well as to be a regulator of membrane fusion events [33, 35], it is plausible that the presence of these abnormal mitochondria in mutant VCP muscle may be the result of a defect in a previously uncharacterized role of VCP in mitochondrial clearance and mitophagy.

Since VCP has been well characterized to indirectly control sarcomere organization by regulating the cellular levels of Unc-45 during muscle fiber development [37], we quantified Unc-45 protein levels in muscle tissue lysates from wild-type and mutant VCP mice. Unc-45 protein levels were found to be

Figure 16.2 VCP mutant mice show loss of myosin-fiber integrity and stabilization of the myosin chaperone protein Unc-45b. (a–d) Transmission electron micrographs of quadriceps muscle ($\times 20\,000$) from nontransgenic (a), VCP-WT (b), VCP-R155H (c), and VCP-A232E (d) mice. Normal mitochondria are indicated by white arrowheads; degenerated mitochondria are indicated by arrows. (e,f) Cross-sectional transmission electron microscopic images of quadriceps muscle from VCP-R155H (e) and VCP-A232E (f) mice. (g) Western-blot analysis of Unc-45b expression in skeletal muscle lysates from 12-month-old nontransgenic (NT), VCP-WT, and mutant (RH, R155H; AE, A232E) mice. (h) Quantitative image analysis of Unc-45b Western blots from three separate experiments. (Reprinted with permission from Custer et al., [54] with permission from Oxford University Press.)

significantly increased in VCP(R155H) and VCP (A232E) mice (Figure 16.2g,h), suggesting the presence of mutant VCP results in the inappropriate stabilization of Unc-45. As shown in other models, elevated expression of Unc-45 leads to irregular myosin assembly and severely disrupted myofilament formation [36, 38]. This, in addition to sarcoplasmic redistribution of TDP-43 and an accumulation of abnormal mitochondria, would certainly be predicted to play a causal role in the progressive myopathic degeneration and weakness found in IBMPFD.

Although the myopathy observed in mutant VCP mice is both significant and severe, we also found pathological degeneration in brain and bone [54]. Mutant VCP mice displayed deficits in learning and memory, and exhibited increased anxiety, which was associated with the redistribution of TDP-43 to the cytoplasm of cells of the frontal cortex, pons, brainstem, and lumbar spinal cord. In addition, mutant VCP mice developed loss of trabecular bone volume and thickness, resulting in decreased bone density and hypomineralization, compared to wild-type and NT mice. Taken together, it is clear that exogenous expression of human VCP(R155H) or VCP(A232E) in the mouse recapitulates the degeneration of muscle, brain, and bone found in IBMPFD patients [26]. Of important note, the heart, liver, kidney, spleen, and intestinal tissues of these animals were found to be overtly free of any pathology, further reproducing the tissue specificity of IBMPFD symptoms [54].

Future roles of animal models

In summary, both of our models of IBMPFD, in the fruit fly and mouse, have yielded considerable insight into the pathogenesis of IBMPFD in specific tissues. Using the fruit fly, we have found a genetic interaction between mutant VCP and TDP-43, revealing TDP-43 to be a significant effector of IBMPFD-associated degeneration, and not simply an indicator of cytotoxic stress. Consequently, we also found cellular mislocalization of TDP-43 in the brain and muscle of mice expressing mutant VCP. In addition, we have found altered Unc-45 levels in response to mutant VCP in muscle, consistent with

the role Unc-45 has been shown to play in myopathic degeneration in other models. Finally, we have found the presence of abnormal mitochondria in the muscle of the mouse, as well as the fruit fly, suggesting this is a conserved, yet previously uncharacterized, property of IBMPFD, which should be investigated in human tissues. Thus, by utilizing multiple animal models of one disease, we have shed light on several potential, previously unknown mechanisms of pathogenesis by VCP mutation.

Although IBMPFD is a rare disease, the symptoms are progressively debilitating with little to no therapeutic treatment currently available [57]. It is, therefore, an important endeavor to further improve understanding of the mechanisms of IBMPFD pathogenesis in order to elucidate druggable targets for therapeutic intervention of this disease. We have identified TDP-43 and Unc-45 as important downstream mediators of IBMPFD. Other targets of VCP, such as nuclear factor κB (NFκB), have also been suggested to play a role in mediating the symptoms associated with IBMPFD [58–60]. Use of animal models will be important to further characterize the mechanism of these targets of mutant VCP in pathogenesis. In addition, animal models will prove to be quite useful in identifying unknown modifiers of VCP function in IBMPFD disease onset and progression.

In addition to the identification of druggable targets of IBMPFD, animal models will also be highly valuable in the screening of newly developed targeted drug therapies. Recently, Bursavich et al. [61] synthesized several novel inhibitors of VCP. Utilizing *in vitro* systems and cell lines to perform high-throughput screens, the ability of these compounds to inhibit the ATPase activity of VCP was assessed. Use of an animal model, such as the fruit fly, could be used as a first step in the characterization of these compounds in an *in vivo* system. Since *Drosophila* grow rapidly and are relatively easy to produce in large numbers quickly, they would be an excellent candidate for high-throughput screening of drug efficacy *in vivo*. Moreover, selective expression of mutant VCP in the fly eye would further improve testing efficiency because the eye is an unessential organ and the effect of expression of toxic genes can be easily observed without affecting the viability of the organism [40]. Once promising compounds have been identified in the fruit fly, they can then be tested in preclinical trials in mice. This would provide information into the efficacy and potential side effects of drugs before being moved into clinical trials with IBMPFD patients.

In conclusion, we have shown that there are many benefits to be gained from the use of multiple animal models of a single disease. Combining animal models is a broad yet specialized approach to fully characterize the mechanism of pathogenesis, identify therapeutic targets, and test the efficacy of developed therapies. This method would allow scientists and clinicians to develop therapies for the treatment of patients more quickly. Currently, drug companies spend an unprecedented amount of money on drug discovery research, with little relative gain. According to a 2001 study by the Tufts Center for the Study of Drug Development, approximately US$802 million and 10–15 years is spent on the development of a single compound that is actually used to treat patients, with a large portion of money and at least 6 years spent on preclinical research [62]. Utilizing multiple animal models for all aspects of preclinical drug-discovery research would greatly streamline the time required for the production of new drugs and, thus, reduce the costs associated with such development. IBMPFD is one of many heritable, neurodegenerative diseases in which there is no known cure and no treatment currently available. Any approach which could speed the development of treatments for persons affected by such diseases is something all researchers, in both the laboratory and clinical setting, should consider.

References

1 Guinto JB, Ritson GP, Taylor JP, Forman MS. (2007) Valosin-containing protein and the pathogenesis of frontotemporal dementia associated with inclusion body myopathy. *Acta Neuropathol* **114**, 55–61.

2 Kimonis VE, Kovach MJ, Waggoner B et al. (2000) Clinical and molecular studies in a unique family with autosomal dominant limb-girdle muscular dystrophy and Paget disease of bone. *Genet Med* **2**(4), 232–241.

3 Kovach MJ, Waggoner B, Leal S.M et al. (2001) Clinical delineation and localization to chromosome 9p13.3-p12 of a unique dominant disorder in four families: hereditary inclusion body myopathy, Paget disease of bone, and frontotemporal dementia. *Mol Genet Metab* **74**(4), 458–475.

4 Kimonis VE, Watts GD. (2005) Autosomal dominant inclusion body myopathy, Paget disease of bone, and frontotemporal dementia. *Alzheimer Dis Assoc Disord* **19** (Suppl. 1), S44–S47.

5 Watts GD, Mehta SG, Zhao C et al. (2005) Mapping autosomal dominant progressive limb-girdle myopathy with bone fragility to chromosome 9p21–p22: a novel locus for a musculoskeletal syndrome. *Hum Genet* **118**, 508–514.

6 Lucas GJ, Mehta SG, Hocking LJ et al. (2006) Evaluation of the role of Valosin-containing protein in the pathogenesis of familial and sporadic Paget's disease of bone. *Bone* **38**(2), 280–285.

7 Schroder R, Watts GD, Mehta SG et al. (2005) Mutant valosin-containing protein causes a novel type of frontotemporal dementia. *Ann Neurol* **57**(3), 457–461.

8 Guyant-Marechal L, Laquerriere A, Duyckaerts C et al. (2006) Valosin-containing protein gene mutations: clinical and neuropathologic features. *Neurology* **67**(4), 644–651.

9 Haubenberger D, Bittner RE, Rauch-Shorny S et al. (2005) Inclusion body myopathy and Paget disease is linked to a novel mutation in the VCP gene. *Neurology* **65**(8), 1304–1305.

10 Hubbers CU, Clemen CS, Kesper K et al. (2007) Pathological consequences of VCP mutations on human striated muscle. *Brain* **130**(2), 381–393.

11 Kimonis VE, Mehta SG, Fulchiero EC et al. (2008) Clinical studies in familial VCP myopathy associated with Paget disease of bone and frontotemporal dementia. *Am J Med Genet* **146**(6), 745–757.

12 Mehta SG, Watts GD, McGillivray B et al. (2006) Manifestations in a family with autosomal dominant bone fragility and limb-girdle myopathy. *Am J Med Genet A* **140**, 322–330.

13 Watts GD, Thomasova D, Ramdeen SK et al. (2007) Novel VCP mutations in inclusion body myopathy associated with Paget disease of bone and frontotemporal dementia. *Clin Genet* **72**(5), 420–426.

14 Weihl CC, Pestronk A, Kimonis VE. (2009) Valosin-containing protein disease: inclusion body myopathy with Paget's disease of the bone and fronto-temporal dementia. *Neuromuscul Disord* **19**(5), 308–315.

15 Weihl CC, Temiz P, Miller SE et al. (2008) TDP-43 accumulation in inclusion body myopathy muscle

suggests a common pathogenic mechanism with frontotemporal dementia. *J Neurol Neurosurg Psychiatry* **79**(10), 1186–1189.

16 Neumann M, Sampathu DM, Kwong LK et al. (2006) Ubiquitinated TDP-43 in frontotemporal lobar degeneration and amyotrophic lateral sclerosis. *Science* **314** (5796), 130–133.

17 Lucas GJ, Daroszewska A, Ralston SH. (2006) Contribution of genetic factors to the pathogenesis of Paget's disease of bone and related disorders. *J Bone Miner Res* **21**Suppl 2, P31–P37.

18 Forman MS, Mackenzie IR, Cairns NJ et al. (2006) Novel ubiquitin neuropathology in frontotemporal dementia with valosin-containing protein gene mutations. *J Neuropathol Exp Neurol* **65**(6), 571–581.

19 Cairns NJ, Bigio EH, Mackenzie IR et al. (2007) Neuropathologic diagnostic and nosologic criteria for frontotemporal lobar degeneration: consensus of the Consortium for Frontotemporal Lobar Degeneration. *Acta Neuropathol* **114**(1), 5–22.

20 Cairns NJ, Neumann M, Bigio EH et al. (2007) TDP-43 in familial and sporadic frontotemporal lobar degeneration with ubiquitin inclusions. *Am J Pathol* **171**, 227–240.

21 Pirici D, Vandenberghe R, Rademakers R et al. (2006) Characterization of ubiquitinated intraneuronal inclusions in a novel Belgian frontotemporal lobar degeneration family. *J Neuropathol Exp Neurol* **65**, 289–301.

22 Bersano A, Del Bo R, Lamperti C et al. (2009) Inclusion body myopathy and frontotemporal dementia caused by a novel VCP mutation. *Neurobiol Aging* **30**(5), 752–758.

23 Djamshidian A, Schaefer J, Haubenberger D et al. (2009) A novel mutation in the VCP gene (G157R) in a German family with inclusion-body myopathy with Paget disease of bone and frontotemporal dementia. *Muscle Nerve* **39**(3), 389–391.

24 Gidaro T, Modoni A, Sabatelli M et al. (2008) An Italian family with inclusion-body myopathy and frontotemporal dementia due to mutation in the VCP gene. *Muscle Nerve* **37**(1), 111–114.

25 Viassolo V, Previtali SC, Schiatti E et al. (2008) Inclusion body myopathy, Paget's disease of the bone and frontotemporal dementia: recurrence of the VCP R155H mutation in an Italian family and implications for genetic counselling. *Clin Genet* **74**, 54–60.

26 Watts GD, Wymer J, Kovach MJ et al. (2004) Inclusion body myopathy associated with Paget disease of bone and frontotemporal dementia is caused by mutant valosin-containing protein. *Nat Genet* **36**(4), 377–381.

27 White SR, Lauring B. (2007) AAA+ ATPases: achieving diversity of function with conserved machinery. *Traffic* **8**, 1657–1667.

28 Rouiller I, DeLaBarre B, May AP et al. (2002) Conformational changes of the multifunction p97 AAA ATPase during its ATPase cycle. *Nat Struct Biol* **9**, 950–957.

29 Zhang X, Shaw A, Bates PA et al. (2000) Structure of the AAA ATPase p97. *Mol Cell* **6**(6), 1473–1484.

30 Dreveny I, Kondo H, Uchiyama K et al. (2004) Structural basis of the interaction between the AAA ATPase p97/VCP and its adaptor protein p47. *EMBO J* **23**, 1030–1039.

31 Dreveny I, Pye VE, Beuron F et al. (2004) p97 and close encounters of every kind: a brief review. *Biochem Soc Trans* **32**(5), 715–720.

32 Woodman PG. (2003) p97, a protein coping with multiple identities. *J Cell Sci* **116**, 4283–4290.

33 Halawani D, Latterich M. (2006) p97: The cell's molecular purgatory? *Mol Cell* **22**, 713–717.

34 Wang Q, Song C, Li CC. (2004) Molecular perspectives on p97-VCP: progress in understanding its structure and diverse biological functions. *J Struct Biol* **146**(1–2) 44–57.

35 Tresse E, Salomons FA, Vesa J et al. (2010) VCP/p97 is essential for maturation of ubiquitin-containing autophagosomes and this function is impaired by mutations that cause IBMPFD. *Autophagy* **6**(2), 217–227.

36 Janiesch PC, Kim J, Mouysset J et al. (2007) The ubiquitin-selective chaperone CDC-48/p97 links myosin assembly to human myopathy. *Nat Cell Biol* **9**(4), 379–390.

37 Kim J, Lowe T, Hoppe T. (2008) Protein quality control gets muscle into shape. *Trends Cell Biol* **18**, 264–272.

38 Wohlgemuth SL, Crawford BD, Pilgrim DB. (2007) The myosin co-chaperone UNC-45 is required for skeletal and cardiac muscle function in zebrafish. *Dev Biol* **303**, 483–492.

39 Halawani D, Leblanc A, Rouiller I et al. (2009) Hereditary inclusion body myopathy-linked p97/VCP mutations in the NH2-domain and the D1 ring modulate p97/VCP ATPase activity and D2 AAA+ ring conformation. *Mol Cell Biol* **29**(16), 4484–4494.

40 Lloyd TE, Taylor JP. (2010) Flightless flies: *Drosophila* models of neuromuscular disease. *Ann N Y Acad Sci* **1184**, e1–e20.

41 Harper A. (2010) Mouse models of neurological disorders--a comparison of heritable and acquired traits. *Biochim Biophys Acta* **1802**, 785–795.

42 Bonini NM, Fortini ME. (2003) Human neurodegenerative disease modeling using *Drosophila*. *Annu Rev Neurosci* **26**, 627–656.

43 Bier E. (2005) *Drosophila,* the golden bug, emerges as a tool for human genetics. *Nat Rev Genet* **6**, 9–23.

44 Fernandez-Funez P, Nino-Rosales ML, de Gouyon B et al. (2000) Identification of genes that modify ataxin-1-induced neurodegeneration. *Nature* **408**, 101–106.

45 Kazemi-Esfarjani P, Benzer S. (2000) Genetic suppression of polyglutamine toxicity in *Drosophila*. *Science* **287**, 1837–1840.

46 Higashiyama H, Hirose F, Yamaguchi M et al. (2002) Identification of ter94, *Drosophila* VCP, as a modulator of polyglutamine-induced neurodegeneration. *Cell Death Differ* **9**(3), 264–273.

47 Ritson GP, Custer SK, Freibaum BD et al. (2010) TDP-43 mediates degeneration in a novel *Drosophila* model of disease caused by mutations in VCP/p97. *J Neurosci* **33**, 7729–7739.

48 Geser F, Martinez-Lage M, Kwong LK, Lee, V. M., and Trojanowski JQ. (2009) Amyotrophic lateral sclerosis, frontotemporal dementia and beyond: the TDP-43 diseases. *J Neurol* **256**, 1205–1214.

49 Neumann M, Mackenzie IR, Cairns NJ et al. (2007) TDP-43 in the ubiquitin pathology of frontotemporal dementia with VCP gene mutations. *J Neuropathol Exp Neurol* **66**(2), 152–157.

50 Salajegheh M, Pinkus JL, Taylor JP et al. (2009) Sarcoplasmic redistribution of nuclear TDP-43 in inclusion body myositis. *Muscle Nerve* **40**, 19–31.

51 Cooper TA, Wan L, Dreyfuss G. (2009) RNA and disease. *Cell* **136**, 777–793.

52 Muller JM, Deinhardt K, Rosewell I et al. (2007) Targeted deletion of p97 (VCP/CDC48) in mouse results in early embryonic lethality. *Biochem Biophys Res Commun* **354**(2), 459–465.

53 Weihl CC, Miller SE, Hanson PI, Pestronk A. (2007) Transgenic expression of inclusion body myopathy associated mutant p97/VCP causes weakness and ubiquitinated protein inclusions in mice. *Hum Mol Genet* **16**(8), 919–928.

54 Custer SK, Neumann M, Lu H et al. (2010) Transgenic mice expressing mutant forms VCP/p97 recapitulate the full spectrum of IBMPFD including degeneration in muscle, brain and bone. *Hum Mol Genet* **19**, 1741–1755.

55 Amato AA, Barohn RJ. (2009) Inclusion body myositis: old and new concepts. *J Neurol Neurosurg Psychiatry* **80**, 1186–1193.

56 Broccolini A, Gidaro T, Morosetti R, Mirabella M. (2009) Hereditary inclusion-body myopathy: clues on pathogenesis and possible therapy. *Muscle Nerve* **40**, 340–349.

57 Kimonis VE, Fulchiero E, Vesa J, Watts G. (2008) VCP disease associated with myopathy, paget disease of bone and frontotemporal dementia: Review of a unique disorder. *Biochim Biophys Acta* **1782**(12), 744–748.

58 Asai T, Tomita Y, Nakatsuka S et al. (2002) VCP (p97) regulates NFkappaB signaling pathway, which is important for metastasis of osteosarcoma cell line. *Jpn J Cancer Res* **93**(3), 296–304.

59 Dai RM, Chen E, Longo DL et al. (1998) Involvement of valosin-containing protein, an ATPase co-purified with IkappaBalpha and 26 S proteasome, in ubiquitin-proteasome-mediated degradation of IkappaBalpha. *J Biol Chem* **273**(6), 3562–3573.

60 Vandermoere F, El Yazidi-Belkoura I, Slomianny C et al. (2006) The valosin-containing protein (VCP) is a target of Akt signaling required for cell survival. *J Biol Chem* **281**, 14307–14313.

61 Bursavich MG, Parker DP, Willardsen JA et al. (2010) 2-Anilino-4-aryl-1, 3-thiazole inhibitors of valosin-containing protein (VCP or p97). *Bioorg Med Chem Lett* **20**, 1677–1679.

62 Kaitin KL (ed.) (2001) Biotech products proliferate, but total development times lengthen. In *Tufts CSDD Impact Report 2001*. Tufts Center for the Study of Drug Development, Medford.

Index

Note: page numbers in italics refer to figures, those in **bold** refer to tables.

Muscle Aging, Inclusion-Body Myositis and Myopathies, First Edition. Edited by Valerie Askanas and W. King Engel.
© 2012 Blackwell Publishing Ltd. Published 2012 by Blackwell Publishing Ltd.